GN00787694

Techniques for Success with Implants in the Esthetic Zone

Techniques for

SUCCESS WITH IMPLANTS

in the Esthetic Zone

Edited by

Arndt Happe, DDS, Dr Med Dent

Assistant Professor and Research Fellow
University of Cologne
Cologne, Germany

Private Practice
Münster, Germany

Gerd Körner, Dr Med Dent

Private Practice
Bielefeld, Germany

Ⓠ QUINTESSENCE PUBLISHING

Berlin, Barcelona, Chicago, Istanbul, London, Mexico City, Milan,
Moscow, Paris, Prague, São Paulo, Seoul, Tokyo, Warsaw

I would like to thank my parents Dr Gabriele and Dr Herwig Happe

For Marlene and Paula

This book was originally published in German under the title *Erfolg mit Implantaten in der ästhetischen Zone: Parodontale, implantologische und restaurative Behandlungsstrategien* in 2018 by Quintessenz Verlags-GmbH, Berlin, Germany.

Library of Congress Cataloging-in-Publication Data

Names: Happe, Arndt, editor. | Körner, Gerd, editor.
Title: Techniques for success with implants in the esthetic zone / edited by Arndt Happe and Gerd Körner.
Other titles: Erfolg mit Implantaten in der ästhetischen Zone. English.
Description: Batavia, IL : Quintessence Publishing Co, Inc, [2019] | Includes bibliographical references and index.
Identifiers: LCCN 2019019189 | ISBN 9780867158229 (hardcover)
Subjects: | MESH: Dental Implantation | Esthetics, Dental
Classification: LCC RK667.I45 | NLM WU 640 | DDC 617.6/93--dc23
LC record available at https://lccn.loc.gov/2019019189

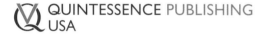

QUINTESSENCE PUBLISHING
USA

© 2019 Quintessence Publishing Co, Inc

Quintessence Publishing Co, Inc
411 N Raddant Road
Batavia, IL 60510
www.quintpub.com

5 4 3 2 1

All rights reserved. This book or any part thereof may not be reproduced, stored in a retrieval system, or transmitted in any form or by any means, electronic, mechanical, photocopying, or otherwise, without prior written permission of the publisher.

Editor: Marieke Zaffron
Design: Sue Zubek
Production: Kaye Clemens and Christine Cianciosi

Printed in China

Contents

Foreword

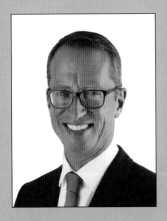

There is a common misconception that implant placement and restoration in the esthetic zone is a "slam dunk," a more or less simple procedure—especially compared with more demanding full-mouth implant-supported reconstructions. The anterior regions are easy to access for surgery and restoration, hard and soft tissue defects are often limited, and patients are likely younger, meaning greater healing potential. However, this doesn't mean the esthetic zone is easy to treat—quite the opposite, especially in extenuating circumstances.

Although anterior treatment sites are easier to access, the esthetic outcomes of implant-supported restorations and the adjacent hard and soft tissue framework require the implant positioning to be extremely accurate. Even minor aberrations in implant location and angulation (as well as prosthetic inaccuracies) may have devastating effects. Preoperative bone and tissue defects may indeed be limited in these cases. However, when these defects do occur, they are in the most visible zone, and their treatment therefore requires significantly more attention to detail and a minimally invasive approach, preferably involving microsurgical techniques to restore these defects indiscernibly. In addition, the fact that implant treatment in the esthetic zone is more prevalent in younger patients actually makes these cases significantly more challenging. The procedures themselves may not be more difficult, but the established esthetic and functional outcomes have to be maintained not just for a few years but potentially for decades.

In the past few years alone, we have gained a tremendous amount of new information on how to treat esthetically debilitated patients in need of implant-support restorations. We have learned from the past, when we were often overzealous and too concerned with trying and implementing the "latest and greatest" techniques—often without sufficient scientific evidence and clinical rigor—rather than truly addressing patients' needs. Therefore, it is extremely difficult to find a comprehensive up-to-date publication that summarizes the current knowledge and clinical techniques and technologies that provide predictable and long-lasting outcomes. In this book, Drs Happe and Körner, with their team of well-known coauthors, have achieved just that and compiled a unique and exhaustive guide for both the beginning as well as the seasoned surgical and restorative implantologist, explaining and illustrating in a most understandable and beautiful manner how implant treatment should be carried out in the esthetic zone today. From treatment planning and fundamental esthetic guidelines to microsurgical techniques and CAD/CAM technologies, the authors guide the reader through current surgical and restorative principles and techniques, ultimately leading up to more complex and challenging implant-supported restorations in the esthetic zone. The thorough list of cited scientific publications exemplifies the evidence-based approach that was chosen to compile the information and select the most appropriate techniques and technologies.

I have been a great admirer of Dr Happe's scientific contributions, deep knowledge, and clinical skills, wonderfully compiled in this book. The comprehensiveness, scientific diligence, and clinical excellence displayed will make this title an indispensable guide for any dentist with ambitions for excellence in implant dentistry. Congratulations to the authors for creating this state-of-the-art piece of literature and to the reader who, without a doubt, will greatly enjoy the journey mapped out by Dr Happe and his coauthors.

Markus B. Blatz, DMD, PhD
Chairman and Assistant Dean for Digital Innovation
Department of Preventive and Restorative Sciences
University of Pennsylvania School of Dental Medicine

Preface

"If there's a book that you want to read, but it hasn't been written yet, then you must be the one to write it."

TONI MORRISON

Since I started placing implants as part of my oral surgery training in the mid-1990s, I have been especially interested in attempting to copy nature as perfectly as possible. Anyone familiar with the subject will appreciate that this has led to some frustrating experiences, especially if you set a high esthetic standard. I quickly found that good results cannot be achieved without taking into consideration the disciplines of periodontology as well as restorative and esthetic dentistry, and so I attended conferences and courses on these subjects. The problem is that a whole universe of information opens up as soon as you start dedicating yourself more to a discipline. Furthermore, you realize that other specialties such as orthodontics, function, and dental technology are also extremely important and must be incorporated, which means you can feel rather overwhelmed in the beginning.

Over time, however, you gain experience and are better able to prioritize the wealth of information and assess the clinical relevance of the different techniques for yourself. This gives rise to certainty, professionalism, and practiced expertise. However, it is not an easy path, and I thank all my readers and mentors for their invaluable support and confidence in me. We often speak in an abstract way about a "learning curve" and readily forget that this is underpinned not only by successes but obviously by failures as well. Failures with implants in the esthetic zone can be extremely frustrating, expensive, and painful for everyone involved.

As a young dental practitioner, I would have greatly appreciated a book devoted specifically to the subject of implant therapy in the esthetic zone—and this was precisely our motivation for producing this title. When Dr Körner and I decided to write it, there were hardly any reference books that dealt specifically with implants in the esthetically sensitive area. Yet, while we were working on the book, several publications by reputable authors appeared that handled exactly this subject—or at least touched on it in one or more chapters. As a consequence, we asked ourselves whether it really made sense to continue working on the project. Naturally, we looked at these works with enormous interest. Each of these books enthused and intrigued us in their own particular way. Nevertheless, it seemed to us that the kind of book we had in mind might be an appropriate addition to the range of existing literature in that it would also incorporate related areas of dentistry. After all, every book reflects the experiences and personality of the author or authors in a very specific way.

I am therefore delighted that we managed to attract fascinating contributors, some of whom were already friends, who agreed to provide their unique expertise and have enormously enhanced the book. With this text, we would like to invite all interested colleagues to engage with our understanding and our philosophy of periodontology, implant therapy, and restorative dentistry but also with our approaches to implant therapy in the esthetic zone. We hope our passion and enjoyment of the work will light a spark in our readers.

Arndt Happe

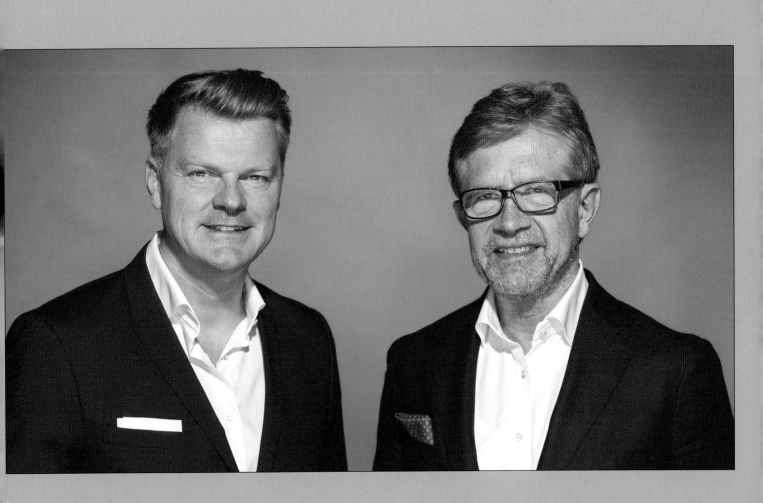

Contributors

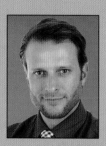

Christian Coachman, DDS, CDT
Founder
Digital Smile Design
São Paulo, Brazil

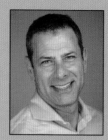

Tal Morr, DMD, MSD
Private Practice Limited to
   Prosthodontics
Miami, Florida

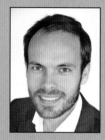

Vincent Fehmer, MDT
Division of Fixed Prosthodontics and
   Biomaterials
Clinic of Dental Medicine
University of Geneva
Geneva, Switzerland

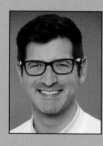

Daniel Rothamel, MD, DMD, PhD
Professor
Department of Maxillofacial and
   Plastic Surgery
University Hospital of Düsseldorf
Düsseldorf, Germany

Head of the Division of Maxillofacial
   Surgery
Protestant Hospital Bethesda
Mönchengladbach, Germany

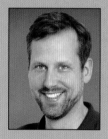

Pascal Holthaus, ZTM
Master Dental Technologist
Münster, Germany

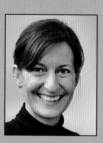

Irena Sailer, Prof Dr Med Dent
Head
Division of Fixed Prosthodontics
   and Biomaterials
Clinic of Dental Medicine
University of Geneva
Geneva, Switzerland

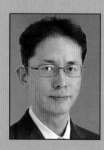

Tomohiro Ishikawa, DDS
Private Practice
Hamamatsu, Japan

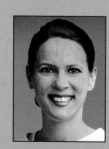

Anja Zembic, PD, DMD
Consultant
Department of Fixed and Removable
   Prosthodontics
University of Zürich
Zürich, Switzerland

"Strength does not come from physical capacity. It comes from an indomitable will."

MAHATMA GANDHI

1

Introduction

/ Arndt Happe, Gerd Körner

Assessment of the esthetic quality of implant treatment has long been ignored in academia. The traditional way to evaluate the success of implants has been to document survival rates, but these only describe whether or not an implant remains functional in the oral cavity. Factors such as clinical immobility and minimal crestal bone level change in defined periods of time have been accepted as measures of osseointegration and consequently of implant success.[1] However, individual criteria for achieving an esthetic appearance in the dentofacial area have been proposed by several authors in the dentistry literature, systematized, and discussed with particular regard to implant treatment.[2–8]

From the patient's point of view, the appearance of the peri-implant soft tissue and the prosthetic superstructures is a very important criterion for successful treatment with implants (Fig 1-1). In 2003, Vermylen et al[8] published a study on patient satisfaction with single-tooth implant restorations and stressed that an esthetically satisfactory outcome was a principal concern of patients receiving this type of treatment.

In ancient Greece, Plato and Aristotle debated the subject of beauty and esthetics and focused on symmetry in this context. Yet how much symmetry or asymmetry is actually perceived? In 2006, Kokich and Kokich[9] examined this topic and compared the esthetic perception of dental deviations among laypeople, dentists, and orthodontists. For this purpose, the smiles of seven women were deliberately manipulated using an image-processing program. Minimal changes were made to crown length, crown width, midline deviation, diastema, papilla height, and the relationship of the mucosa to the lips. The images were then assessed by orthodontists, dentists, and laypeople. It emerged that the orthodontists' assessment of the dental condition was more critical than that of the dentists and laypeople. All three groups were able to identify unilateral discrepancies in crown width of 2 mm. A unilateral alteration of the gingival margin at a central incisor was

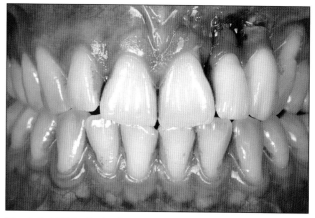

Fig 1-1 / While the implants at the maxillary left lateral incisor and canine sites have been functioning for several years, the result is not a success for the patient because the esthetics are so poor.

recognized by trained dentists when the discrepancy was only 0.5 mm. Laypeople did not notice this change until the difference was 1.5 mm. None of the study groups classified a diastema as unattractive. A unilateral reduction of papilla height was judged less attractive than the same change bilaterally. Orthodontists as well as laypeople rated gingival exposure of more than 3 mm as unattractive.[9]

Gehrke et al[10] conducted a similar study to investigate the influence of papilla length and position of interproximal contact in symmetric and asymmetric situations, comparing the esthetic sensitivity of dentists and laypeople. Starting from a reference image of an anterior dentition that had been digitally idealized, further image processing was carried out to make changes to papilla length and position of the coronal contact point. The digitally manipulated photographs of the anterior dentition were assessed by 105 dental practitioners and 106 laypeople using a questionnaire, and these questionnaires were then analyzed. The authors concluded that the phenomenon of papillary loss associated with the "black triangle" in the midline was recognized early by laypeople and dentists alike but judged differently in terms of its esthetic impact.

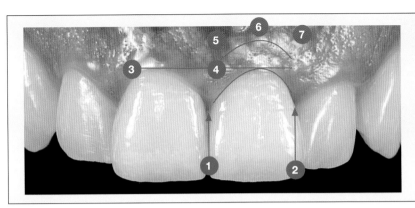

Pink esthetic score

1. Mesial papilla
2. Distal papilla
3. Height of marginal mucosa
4. Soft tissue contour (emergence)
5. Alveolar juga (convexity, volume)
6. Soft tissue color
7. Soft tissue texture

Fig 1-2 / Pink esthetic score: index for assessment of peri-implant soft tissue according to Fürhauser et al.[13]

Laypeople tolerated the gradual loss of the papilla, provided the remaining interproximal space was completely filled with mucosa due to lengthening of the contact point, thus avoiding a black triangle. Clinicians were significantly more critical in their assessment of asymmetric changes to contact point or papillary length.

In 2004, Belser et al[11] criticized the fact that the appearance of implant prosthetic restorations had been neglected in clinical trials and, in their review article on the outcome of anterior implant restorations, concluded that although "the use of dental implants in the esthetic zone is well-documented in the literature . . . most of these studies do not include well-defined esthetic parameters."[11] This indicates that the esthetic outcome is for the most part poorly documented in scientific studies and is not a criterion of success.

Dental Scores

Various measurable criteria have been sought in dentistry to provide an objective method of addressing this esthetic deficit. In 2005, Meijer et al[12] proposed a white esthetic score (WES) to assess the esthetic result of implant restorations. This index was intended to evaluate and document the appearance of crown and soft tissue based on nine parameters. At the same time, Fürhauser et al[13] published an index designed solely to assess the peri-implant soft tissue, known as the *pink esthetic score* (PES) (Fig 1-2). This involves evaluating seven parameters that describe the soft tissue situation and rating them from 0 to 2 so that a maximum score of 14 points can be achieved. In 2009, Belser et al[14] proposed their own simplified index that assesses both the soft tissue

and the prosthetic superstructure. Their combined PES/WES score includes five parameters each for crown and peri-implant soft tissue, allowing a maximum score of 10.

Patient-Related Factors

It is currently a matter of course for the diagnostic assessment of new patients to include some form of screening to check for various diseases. For instance, there is the periodontal screening index (PSI) for identifying or excluding periodontitis, and temporomandibular screening to evaluate the situation of the temporomandibular joints and involved musculature has also been proposed.[15] However, it makes sense for patients to also be screened for esthetic risk factors prior to implantology treatment so that at-risk patients can be identified. One classification for risk assessment of implant treatment that has become established internationally is known as the *SAC classification*, which divides cases into straightforward, advanced, and complex.[16]

Lip dynamics

The smile line naturally plays a role in this risk assessment. According to Fradeani,[17] a *low smile line* reveals a maximum of 75% of the maxillary anterior teeth, a *medium smile line* reveals 75% to 100% of the maxillary anterior teeth plus the papillary apices, and a *high smile line* exposes 100% of the maxillary anterior teeth plus the facial soft tissues. About 20% of people have a low smile line, 70% have a medium smile line, and 10% have a high smile line. Women have a greater tendency toward high smile

3

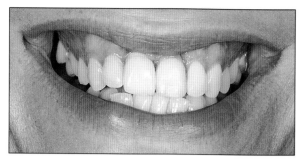

Fig 1-3 / A patient with a high smile line exposes the esthetically and functionally inadequate peri-implant soft tissue situation in the region of the maxillary central incisors.

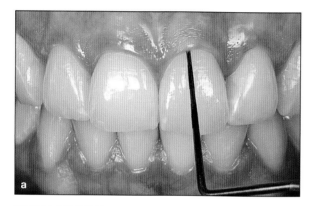

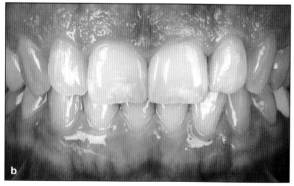

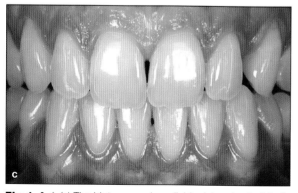

Fig 1-4 / (a) The biotype can be reliably determined clinically with the aid of a periodontal probe. Two different illustrative tissue types: (b) thick biotype with tough, fibrous tissue and flat papillary contour (scalloping); (c) thin biotype with delicate, transparent tissue and high papillary contour.

lines.[18] Because patients with a high smile line expose their facial soft tissue, recessions or other esthetically problematic alterations in this area are instantly visible, whereas they remain unnoticed in patients with a low smile line (Fig 1-3).

Tissue phenotype

Another typical patient-related factor is the periodontal tissue phenotype, also known as the *periodontal morphotype* or *periodontal biotype*. According to Müller et al,[19] the thickness of marginal periodontal tissue (masticatory mucosa) is less than 1 mm in roughly 75% of patients. Only about 25% have a tissue thickness of more than 1 mm. Kois[4] and Kan et al[20] postulated that the different tissue types also react differently to an iatrogenic or inflammatory trauma, which therefore has an influence on the predictability of treatment protocols. Clinical experience shows that thin tissue tends to react to surgical trauma with scarring and recession with more frequency than does thick, fibrous soft tissue.

Kan et al[20] showed in a clinical trial that the dimension of the peri-implant tissue around single-tooth implants (eg, the tissue thickness in the interproximal papillary area) is larger in patients with thick biotypes, thereby influencing the esthetic appearance. Regarding immediate implant placement, patients with a thin periodontal biotype clearly have a stronger tendency to severe recession than patients with a thick biotype.[21]

As a rule, it is not realistic to measure the thickness of the tissue type directly. In clinical practice, this measurement is instead based on the transparency of the periodontal probe through the gingival margin (Fig 1-4a). De Rouck et al[22] proposed this method in 2009 and demonstrated a strong correlation with direct measurement in 100 patients. In 2010, Kan et al[23] showed in a prospective clinical trial that visual determination of the biotype alone, without the aid of a periodontal probe, is not a reliable method. Tissue thickness also has a considerable influence when selecting restorative materials (see chapter 11).

Interdental papillae and scalloping

The interdental papillae or so-called *scalloping* play an important role in all of the scores used to assess the peri-implant soft tissue. Scalloping describes how great the difference in level is between the facial gingival margin and the apex of the papilla and therefore how much the gingival contour undulates. In implantology, flat and wide papillae (Fig 1-4b) are easier to reconstruct than high and narrow papillae[4] (Fig 1-4c). Jemt[24] proposed a papilla index to assess and systematize the papillary situation:

- Score 0: No papilla present
- Score 1: Less than half of the embrasure filled
- Score 2: Half or more of the embrasure filled
- Score 3: All of the embrasure filled (ie, optimal papilla)
- Score 4: Hyperplastic papilla

In 2001, Choquet et al[25] reported that reconstruction of papillae in single-tooth implant restorations is highly dependent on the vertical location of the peri-implant bone and can only be performed predictably if the distance between the contact point of the crowns and the bone is 5 mm or less. Kan et al[20] also showed that the tissue height in the area of the papillae is highly dependent on the attachment of adjacent teeth in the case of single-tooth implants; they additionally investigated the influence of the individual tissue phenotype. It emerged that thick tissue phenotypes are likely to have greater tissue height than thin phenotypes. As a result of these interdependences, loss of attachment at adjacent teeth means significant limitations for peri-implant soft tissue. As the foundation, bone codetermines the vertical position of the soft tissue. Therefore, a compromised bony situation that cannot be surgically remedied and affects adjacent teeth will always lead to soft tissue compromise later on. For the most part, these are local prognostic factors.

Predictable reconstruction of a papilla is particularly problematic between adjacent implants,[26] especially if three-dimensional (3D) bone augmentation measures are required.[27] While crown shape and localization of the contact point also influence the esthetic prognosis of implant restorations, lack of an interdental papilla often spells esthetic failure. Whereas the lack of this papilla can be concealed by a long contact surface in the case of rectangular teeth, this is not possible with triangular teeth and quickly leads to a black triangle in this area.[4]

Biologic Factors

An understanding of biologic principles with respect to peri-implant tissues is essential when planning for esthetic

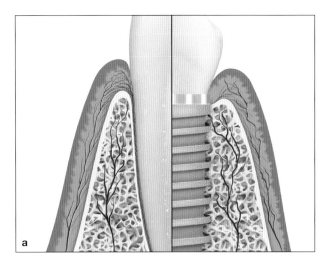

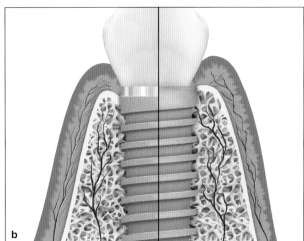

Fig 1-5 / (a) Unlike natural teeth, implants have no attachment: The collagen fibers of the connective tissue do not integrate with the implant, and no supracrestal fibrous tissue exists. Because the implant has no periodontal space, its vessels are absent, and the peri-implant tissue is poorer in blood vessels. Then there is the added influence of the microgap. All of these circumstances make it difficult to reconstruct soft tissues and papillae around implants. (b) Comparison of structures around implants with non-platform-switched connection (left) and platform switching (right).

implant restorations (Fig 1-5). These principles are primarily patient independent. For instance, consider postrestorative remodeling. After reopening of two-part, two-stage implant systems, a biologic width is established around implants in the same way as the biologic width of natural teeth.[28,29] This means that the crestal bone is positioned 1.3 to 2.6 mm apical to the interface or the microgap between implant and abutment.[30,31] The supporting bone, which ultimately determines the position of the soft tissue, therefore retracts. This can lead buccally to recessions and interproximally to insufficient papilla height (Figs 1-6a to 1-6f).[26] The

5

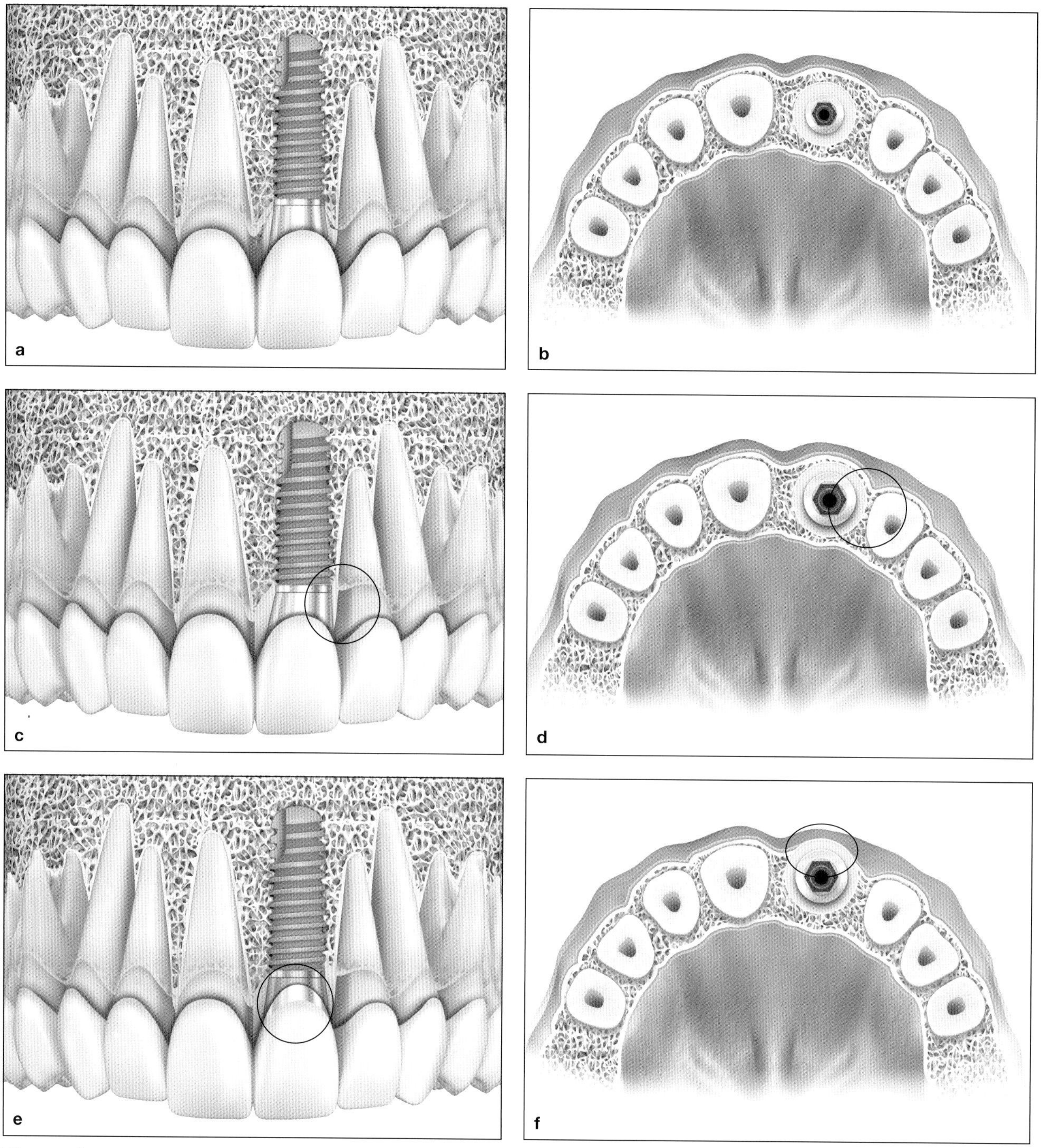

Fig 1-6 / *(a and b)* Anatomy around non-platform-switched implants. *(c and d)* Excessively large diameter and malpositioning distally lead to loss of papilla. *(e and f)* Excessively large diameter and malpositioning buccally lead to recession.

latter effect usually does not occur with single-tooth implants because the attachment of adjacent teeth determines papilla height. However, it is a major problem with adjacent implants and makes the reconstruction of papillae between adjacent implants highly unpredictable (Figs 1-6g to 1-6j and Fig 1-7).[26] These circumstances and their influence on esthetics were described graphically by Grunder et al[26] as early as 2005 and motivated the use of platform switching to exert a positive effect on the peri-implant bone situation. As a result, components reduced in diameter came to be used to move the microgap away from the bone in a central direction (see Fig 1-5b).

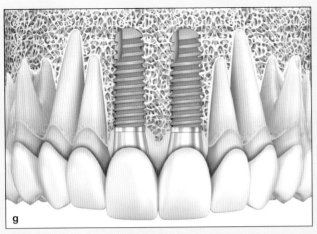

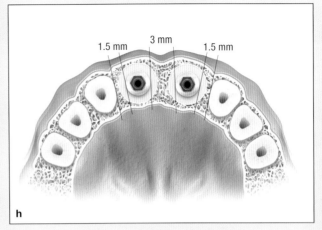

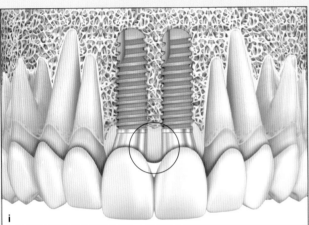

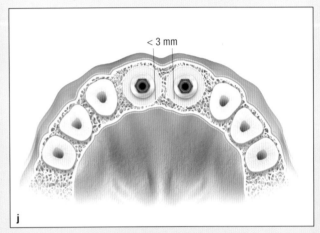

Fig 1-6 *cont.* / *(g and h)* Recommended distances for adjacent implants. *(i and j)* Adjacent implants placed too close together lead to loss of papilla. (Adapted with permission from Grunder et al.[26])

Fig 1-7 / *(a)* Implant design with smooth (ie, machined) 1.4-mm shoulder. *(b)* All-ceramic restorations after full-mouth reconstruction, including implants placed at the maxillary right lateral incisor and canine sites and the mandibular right canine site. The interproximal soft tissue between the maxillary lateral incisor and canine is deficient. (Laboratory work performed by A. Nolte.)

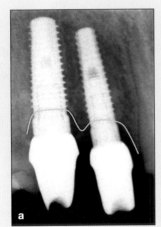

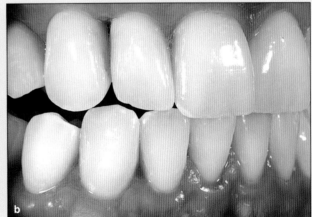

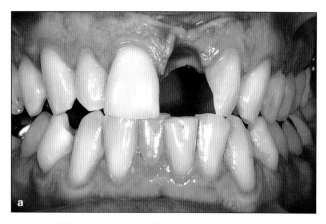
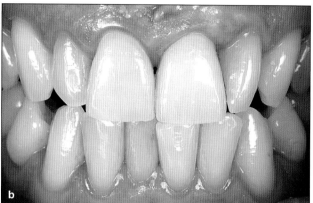
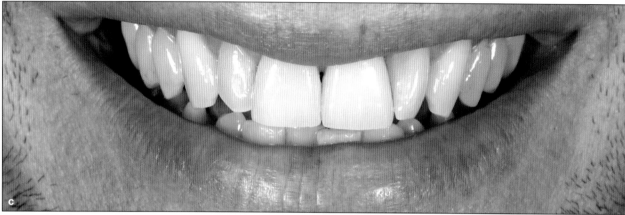

Fig 1-8 / *(a)* Single-tooth gap at the maxillary left central incisor with adverse preoperative situation due to 3D ridge defect, scarring, triangular tooth shape, and loss of mesial attachment at the rotated maxillary left lateral incisor. *(b)* Implant restoration 10 years after placement of an all-ceramic crown. *(c)* The patient has a medium smile line. (Laboratory work performed by A. Nolte.)

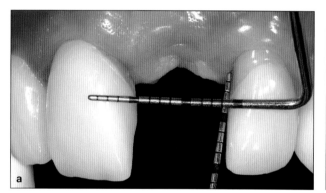
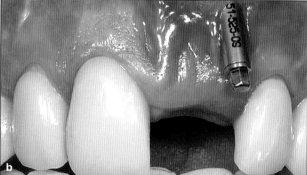

Fig 1-9 / *(a)* Adverse preoperative situation at the left central incisor due to a vertical defect at the central incisor and loss of attachment at the lateral incisor. *(b)* Vertical augmentation by distraction osteogenesis.

Loss of attachment to adjacent teeth poses another limitation. Here again bone height or attachment level determines the expected soft tissue height, which can cause interproximal deficits if there is preexisting periodontal damage (Fig 1-8). The soft tissue situation at the adjacent teeth can only rarely be improved with considerable time and effort (Figs 1-9 and 1-10).

Table 1-1 summarizes vertical soft tissue limitations.[7,32] A multicenter study by Tarnow et al[33] showed that the soft tissue height between implants is 3.4 mm on average, with

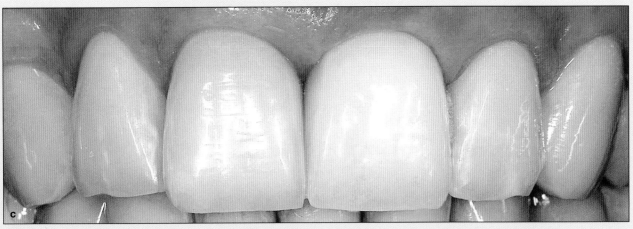

Fig 1-9 *cont.* / *(c)* Final appearance after restoration with an implant and veneers. (Laboratory work performed by K. Müterthies.)

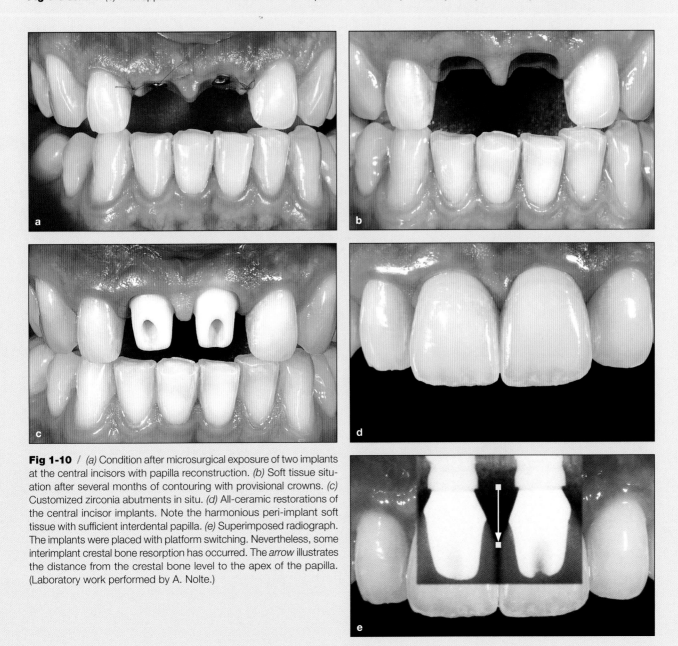

Fig 1-10 / *(a)* Condition after microsurgical exposure of two implants at the central incisors with papilla reconstruction. *(b)* Soft tissue situation after several months of contouring with provisional crowns. *(c)* Customized zirconia abutments in situ. *(d)* All-ceramic restorations of the central incisor implants. Note the harmonious peri-implant soft tissue with sufficient interdental papilla. *(e)* Superimposed radiograph. The implants were placed with platform switching. Nevertheless, some interimplant crestal bone resorption has occurred. The *arrow* illustrates the distance from the crestal bone level to the apex of the papilla. (Laboratory work performed by A. Nolte.)

Table 1-1 Vertical soft tissue limitations*

Class	Restorative surroundings	Minimum distance	Vertical soft tissue limitation
1	Tooth-tooth	1.0 mm	5.0 mm
2	Tooth-pontic	–	6.5 mm
3	Pontic-pontic	–	6.0 mm
4	Tooth-implant	1.5 mm	4.5 mm
5	Implant-pontic	–	5.5 mm
6	Implant-implant	3.0 mm	3.5 mm

–, not applicable.
*Data from Salama et al.[7] Reprinted with permission from Salama et al.[32]

a wide variation. The authors took measurements of 33 patients and 136 papillae and reported papilla heights of up to 7 mm. However, the most common heights were 2 mm (16.9%), 3 mm (35.3%), and 4 mm (37.5%). Unfortunately, the publication provided no information on the patients' tissue types or the surgical protocol used. One-part and two-part implant systems as well as single-stage and two-stage procedures have also been compared.

Tymstra et al[27] studied 10 patients with adjacent implants in the anterior dentition who required bone augmentation before implants could be placed. After prosthodontic restoration, the esthetic outcome was assessed by patients and dentists on a scale from 0 to 10. The results showed that the patients' satisfaction with the esthetic outcome was higher than that of the dentists. Overall, it was concluded that the papillary situation is often unsatisfactory when adjacent implants are placed following prior augmentation.

However, buccal recession at implants is also a problem that can cause esthetic difficulties. In a 1-year study involving a total of 63 implants, Small and Tarnow[34] investigated the changes to the peri-implant soft tissue after the exposure procedure. In their study, 80% of the implants exhibited buccal recession, which was 0.75 mm on average after 3 months, 0.85 mm after 6 months, and 1.05 mm after 12 months. The authors concluded that clinicians should wait a minimum of 3 months after exposure before fabricating the definitive prosthesis for implants in the esthetic zone.

In a prospective 1-year study with 11 patients, Cardaropoli et al[35] also investigated the tissue changes around single-tooth implants in the anterior maxilla and reported buccal recessions of 0.6 mm after 1 year and papillary growth within the same observation period. These results coincide with those of Grunder,[36] who in a 1-year study

on 10 patients measured an average of 0.5 mm of buccal recession for 70% of the implants and found increased papillary volume at all implant sites.

Surgical Factors

Uncorrected alveolar ridge defects are a common cause of esthetic problems. The literature makes it clear that despite a variety of treatment options, correction of 3D ridge defects is difficult and cannot always be fully achieved.[37,38] Especially in the esthetically sensitive anterior dentition, microsurgical techniques are recommended to attain an esthetically attractive, natural soft tissue appearance[39,40] (Fig 1-11). Particularly in the interdental papillary area, deficits in the millimeter range can mean the difference between esthetic success and failure. Microsurgical techniques are already well established in periodontal surgery and result in less tissue trauma and better healing.[41,42] It is particularly important in the esthetic zone to avoid complications of implant placement or augmentation that can impair the esthetics.

The therapeutic concept of immediate implant placement was reevaluated after Botticelli et al[43] and Araújo et al[44] showed in an animal model that while the placement of implants into extraction sockets did not lead to preservation of bony structures, the remodeling processes of the bony socket nevertheless proceeded.[45] According to Schropp et al,[46] the horizontal loss of volume after extraction can be as high as 50% 1 year postextraction. However, augmentation of the buccal areas of the socket with xenograft material can markedly reduce this loss of volume.[47] It is therefore advisable to immediately place

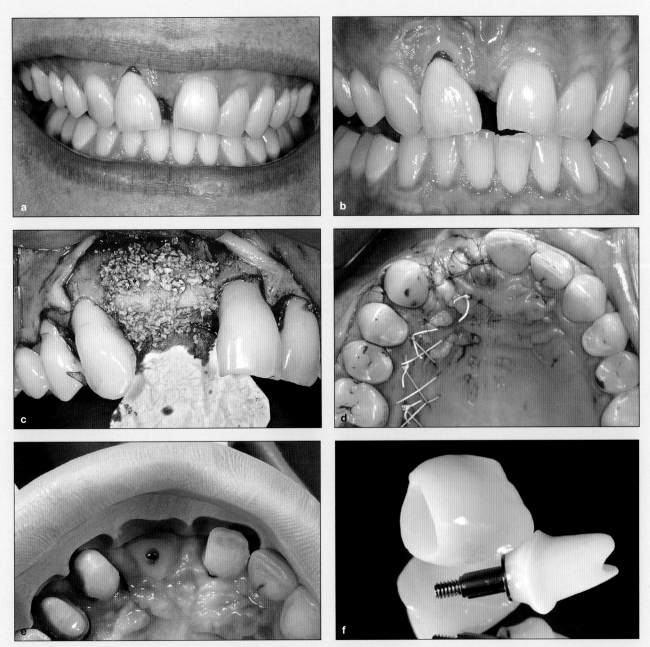

Fig 1-11 / *(a)* Unharmonious smile caused by diastema, agenesis of the maxillary right lateral incisor, and recession at the right central incisor, which is not worth preserving. *(b)* Unfavorable preoperative view due to ridge defect, scars, and difficult overall esthetic situation. The right central incisor will be replaced by an implant. *(c)* 3D augmentation of the implant site. Vertical releasing incisions are not used to avoid producing additional scars and because the blood supply to the flap is more favorable. *(d)* Microsurgical suturing. A connective tissue graft was harvested palatally for soft tissue augmentation at the implant site. *(e)* Preparation of the adjacent teeth according to the wax-up created in advance, checked with a silicone key. *(f)* All-ceramic implant restoration with marginally veneered, customized zirconia abutment and all-ceramic crown.

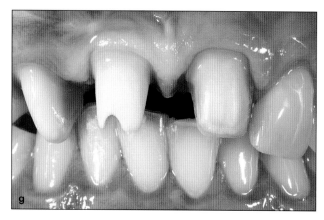
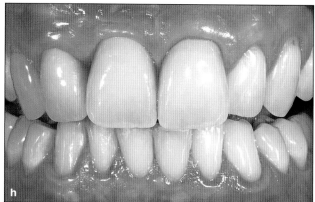

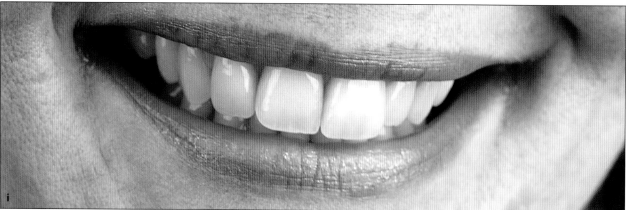

Fig 1-11 *cont.* / *(g)* Clinical situation with all-ceramic abutment in situ. *(h)* Final appearance 6 months after restoration. *(i)* Smile after treatment. (Laboratory work performed by A. Nolte.)

implants only if the buccal lamella is intact and in thicker periodontal biotypes; furthermore, the implant should be inserted in the palatal/lingual region of the socket, and the buccal area should be augmented using validated methods[45] (see chapter 4). Aside from bone augmentation, connective tissue grafts are also recommended to compensate for imminent or existing volume deficits.[48–50]

3D positioning of the implant is a fundamentally important factor in the esthetic outcome (see chapter 5). This must be guided by the planned restoration.[3] Chen et al[47] studied the influence of gingival biotype, implant position, and the design of two different implant systems on the degree of buccal recession at 42 immediate implant sites. They concluded that implant position has the greatest influence. What this means clinically is that the implant should be placed slightly palatally, and a buccal angulation must be avoided. If the implant is placed too far buccally or there is an excessive buccal angulation of the implant axis, later attempts at corrective surgery in terms of covering recession are not very promising.

Restorative and Material-Related Factors

The restorative materials have a major influence on the esthetic appearance of implant restorations. Abutments made of titanium can show through the vestibular soft tissues, and these effects are particularly noticeable in

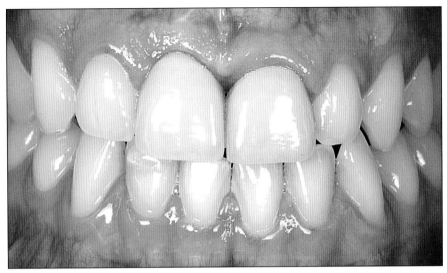

Fig 1-12 / The soft tissue in the region of the right central incisor shows recession and transparency to the abutment material.

the thin marginal soft tissue region.[51] In their much-quoted article on the PES, Führhauser et al[13] reported that 60% of the studied restorations exhibited distinct color deviations in the peri-implant soft tissue. Jung et al[52] conducted an in vitro study in an animal model to analyze the color change in oral mucosa caused by translucent materials. Titanium and zirconia, each without veneer and veneered with dental ceramic, were tested under different tissue thicknesses. The mucosal color differences were measured using a spectrophotometer. The results showed that titanium causes significant color differences even at a tissue thickness of 3 mm (Fig 1-12). By contrast, zirconia ceases to cause color differences above a tissue thickness of 2 mm. Based on the results, it may be concluded that all-ceramic abutments produce better esthetic outcomes, especially in patients with thin facial tissue.

A clinical trial conducted at Harvard University using a spectrophotometer showed that anterior implants with titanium abutments produced visibly perceptible discoloration of the soft tissue compared with the natural adjacent teeth.[51] The same study group[53] demonstrated in a second clinical trial that the colors light orange and light pink are most suitable for color masking of abutments. They also showed that white performs poorly as an abutment color.

In a prospective, randomized, controlled trial conducted at Zurich University involving 30 patients, porcelain-fused-to-metal restorations were compared directly with all-ceramic restorations on implants.[54] The results showed that both materials cause color changes. However, the all-ceramic restorations performed markedly better. Because the light optical effect of abutments can influence the esthetics of implant restorations depending on tissue thickness, an entire chapter is dedicated to this topic (see chapter 11).

Conclusion

The following are key factors for the esthetic success of implant restorations:

1. Correct 3D position of the implant
2. Appropriate bone architecture and stable bone volume
3. Adequate thickness and quality of soft tissue
4. Transmucosal form, material, and surface of abutment and restoration
5. Development and preservation of the soft tissue contour

Each of these aspects is described in detail in the following chapters, and practice-based concepts with the appropriate evidence are presented. Typical risk factors with respect to the esthetic outcome are summarized in Table 1-2.[55,56]

13

Table 1-2 Classification for risk assessment of implant treatments*

Esthetic risk	Low	Medium	High
Patient-related factors			
General state of health	Healthy, cooperative (ASA 1)[†]	Mild illnesses without impairments (ASA 2)	Multimorbid, impaired immune system (ASA 3 and above)
Nicotine consumption	Nonsmoker	Light smoker (< 10 cigarettes/day)	Heavy smoker (≥ 10 cigarettes/day)
Oral hygiene	Excellent	Satisfactory	Deficient
Anatomical factors			
Adjacent implants	None	–	Present
Width of the gap	Anatomical gap width[‡]	–	Gap too small
Soft tissue factors			
Smile line	Low	Medium	High
Periodontal biotype	Thick	Medium	Thin
Width of keratinized gingiva/mucosa	4 mm	2 mm	< 2 mm
Soft tissue quality	Intact/healthy	Scars	Severe scarring, discoloration
Papillary contour	Flat	Medium	High
Dental factors			
Type of tooth shape	Rectangular	–	Triangular
Interdental contacts	Flat	–	Punctate
Restoration status of adjacent teeth	Natural healthy teeth	–	Restored
Attachment at adjacent teeth	No loss of attachment	–	Loss of attachment
Position of contact point	< 5 mm above the bone	5.5–6.5 mm from the bone	> 7 mm from the bone
Bony factors			
Horizontal bone	No horizontal defect	Mild horizontal defect	Severe horizontal defect
Vertical bone	No vertical defect	No vertical defect	Vertical defect
Extent of defect	–	1 tooth	> 1 tooth

–, not applicable.
*Adapted from Belser et al[55] and Renouard and Rangert.[56]
[†]ASA Physical Status Classification of the American Society of Anesthesiologists.
[‡]Central incisor, canine, and premolar at least 7 mm, lateral incisor at least 5 mm.

References

1. Albrektsson T, Sennerby L. State of the art in oral implants. J Clin Periodontol 1991;18:474–481.
2. Chiche GJ, Pinault A. Esthetics of Anterior Fixed Prosthodontics. Chicago: Quintessence, 1994.
3. Garber DA. The esthetic dental implant: Letting restoration be the guide. J Oral Implantol 1996;22:45–50.
4. Kois JC. Predictable single tooth peri-implant esthetics: Five diagnostic keys. Compend Contin Educ Dent 2001;22:199–206.
5. Kokich VO Jr, Kiyak HA, Shapiro PA. Comparing the perception of dentists and lay people to altered dental esthetics. J Esthet Dent 1999;11:311–324.
6. Magne P, Belser U. Bonded Porcelain Restorations in the Anterior Dentition: A Biomimetic Approach. Chicago: Quintessence, 2002.
7. Salama M, Salama H, Garber D. Guidelines for aesthetic restorative options and implant site enhancement. Pract Proced Aesthet Dent 2002;14:125–130.
8. Vermylen K, Collaert B, Lindén U, Björn AL, De Bruyn H. Patient satisfaction and quality of single-tooth restorations. Clin Oral Implants Res 2003;14:119–124.
9. Kokich VG, Kokich VO. Ästhetische Korrekturen im Frontzahnbereich – Teil 1: Wann und warum? Inf Orthod Kieferorthop 2006;38:236–246.
10. Gehrke P, Degidi M, Lulay-Saad Z, Dhom G. Reproducibility of the implant crown aesthetic index: Rating aesthetics of single-implant crowns and adjacent soft tissues with regard to observer dental specialization. Clin Implant Dent Relat Res 2009;11:201–213.
11. Belser UC, Schmid B, Higginbottom F, Buser D. Outcome analysis of implant restorations located in the anterior maxilla: A review of the recent literature. Int J Oral Maxillofac Implants 2004;19(suppl):30–42.

12. Meijer HJ, Stellingsma K, Meijndert L, Raghoebar GM. A new index for rating aesthetics of implant-supported single crowns and adjacent soft tissues: The Implant Crown Aesthetic Index. Clin Oral Implants Res 2005;16:645–649.

13. Fürhauser R, Florescu D, Benesch T, Haas R, Mailath G, Watzek G. Evaluation of soft tissue around single-tooth implant crowns: The pink esthetic score. Clin Oral Implants Res 2005;16:639–644.

14. Belser UC, Grütter L, Vailati F, Bornstein MM, Weber HP, Buser D. Outcome evaluation of early placed maxillary anterior single-tooth implants using objective esthetic criteria: A cross-sectional, retrospective study in 45 patients with a 2- to 4-year follow-up using pink and white esthetic scores. J Periodontol 2009;80:140–151.

15. Ahlers MO, Jakstat HA. Evidence-based development of a diagnosis-dependent therapy planning system and its implementation in modern diagnostic software. Int J Comput Dent 2005;8:203–219.

16. Dawson A, Chen S (eds). The SAC Classification in Implant Dentistry. Berlin: Quintessence, 2009.

17. Fradeani M. Esthetic Rehabilitation in Fixed Prosthodontics. Volume 1: Esthetic Analysis: A Systematic Approach to Prosthetic Treatment. Chicago: Quintessence, 2004.

18. Owens EG, Goodacre CJ, Loh PL, et al. A multicentre interracial study of facial appearance. Part 1: A comparison of extraoral parameters. Int J Prosthodont 2002;15:273–282.

19. Müller HP, Heinecke A, Schaller N, Eger T. Masticatory mucosa in subjects with different periodontal phenotypes. J Clin Periodontol 2000;27:621–626.

20. Kan JY, Rungcharassaeng K, Umezu K, Kois JC. Dimensions of peri-implant mucosa: An evaluation of maxillary anterior single implants in humans. J Periodontol 2003;74:557–562.

21. Evans CD, Chen ST. Esthetic outcomes of immediate implant placements. Clin Oral Implants Res 2008;19:73–80.

22. De Rouck T, Eghbali R, Collys K, De Bruyn H, Cosyn J. The gingival biotype revisited: Transparency of the periodontal probe through the gingival margin as a method to discriminate thin from thick gingiva. J Clin Periodontol 2009;36:428–433.

23. Kan JY, Morimoto T, Rungcharassaeng K, Roe P, Smith DH. Gingival biotype assessment in the esthetic zone: Visual versus direct measurement. Int J Periodontics Restorative Dent 2010;30:237–243.

24. Jemt T. Regeneration of gingival papillae after single-implant treatment. Int J Periodontics Restorative Dent 1997;17:326–333.

25. Choquet V, Hermans M, Adriaenssens P, Daelemans P, Tarnow DP, Malevez C. Clinical and radiographic evaluation of the papilla level adjacent to single-tooth dental implants. A retrospective study in the maxillary anterior region. J Periodontol 2001;72:1364–1371.

26. Grunder U, Gracis S, Capelli M. Influence of the 3-D bone-to-implant relationship on esthetics. Int J Periodontics Restorative Dent 2005;25:113–119.

27. Tymstra N, Meijer HJ, Stellingsma K, Raghoebar GM, Vissink A. Treatment outcome and patient satisfaction with two adjacent implant-supported restorations in the esthetic zone. Int J Periodontics Restorative Dent 2010;30:307–316.

28. Gargiulo AW, Wentz FM, Orban B. Mitotic activity of human oral epithelium exposed to 30 per cent hydrogen peroxide. Oral Surg Oral Med Oral Pathol 1961;14:474–492.

29. Berglundh T, Lindhe J. Dimension of the periimplant mucosa. Biological width revisited. J Clin Periodontol 1996;23:971–973.

30. Hermann JS, Buser D, Schenk RK, Schoolfield JD, Cochran DL. Biologic width around one- and two-piece titanium implants. Clin Oral Implants Res 2001;12:559–571.

31. Hermann JS, Schoolfield JD, Schenk RK, Buser D, Cochran DL. Influence of the size of the microgap on crestal bone changes around titanium implants. A histometric evaluation of unloaded non-submerged implants in the canine mandible. J Periodontol 2001;72:1372–1383.

32. Salama M, Ishikawa T, Salama H, Funato A, Garber D. Advantages of the root submergence technique for pontic site development in esthetic implant therapy. Int J Periodontics Restorative Dent 2007;27:521–527.

33. Tarnow D, Elian N, Fletcher P, et al. Vertical distance from the crest of bone to the height of the interproximal papilla between adjacent implants. J Periodontol 2003;74:1785–1788.

34. Small PN, Tarnow DP. Gingival recession around implants: A 1-year longitudinal prospective study. Int J Oral Maxillofac Implants 2000;15:527–532.

35. Cardaropoli G, Lekholm U, Wennstrom JL. Tissue alterations at implant-supported single-tooth replacements: A 1-year prospective clinical study. Clin Oral Implants Res 2006;17:165–171.

36. Grunder U. Stability of the mucosal topography around single-tooth implants and adjacent teeth: 1-year results. Int J Periodontics Restorative Dent 2000;20:11–17.

37. Aghaloo TL, Moy PK. Which hard tissue augmentation techniques are the most successful in furnishing bony support for implant placement? Int J Oral Maxillofac Implants 2007;22(suppl):49–70.

38. Esposito M, Grusovin MG, Coulthard P, Worthington HV. The efficacy of various bone augmentation procedures for dental implants: A Cochrane systematic review of randomized controlled clinical trials. Int J Oral Maxillofac Implants 2006;21:696–710.

39. Zadeh HH, Daftary F. Minimally invasive surgery: An alternative approach for periodontal and implant reconstruction. J Calif Dent Assoc 2004;32:1022–1030.

40. Shanelec DA. Anterior esthetic implants: Microsurgical placement in extraction sockets with immediate plovisionals. J Calif Dent Assoc 2005;33:233–240.

41. Cortellini P, Tonetti MS. Microsurgical approach to periodontal regeneration. Initial evaluation in a case cohort. J Periodontol 2001;72:559–569.

42. Burkhardt R, Lang NP. Coverage of localized gingival recessions: Comparison of micro- and macrosurgical techniques. J Clin Periodontol 2005;32:287–293.

43. Botticelli D, Berglundh T, Lindhe J. Hard-tissue alterations following immediate implant placement in extraction sites. J Clin Periodontol 2004;31:820–828.

44. Araújo MG, Sukekava F, Wennström JL, Lindhe J. Ridge alterations following implant placement in fresh extraction sockets: An experimental study in the dog. J Clin Periodontol 2005;32:645–652.

45. Hämmerle CH, Chen ST, Wilson TG Jr. Consensus statements and recommended clinical procedures regarding the placement of implants in extraction sockets. Int J Oral Maxillofac Implants 2004;19(suppl):26–28.

46. Schropp L, Wenzel A, Kostopoulos L, Karring T. Bone healing and soft tissue contour changes following single-tooth extraction: A clinical and radiographic 12-month prospective study. Int J Periodontics Restorative Dent 2003;23:313–323.

47. Chen ST, Darby IB, Reynolds EC. A prospective clinical study of non-submerged immediate implants: Clinical outcomes and esthetic results. Clin Oral Implants Res 2007;18:552–562.

48. Mankoo T. Contemporary implant concepts in aesthetic dentistry—Part 2: Immediate single-tooth implants. Pract Proced Aesthet Dent 2004;16:61–68.

15

49. Chung S, Rungcharassaeng K, Kan JY, Roe P, Lozada JL. Immediate single tooth replacement with subepithelial connective tissue graft using platform switching implants: A case series. J Oral Implantol 2011;37:559–569.

50. Grunder U. Crestal ridge width changes when placing implants at the time of tooth extraction with and without soft tissue augmentation after a healing period of 6 months: Report of 24 consecutive cases. Int J Periodontics Restorative Dent 2011;31:9–17.

51. Park SE, Da Silva JD, Weber HP, Ishikawa-Nagai S. Optical phenomenon of peri-implant soft tissue. Part I. Spectrophotometric assessment of natural tooth gingiva and peri-implant mucosa. Clin Oral Implants Res 2007;18:569–574.

52. Jung RE, Sailer I, Hämmerle CH, Attin T, Schmidlin P. In vitro color changes of soft tissues caused by restorative materials. Int J Periodontics Restorative Dent 2007;27:251–257.

53. Ishikawa-Nagai S, Da Silva JD, Weber HP, Park SE. Optical phenomenon of peri-implant soft tissue. Part II. Preferred implant neck color to improve soft tissue esthetics. Clin Oral Implants Res 2007;18:575–580.

54. Jung RE, Holderegger C, Sailer I, Khraisat A, Suter A, Hämmerle CH. The effect of all-ceramic and porcelain-fused-to-metal restorations on marginal peri-implant soft tissue color: A randomized controlled clinical trial. Int J Periodontics Restorative Dent 2008;28:357–365.

55. Belser U, Buser D, Wismeijer D. ITI Treatment Guide. Vol 1: Implant Therapy in the Esthetic Zone for Single-Tooth Replacements. Berlin: Quintessence, 2007.

56. Renouard F, Rangert B. Risk Factors in Implant Dentistry: Simplified Clinical Analysis for Predictable Treatment, ed 2. Paris: Quintessence, 2007.

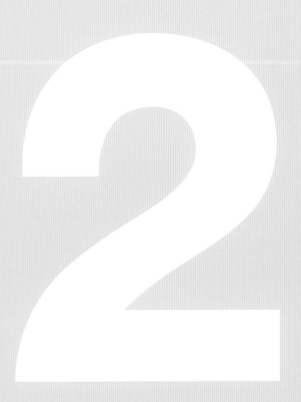

"When a flower doesn't bloom, you fix the environment in which it grows, not the flower."

ALEXANDER DEN HEIJER

2 Requirements

/ Arndt Happe

here are certain requirements that must be met by practices that offer implant dentistry. These relate to building design as well as the level of organization in the practice and the qualifications of practitioners and support staff.

Implant and periodontal surgery requires appropriate surgical skills from the dental practitioner and demands high standards of hygiene and organization from the team. Sterile care must be guaranteed to ensure safe and successful treatment (Fig 2-1). Dentists and assistants should regularly attend postgraduate courses so that the latest hygiene regulations are rigorously put into practice. Appropriate quality management is another prerequisite.

Beyond high hygiene standards, it must be remembered that patients come to the practice with certain anxieties and expectations. For areas such as waiting and consulting rooms, consider warm materials and color schemes. First impressions play a key role in building a trusting relationship between the patient and the clinician. The environment is part of external communication and should convey a sense of quality and be esthetically appealing. It is beneficial to keep a separate room for consultations, and this space should have room for the patient as well as spouses or caretakers who may accompany them to appointments (Figs 2-2 and 2-3). Rooms used for medical functions, on the other hand, should exude professional order and cleanliness (Figs 2-4 to 2-6).

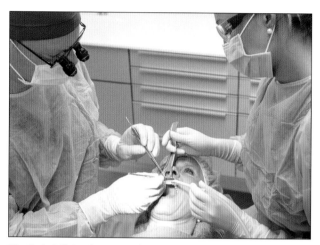

Fig 2-1 / Outpatient operations require certain hygiene standards, which are a prerequisite for safe and successful treatment.

Precare and Aftercare

In addition to the clinician's surgical expertise and scrupulous compliance with hygiene standards, the precare and aftercare of patients is a key point in the treatment approach. Good and excellent results can only be achieved in the long term if patients receive precare and aftercare as part of a systematic preventive concept. All of the therapeutic approaches depicted in this book require

the tissues of the oral cavity to be healthy and free of inflammation. Not only must the patient be instructed on how to practice oral hygiene, but the clinical situation must allow for this cleaning. If it does not, this must be remedied during precare.

The dental practice must provide the premises, equipment, and staff resources for this purpose. Trained staff (eg, dental hygienists, dental assistants) and an efficient recall system are important requirements for therapeutic success. If a referral system is being used, it is essential to ensure that patients receive appropriate care in the referring practice before and after the implant therapy.

The absence of periodontal and peri-implant inflammatory processes is a basic precondition for a sustained esthetic and—above all—healthy outcome. Tissue stability can only be expected if the peri-implant tissues as well as the periodontal tissues of adjacent teeth are free from inflammation. The spectrum of bacteria and the pathogenesis of periodontitis and peri-implantitis are known to be very similar.[1] The overwhelming majority of periodontal and peri-implant diseases are caused by

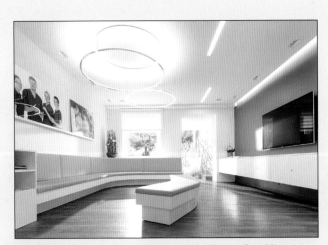

Fig 2-2 / Example of a waiting room that is comfortable yet professional.

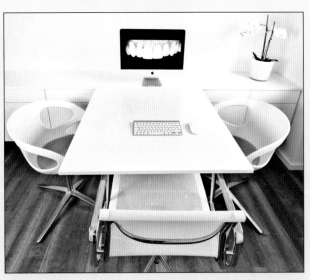

Fig 2-3 / Consulting room for treatment planning and interviews with patients. This is a private space with room for several people.

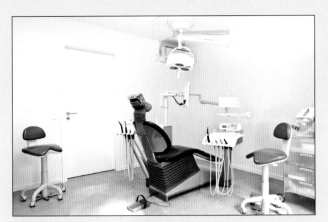

Fig 2-4 / Treatment room for dental treatments and implantology procedures.

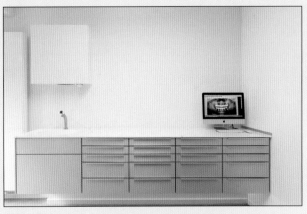

Fig 2-5 / Clear, streamlined, and well-arranged layout of the treatment room surfaces conducive to patient care.

Fig 2-6 / Functional space should be available for storing sterile supplies.

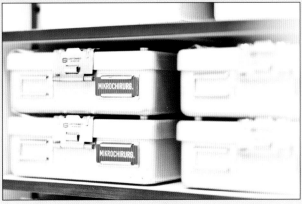

colonization with microorganisms that form a biofilm on nonexfoliating surfaces, including teeth and implants. This biofilm causes a local inflammatory reaction of the surrounding soft tissues (ie, gingiva and peri-implant mucosa). If the biofilms are not removed regularly by proper oral hygiene measures at home, this results in overgrowth of microorganisms pathogenic to the periodontium, which ultimately leads to chronic inflammation of the soft tissues (ie, gingivitis or peri-implant mucositis). In patients who are predisposed to periodontal disease, this chronic inflammation can result in the formation of periodontitis or peri-implantitis.[2,3]

The etiopathogenesis of periodontitis and peri-implantitis illustrates the key role of the biofilm in the development of these diseases. Patients with poor oral hygiene have a significantly higher risk of developing peri-implantitis.[4] Patients who suffer from periodontitis also have a significantly higher risk.[2,4] Like periodontitis and peri-implantitis, smoking is an additional risk factor that must be taken into consideration.

The statistical risk of developing peri-implantitis is increased by several factors.[4–8] The *odds ratio* (OR) for each factor describes its relative impact on peri-implantitis (eg, an OR of 2 would indicate that this factor results in a doubled likelihood of developing peri-implantitis):

- Poor oral hygiene: OR = 14.3
- Treated periodontitis: OR = 3.1 to 4.7
- Residual pockets of 5 mm or more: OR = 5
- Smoking: OR = 3.6 to 4.6
- No preventive measures or aftercare: OR = 5.9
- Previous history of periodontitis and lack of aftercare: OR = 11

These values illustrate that precare and aftercare as well as patient education play an important role in the success of implant treatment.

Precare

One purpose of precare is to thoroughly inform patients what part they themselves have to play in the long-term success of their implant therapy and what oral hygiene measures they should implement at home to remove the biofilm regularly and adequately. Secondly, precare should result in tissue that is free of inflammation. Patients with preexisting periodontal damage generally have an increased risk of developing peri-implantitis.[9–12] There is

a scientific consensus that existing periodontitis must be treated before implant placement.[2,3]

In a clinical trial, it was found that patients with preexisting periodontal damage with just one localized probing depth $\geq$ 5 mm at natural abutments have a significantly higher risk of peri-implantitis than patients with preexisting periodontal damage without such deep residual pockets.[8] More than 50% of adults suffer from periodontitis, and 11% are affected by a particularly severe form; this demonstrates how many potential implant patients actually carry an increased risk of peri-implantitis due to preexisting damage to their periodontium.[2] Patients must be educated on the relationships between plaque, peri-implantitis, and long-term prognosis. Patients with periodontal damage (as well as patients who smoke or patients who have diabetes) must be told about their increased risk.[3] For patients who smoke, tobacco/nicotine withdrawal should be considered, where appropriate, or the individual risk should be assessed.[7]

As part of precare, teeth not worth preserving must be extracted and periodontal infections controlled by systematic periodontal therapy. The periodontal situation must be reevaluated before the actual implant planning and after an appropriate healing phase.

The consensus conference of the European Workshop in Periodontology issued the following recommendations on steps to take prior to implant therapy[13]:

- Patients should be informed about the risk of peri-implantitis and the need for preventive measures.
- An individual risk analysis should be prepared that identifies systemic and local risks. Where appropriate, this will include tobacco withdrawal, smoking cessation, and elimination of periodontal pockets.
- Because plaque control is the basis for prevention of peri-implantitis, patients must receive regular instruction and be educated on suitable oral hygiene measures.
- Planning of implant restorations should consider the fact that cemented restorations carry a higher risk of peri-implant infections due to cement residue. Customized abutments allow paramarginal placement of the cement line, if appropriate, and therefore make it easier to check for cement residue.

Aftercare

Colonization by microorganisms begins immediately after the implant has been exposed to the oral cavity during the exposure step. Only 1 to 2 weeks after placement of an implant abutment, the same potentially periodontally pathogenic microorganisms as those found in periodontal pockets can be detected on an implant.[14,15] Regular removal of the biofilm forms the basis of oral hygiene aftercare of implant restorations. To achieve this, a system needs to be set up that facilitates adequate and individualized maintenance of implant patients.

The etiopathogenesis of peri-implantitis, which is characterized by loss of crestal bone, demonstrates that mucositis always precedes peri-implantitis. Because the therapeutic options for treating peri-implantitis are still unsatisfactory, it is crucial to prevent the disease and to specifically prevent mucositis as the precursor of peri-implantitis.[3,13] The prevalence of mucositis is given as 43% in the literature, and that of peri-implantitis as 22%.[2] The consensus conference of the European Workshop in Periodontology provides the following recommendations on aftercare following implant therapy[13]:

- The recall interval should be decided according to the patient's individual needs (eg, every 3, 6, or 12 months). Patient cooperation is required.
- Short recall intervals should be selected, especially if patients have been treated in the past for aggressive periodontitis.
- During recall sessions, peri-implant tissue should regularly be examined; this involves recording probing results with a special focus on the criterion of bleeding on probing.

Preventive measures should be taken to ensure that the relatively soft titanium of implants and abutments is not roughened during cleaning. Although ceramic abutments tend to be preferred in the esthetic zone, it is necessary to understand the risks associated with roughened titanium abutments. Prefabricated, machined, commercially available titanium abutments have a surface roughness (Ra) of 0.15 to 0.24 μm.[16–18] If the abutments are roughened to Ra 0.8 μm, the accumulation of plaque increases 25-fold compared with machined abutments, and the pathogenicity of the plaque also increases.[19] These numbers illustrate the importance of proper surface treatment of implant restorations.

The following methods or instruments are clinically relevant to the cleaning of dental implants:

- Ultrasonic scaler
- Ultrasonic scaler with plastic tip

- Compressed air or sonic scaler (air scaler)
- Steel curette
- Titanium curette
- Polytetrafluoroethylene curette
- Plastic curette
- Air polishing device
- Polishing cups
- Brushes
- Composite abrasives

The methods recommended by the author are plastic curettes and air polishing devices with subsequent rubber cup polishing (Figs 2-7 and 2-8). In vitro, the plastic curette cleaned more efficiently than the air polishing device.[20] In vivo, the air polishing device, plastic curette, and rubber polisher minimally roughened the surface, and the subsequent retention of plaque to cleaned abutments was similar for all methods.[21] These methods are therefore effective and leave the implant surface mostly unchanged. Sonic, ultrasonic, and metallic instruments, on the other hand, significantly roughened the implant surface in vitro and in vivo.[22,23]

Cafiero et al[24] also studied different cleaning methods for titanium surfaces, including the use of rubber cups and brushes in combination with cleaning pastes with abrasive particles of zircon or perlite (volcanic glass) as well as an air polishing device with glycine powder on two different settings (low and high air pressure). The polishing paste containing zircon particles produced the highest surface roughness values of Ra 0.30 to 0.33 μm, and the polishing paste with perlite produced lower values (Ra 0.25 to 0.28 μm). The air polishing device led to surface roughness levels of Ra 0.23 μm at the low pressure setting and Ra 0.16 μm at the high pressure setting.

The following methods and instruments cause very significant roughening of the implant neck:

- Ultrasonic scaler (Ra = 2.08 μm)
- Steel curette (Ra = 1.32 μm)
- Titanium curette (Ra = 0.8 μm)
- Sonic scaler (air scaler) (Ra = 0.68 to 0.8 μm)

The following methods or instruments cause minimal roughening of the implant neck:

- Nonabrasive polishing cups (Ra = 0.48 to 0.57 μm)
- Nonabrasive brushes (Ra = 0.43 to 0.57 μm)
- Polytetrafluoroethylene curette (Ra = 0.53 μm)
- Plastic curette (Ra = 0.49 μm)
- Ultrasonic scaler with plastic tip (Ra = 0.44 to 0.52 μm)

21

The following methods or instruments cause no roughening or cause additional smoothing of the implant neck:

* Abrasive rubber polisher, such as those used for amalgam polishing (Ra = 0.22 to 0.36 µm)
* Abrasive polishing pastes with zircon (Ra = 0.30 to 0.33 µm)
* Abrasive polishing pastes with perlite (Ra = 0.25 to 0.28 µm)
* Air polishing device with glycine powder (Ra = 0.17 to 0.23 µm)

Dental Photography

Photographic documentation of dental treatments has never been simpler than it is today. Any radiographic software can currently manage digital clinical images. Similar to radiographs and models, digital clinical photographs should now be used as a matter of course for clinical diagnostics during treatments in the esthetic zone. Systematic documentation of implant treatments, especially in the esthetic zone, is advisable for a variety of reasons, including communication, documentation, analysis and planning, forensic reasons, and even marketing.

Communicating with patients

Clinical photographs can help to advise patients and improve their awareness of their individual problem. Unlike looking in a hand mirror in the dentist's chair, a discussion with a screen in a consulting room can create a very different atmosphere. Rather than being reduced to a person on whom procedures are being performed, the patient becomes fully involved in decision making about his or her own treatment and options for care.

Documentation and comparison of findings

Changes to mucosal appearance, retraction of tissue, migration of teeth, and more can be digitally documented and therefore allow comparison to be made with preoperative findings.

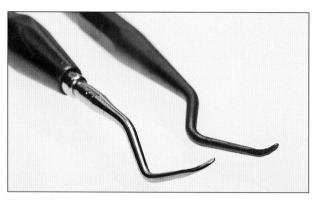

Fig 2-7 / Unlike a titanium curette *(left)*, rough plastic curettes *(right)* do not significantly roughen the neck of the implant.

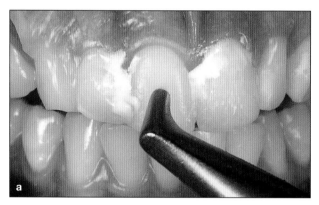

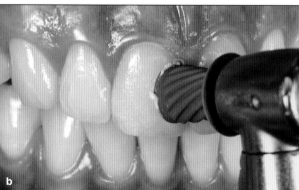

Fig 2-8 / *(a)* Air-flow with glycine powder for cleaning the restoration and removing the biofilm. *(b)* Polishing cup for polishing the surface of the restoration.

Esthetic analysis and planning

A separate chapter is dedicated to esthetic analysis with the aid of dental photographs (see chapter 5). Intensive and systematic analysis of the documented findings enables the practitioner to gain a nuanced view of the problems and an overview of the big picture without getting lost in details. With the aid of images and models, clinicians can devise treatment plans at their desk even without the patient present. These planning processes can be

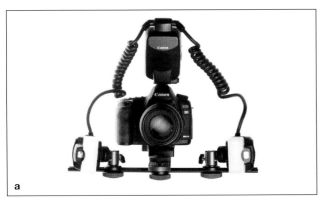
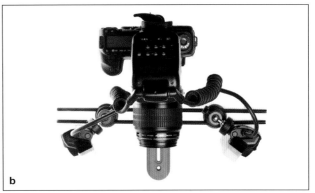
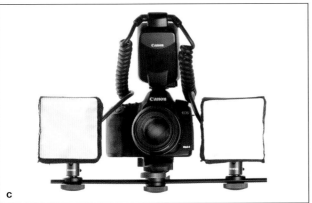
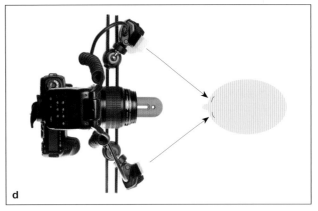

23

Fig 2-9 / *(a)* Canon digital single-lens reflex camera with side flash system on a rig setup (Novoflex). *(b)* Top view of the camera system. *(c)* Side flashes with miniature soft boxes fitted for flatter flash lighting. *(d)* Light direction with side flashes.

captured in images so that they can also be used as a medium of communication between the dentist and the dental technician. This also facilitates cooperation between specialists in different locations.

Forensic aspects

Documentation of initial findings, intraoperative findings, and results can provide a degree of certainty in the event of legal disputes. An image can often clarify matters related to queries from insurers and assessors.

Marketing

Treatment results can be presented and made available to patients and prospective patients in before-and-after records, which provide a quick and dramatic comparison. These can also be used for patient referrals.

Clinical Photographic Documentation

Equipment

Macro lenses and special flash systems for macro photography are used in dental photography. The following are photographic systems and setups recommended by the author (Figs 2-9 and 2-10):

Canon setup

- Canon 5D mark IV
- Canon 100-mm macro lens
- Canon macro-flash MT-24EX Macro Twin Lite Flash on track system with soft boxes (see Fig 2-9c)

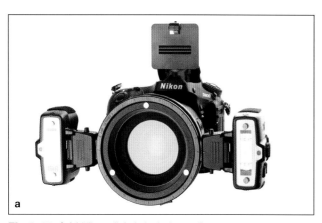

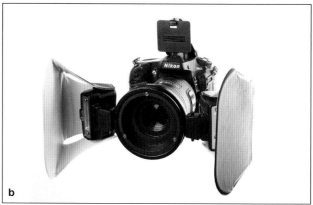

Fig 2-10 / *(a)* Nikon digital single-lens reflex camera with side flash system. *(b)* Reflectors on the flashes for flatter flash lighting.

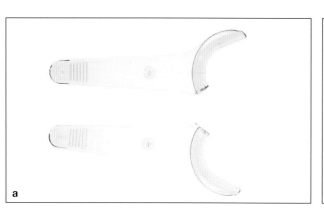

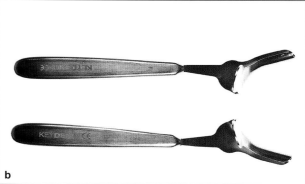

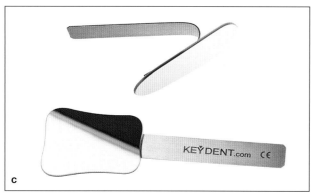

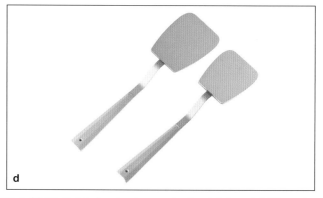

Fig 2-11 / *(a)* These customized plastic lip retractors have been trimmed. *(b)* Sterilizable lip retractors made of metal. *(c and d)* Mirrors for intraoral images: rectangular-shaped for occlusal pictures and tongue-shaped for lateral shots.

Nikon setup

- Nikon D800
- Nikon 100 macro lens
- Nikon macro-flash R1C1
- Reflectors (see Fig 2-10b)

The use of side flashes (also known as *twin flashes*) makes sense in the esthetic zone because it gives the teeth a more defined appearance. As the light hits the teeth from the side (see Fig 2-9d), internal characteristics of the teeth are accentuated more strongly. Soft boxes or reflectors alter the reflections on the tooth surface as well as on the soft tissue. The light of the flash becomes softer and flatter. Retractors and mirrors are also required to take useful clinical photographs (Figs 2-11 and 2-12). Teeth can be exposed and set against a black background (Figs 2-13 and 2-14).

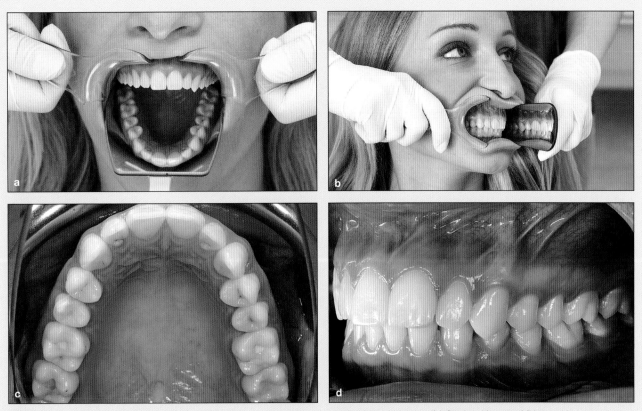

Fig 2-12 / *(a)* Technique for taking occlusal images. *(b)* Technique for taking lateral images. *(c)* Occlusal image. *(d)* Lateral image.

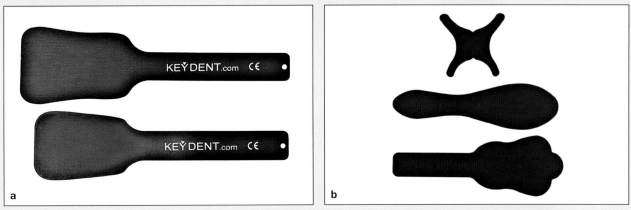

Fig 2-13 / *(a)* Black backgrounds (contrastors) made of anodized aluminum. These can be sterilized. *(b)* Metallic, silicone-coated contrastors.

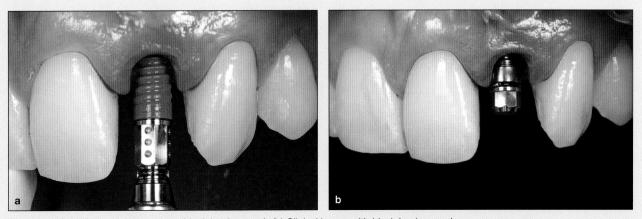

Fig 2-14 / *(a)* Clinical image without black background. *(b)* Clinical image with black background.

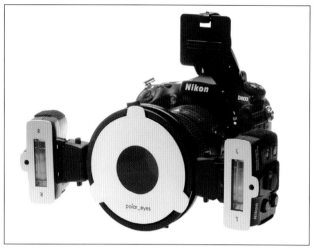

Fig 2-15 / Camera system with polarizing filter.

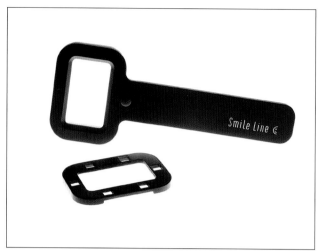

Fig 2-16 / Polarizing filters for use on patients.

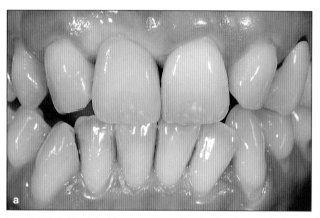

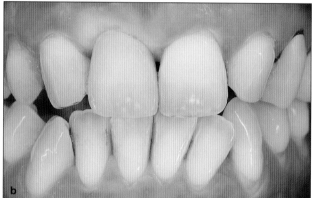

Fig 2-17 / (a) Clinical image without filter (try-in of an implant crown). (b) Clinical image with polarizing filter.

Polarizing filters

Reflections of light on the teeth can conceal details and cause problems when communicating with the laboratory. Polarizing filters placed in front of the macro flash and lens can remove all of the reflections caused by the flash on teeth and tissues (Figs 2-15 to 2-17). This makes internal characteristics easier to see. Separately from dental photography, there are also polarizing filters with suitable lighting that can be used directly on patients to assess individual characteristics. However, photographs with polarizing filters are not appropriate for assessing surface characteristics because they erase the reflections necessary for this aspect of analysis. The two techniques together allow the internal and external characteristics to be captured and evaluated.

Portrait photography

Portraits taken with the previously mentioned photographic systems and used for clinical documentation are sufficient for esthetic analysis. More professional photographs, which can also be used for patient communication, can be taken relatively simply with commercially available studio flashes (eg, Bowens Gemini 200 studio kit). These are placed on tripods or mounted on the ceiling with track systems. A studio flash passes along the side of the patient and lights one side and the wall behind the patient, while the other flash lights up the other side of the patient's face as well as the whole face. The position and setting of the flashes should be tested with trial photographs. The exposure settings on the camera and the exact setting of the flash unit should also be tried out for optimal results (Fig 2-18).

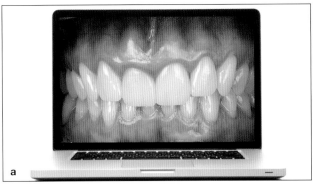
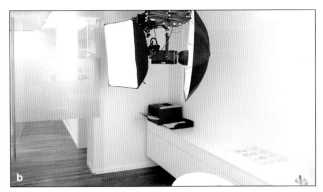
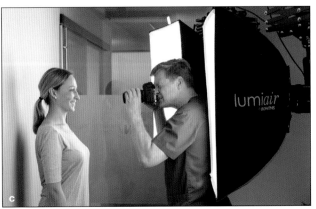
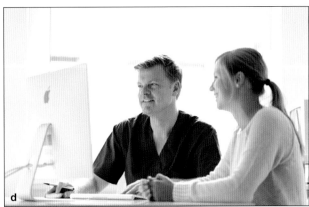

Fig 2-18 / *(a)* Digital photographs can greatly simplify communication with patients. *(b)* Studio flash unit with ceiling mounting in a dental practice. *(c)* Given the right setup, professional patient portraits can be taken with relatively minimal investment. *(d)* Viewing the photographs together with the patient rather than chairside is a more comfortable experience for the patient.

References

1. Mombelli A, Lang NP. The diagnosis and treatment of peri-implantitis. Periodontol 2000 1998;17:63–76.
2. Tonetti MS, Chapple IL, Jepsen S, Sanz M. Primary and secondary prevention of periodontal and peri-implant diseases: Introduction to, and objectives of the 11th European Workshop on Periodontology consensus conference. J Clin Periodontol 2015;42(suppl 16):S1–S4.
3. Lindhe J, Meyle J, Group DoEWoP. Peri-implant diseases: Consensus Report of the Sixth European Workshop on Periodontology. J Clin Periodontol 2008;35(8 suppl):282–285.
4. Ferreira SD, Silva GL, Cortelli JR, Costa JE, Costa FO. Prevalence and risk variables for peri-implant disease in Brazilian subjects. J Clin Periodontol 2006;33:929–935.
5. Costa FO, Takenaka-Martinez S, Cota LO, Ferreira SD, Silva GL, Costa JE. Peri-implant disease in subjects with and without preventive maintenance: A 5-year follow-up. J Clin Periodontol 2012;39:173–181.
6. Heitz-Mayfield LJ. Peri-implant diseases: Diagnosis and risk indicators. J Clin Periodontol 2008;35(8 suppl):292–304.
7. Heitz-Mayfield LJ, Huynh-Ba G. History of treated periodontitis and smoking as risks for implant therapy. Int J Oral Maxillofac Implants 2009;24(suppl):39–68.
8. Cho-Yan Lee J, Mattheos N, Nixon KC, Ivanovski S. Residual periodontal pockets are a risk indicator for peri-implantitis in patients treated for periodontitis. Clin Oral Implants Res 2012;23:325–333.
9. Matarasso S, Rasperini G, Iorio Siciliano V, Salvi GE, Lang NP, Aglietta M. A 10-year retrospective analysis of radiographic bone-level changes of implants supporting single-unit crowns in periodontally compromised vs. periodontally healthy patients. Clin Oral Implants Res 2010;21:898–903.
10. Karoussis IK, Salvi GE, Heitz-Mayfield LJ, Brägger U, Hämmerle CH, Lang NP. Long-term implant prognosis in patients with and without a history of chronic periodontitis: A 10-year prospective cohort study of the ITI Dental Implant System. Clin Oral Implants Res 2003;14:329–339.
11. Roos-Jansåker AM, Lindahl C, Renvert H, Renvert S. Nine- to fourteen-year follow-up of implant treatment. Part II: Presence of peri-implant lesions. J Clin Periodontol 2006;33:290–295.
12. Roccuzzo M, De Angelis N, Bonino L, Aglietta M. Ten-year results of a three-arm prospective cohort study on implants in periodontally compromised patients. Part 1: Implant loss and radiographic bone loss. Clin Oral Implants Res 2010;21:490–496.
13. Jepsen S, Berglundh T, Genco R, et al. Primary prevention of peri-implantitis: Managing peri-implant mucositis. J Clin Periodontol 2015;42(suppl 16):S152–S157.

14. Quirynen M, Vogels R, Peeters W, van Steenberghe D, Naert I, Haffajee A. Dynamics of initial subgingival colonization of 'pristine' peri-implant pockets. Clin Oral Implants Res 2006;17:25–37.
15. Mombelli A, Marxer M, Gaberthuel T, Grunder U, Lang NP. The microbiota of osseointegrated implants in patients with a history of periodontal disease. J Clin Periodontol 1995;22:124–130.
16. Quirynen M, van der Mei HC, Bollen CM, et al. An in vivo study of the influence of the surface roughness of implants on the microbiology of supra- and subgingival plaque. J Dent Res 1993;72:1304–1309.
17. Sawase T, Wennerberg A, Hallgren C, Albrektsson T, Baba K. Chemical and topographical surface analysis of five different implant abutments. Clin Oral Implants Res 2000;11:44–50.
18. Hermann JS, Buser D, Schenk RK, Higginbottom FL, Cochran DL. Biologic width around titanium implants. A physiologically formed and stable dimension over time. Clin Oral Implants Res 2000;11:1–11.
19. Quirynen M, Bollen CM, Papaioannou W, Van Eldere J, van Steenberghe D. The influence of titanium abutment surface roughness on plaque accumulation and gingivitis: Short-term observations. Int J Oral Maxillofac Implants 1996;11:169–178.
20. Augthun M, Tinschert J, Huber A. In vitro studies on the effect of cleaning methods on different implant surfaces. J Periodontol 1998;69:857–864.
21. McCollum J, O'Neal RB, Brennan WA, Van Dyke TE, Horner JA. The effect of titanium implant abutment surface irregularities on plaque accumulation in vivo. J Periodontol 1992;63:802–805.
22. Mengel R, Buns CE, Mengel C, Flores-de-Jacoby L. An in vitro study of the treatment of implant surfaces with different instruments. Int J Oral Maxillofac Implants 1998;13:91–96.
23. Matarasso S, Quaremba G, Coraggio F, Vaia E, Cafiero C, Lang NP. Maintenance of implants: An in vitro study of titanium implant surface modifications subsequent to the application of different prophylaxis procedures. Clin Oral Implants Res 1996;7:64–72.
24. Cafiero C, Aglietta M, Iorio-Siciliano V, Salvi GE, Blasi A, Matarasso S. Implant surface roughness alterations induced by different prophylactic procedures: An in vitro study. Clin Oral Implants Res 2017;28:e16–e20.

28

Microsurgery is not a technique.
It's a mindset.

3

Microsurgery

/ Arndt Happe, Gerd Körner

The term *microsurgery* denotes an operating technique that developed out of minimally invasive surgery of the hand—vascular surgery in particular. To perform microsurgery, the surgeon works with some form of optical magnification such as a loupe (2- to 5-fold magnification; Fig 3-1) or with an operating microscope.

Extremely slim needle-and-thread combinations down to size 11-0 can technically be manufactured; these are used particularly in vascular microsurgery and neurosurgery. As a rule, suture thicknesses of 6-0 and 7-0 are used for dental microsurgery. After the implementation of microsurgical techniques led to a paradigm shift in periodontal surgery, these techniques were soon adapted for use in implant surgery as well.[1-4]

Using fluorescence angiography, Burkhardt and Lang[5] showed in a comparative split-mouth clinical trial that vascularization immediately after the procedure and 1 week postoperatively was significantly better at the sites treated with microsurgery than at the sites treated with a macrosurgical approach. The thin surgical instruments evidently minimize injuries to microvascular structures, by extension minimizing complications such as those caused by necrosis. Precise approximation of wound margins can be achieved thanks to delicate instruments and extremely fine suture materials. These effects can be used to reduce scarring in the esthetic zone but also to perform certain plastic-periodontal operations that would not be possible with macrosurgical techniques. For these reasons, microsurgery also provides predictable results in bone augmentation procedures, in which flap necrosis and dehiscence with subsequent exposure of the augmentation material are typical complications.[6]

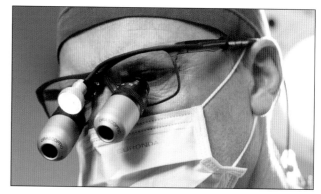

Fig 3-1 / Loupe with 3×, 4×, and 5× magnification and light-emitting diode (LED) light.

Instruments

The following instruments are used by the authors for microsurgery (Figs 3-2 to 3-13):

- Microneedle holder straight (Laschal PCF-N_7TCL/R/M1)
- Suture scissors (Laschal #71-15-30C/R)
- Microsurgical tying forceps with rat tooth (Laschal PLAF/R/1X2)
- Microsurgical scalpel handle (American Dental Systems Mamadent Mikro 071)
- Tunneling knife (American Dental Systems Mamadent Mikro 006)
- Large raspatory (American Dental Systems Mamadent Mikro 007)
- Microsurgical raspatory (American Dental Systems Mamadent Mikro 070)
- Titanium plugger (American Dental Systems Mamadent Mikro 074)

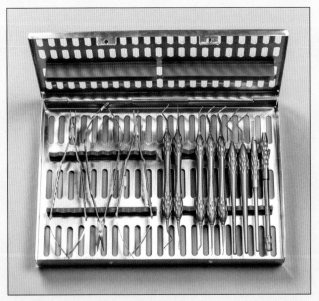

Fig 3-2 / Microsurgery instrument tray.

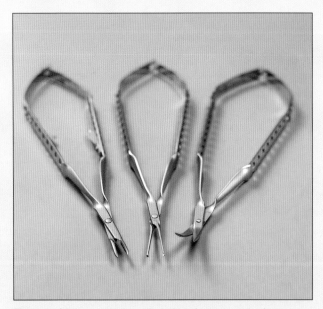

Fig 3-3 / Microsurgical needle holder, forceps, and scissors.

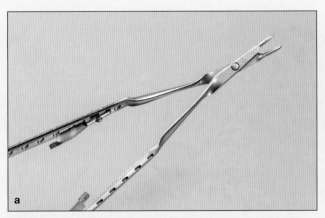

a

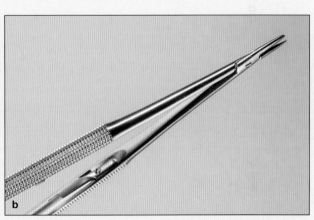

b

Fig 3-4 / *(a and b)* Examples of straight microneedle holders.

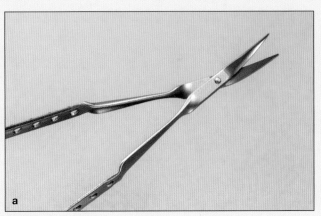

a

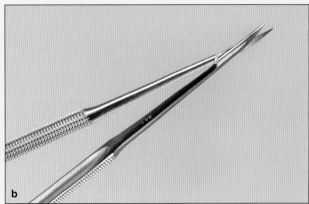

b

Fig 3-5 / *(a and b)* Examples of microsuture scissors.

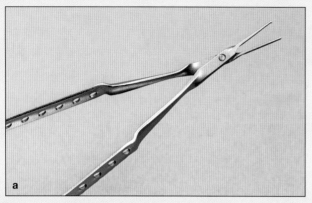 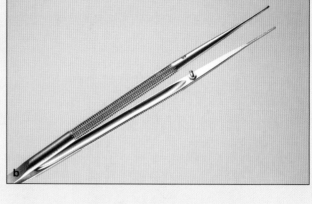

Fig 3-6 / *(a and b)* Examples of atraumatic forceps for microsurgery.

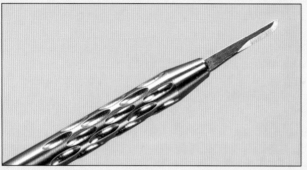

Fig 3-7 / Microsurgical scalpel handle.

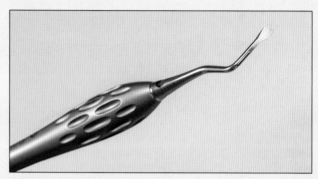

Fig 3-8 / Tunneling knife.

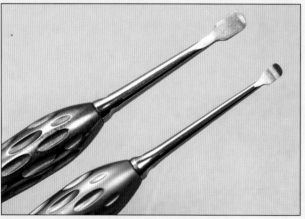

Fig 3-9 / Raspatory: large, straight end.

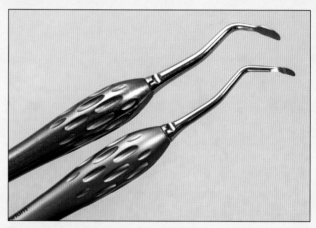

Fig 3-10 / Raspatory: large, curved end.

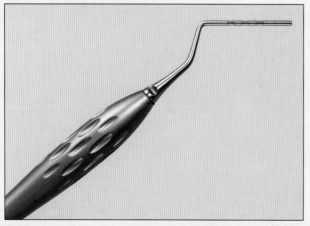

Fig 3-11 / Titanium plugger for immediate implant placement.

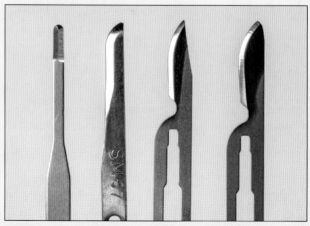

Fig 3-12 / Scalpels: *(left to right)* microblade, SM 67, 15c, 15.

Fig 3-13 / Two needle-and-thread combinations: 6-0 *(left)*; 4-0 *(right)*.

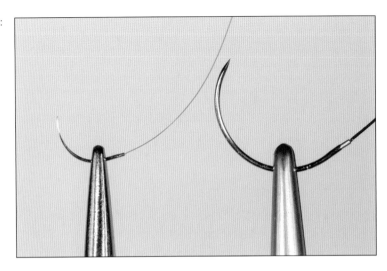

Suturing Materials

Microsurgical suturing materials must have the following characteristics:

- Sterility
- High tear resistance
- Biocompatibility
- Strength to hold knots firmly
- No capillarity

Only atraumatic suture materials are generally used in microsurgery. A characteristic of these needles is that the transition to the suture thread occurs without any change in diameter and the thread completely fills the puncture channel (see Fig 3-13).

If possible, resorbable suture material should be avoided. This is because hydrolysis splits the material in tissue into glycol and lactate, which are broken down during intermediary metabolism. This reaction can result in delayed wound healing. If there is a clinical necessity to use resorbable sutures, it is necessary to consider the resorption time (eg, 60 to 90 days or faster with explicitly fast-resorbable materials) and the lifetime of the material.

The use of multifilament sutures is obsolete in microsurgery; if possible, these sutures should not be used. They have a tendency to a wick effect: As a result of the rough surface of multifilament suture materials, fluid as well as bacteria are drawn into the wound area like a wick.[7] This applies especially to suture materials made of natural silk and becomes more problematic the longer the material remains in situ.[8]

It is best to use nonresorbable monofilament suture material (Fig 3-14) for microsurgical wound suturing because it minimizes postoperative complications caused by trauma, plaque deposits, and resorption processes. The esthetic outcome in terms of scars and recessions is also much better clinically when monofilament sutures are used.

Polyvinyl fluoride (eg, Seralene, Serag Wiessner; Fig 3-15) is the most biocompatible suture material. It is hydrophobic and is not altered by hydrolysis in the body, unlike polyamides. Monofilament polypropylene is relatively stiff. This means that handling and the firm hold of knots become problematic unless the thickness is above 6-0. The next most biocompatible material is polyamide/nylon (eg, Seralon, Serag Wiessner or Ethilon, Johnson & Johnson), followed by polyester (eg, Ethibond, Johnson & Johnson) and finally expanded polytetrafluoroethylene (ePTFE; Gore-Tex, W.L. Gore; Cytoplast, Osteogenics; Keydent, American Dental Systems).[7]

However, the advantage of monofilament ePTFE material is that it is elastic and therefore offers a special material property not exhibited by other materials, which tend to be stiffer (Fig 3-16). This can be beneficial to wound closure. The authors use ePTFE especially as a strategic holding suture in the form of horizontal mattress sutures (eg, to guarantee flatter apposition of the wound margins for augmentation procedures).

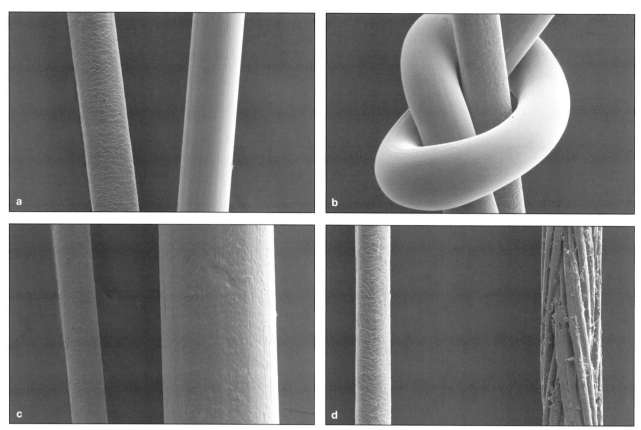

Fig 3-14 / *(a)* 6-0 suture material (Seralene, Serag Wiessner; *right*) compared with a human hair under scanning electron microscope; 200× magnification. *(b)* 6-0 suture material knotted around a human hair. *(c)* 4-0 polytetrafluoroethylene suture material (Cytoplast, Osteogenics; *right*) compared with a human hair (200× magnification). *(d)* 6-0 braided resorbable material made of polyglactin (PGA Resorba, Osteogenics; *right*) compared with a human hair (200× magnification). (Courtesy of Dr Andreas Schäfer, NanoAnalytics, Münster, Germany.)

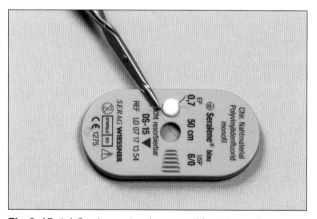

Fig 3-15 / A Seralene suture is removed from the pack.

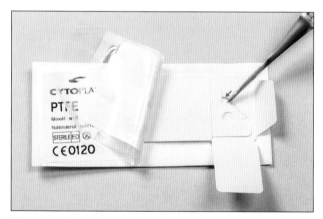

Fig 3-16 / A PTFE suture is removed from the pack.

By this technique, the flap is set up so that full and flat contact of the wound margins is achieved; this contact is retained even on slight retraction of the flap (eg, from pulling). At the same time, microsurgical interrupted sutures ensure relatively atraumatic, precise approximation so that rapid vascular connection and hence rapid wound healing are guaranteed. Figures 3-17 to 3-19 show handling and elements of the needle-and-suture combinations.

Thread thickness only denotes the diameter (and parameters that depend on it) of surgical suture material. Two different measuring systems are used for this purpose: the American USP (United States Pharmacopeia)

Fig 3-17 / The needle should be gripped in the posterior third *(a)*, but not in the swaging zone *(b)*.

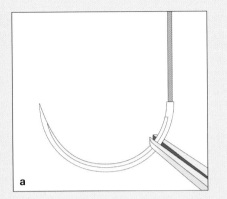
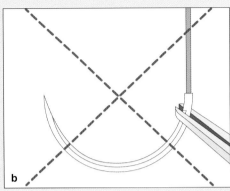

Fig 3-18 / Elements of a needle-and-suture combination.

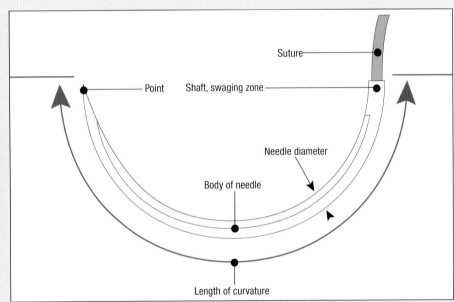

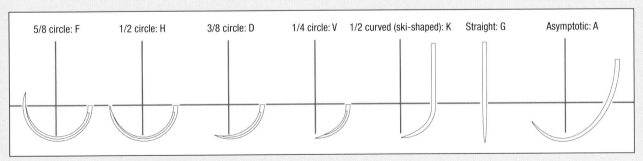

Fig 3-19 / Different surgical needles.

Table 3-1 Thread thicknesses of surgical suture material

USP	Metric	Range (mm)
11-0	0.1	0.010–0.019
10-0	0.2	0.020–0.029
9-0	0.3	0.030–0.039
8-0	0.4	0.040–0.049
7-0	0.5	0.050–0.059
6-0	0.7	0.070–0.079
5-0	1.0	0.100–0.149
4-0	1.5	0.150–0.199
3-0	2.0	0.200–0.249
2-0	2.5	0.250–0.299
1-0	3.0	0.300–0.349
0	3.5	0.350–0.399
1	4.0	0.400–0.499
2	5.0	0.500–0.599
3+4	6.0	0.600–0.699
5	7.0	0.700–0.799
6	8.0	0.800–0.899
7	9.0	0.900–0.999
8	10.0	1.000–1.099

②	Do not reuse
STERILE | EO	Method of sterilization: Ethylene oxide
STERILE | R	Method of sterilization: Irradiation
⧖	Use by (expiration date)
⋀	Date of manufacture
LOT	Batch (lot) number
[i] ⚠	See instructions for use
REF	Order number
CE 1275	CE mark and identification number of notified body (certification institute)

Fig 3-20 / Key to pictograms on suture packs.

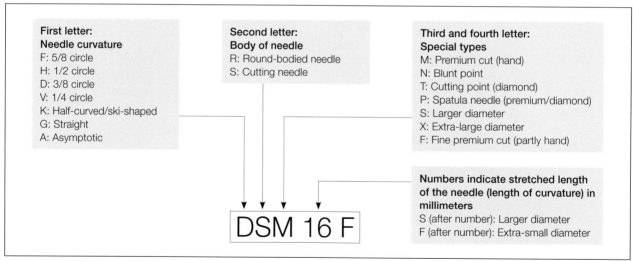

First letter:
Needle curvature
F: 5/8 circle
H: 1/2 circle
D: 3/8 circle
V: 1/4 circle
K: Half-curved/ski-shaped
G: Straight
A: Asymptotic

Second letter:
Body of needle
R: Round-bodied needle
S: Cutting needle

Third and fourth letter:
Special types
M: Premium cut (hand)
N: Blunt point
T: Cutting point (diamond)
P: Spatula needle (premium/diamond)
S: Larger diameter
X: Extra-large diameter
F: Fine premium cut (partly hand)

Numbers indicate stretched length of the needle (length of curvature) in millimeters
S (after number): Larger diameter
F (after number): Extra-small diameter

DSM 16 F

Fig 3-21 / Key to identification of needles.

system and the EP (European Pharmacopoeia) system (metric system) (Table 3-1). The thread thickness printed on a pack is always the minimum thickness; the actual suture thickness is usually in the upper millimeter range. Other information about the suture material appears on the packaging (Figs 3-20 and 3-21).

Clinical Examples

The clinical examples shown in Figs 3-22 to 3-24 illustrate typical use of microsurgical instruments for implant placement in the anterior maxillary dentition.[9]

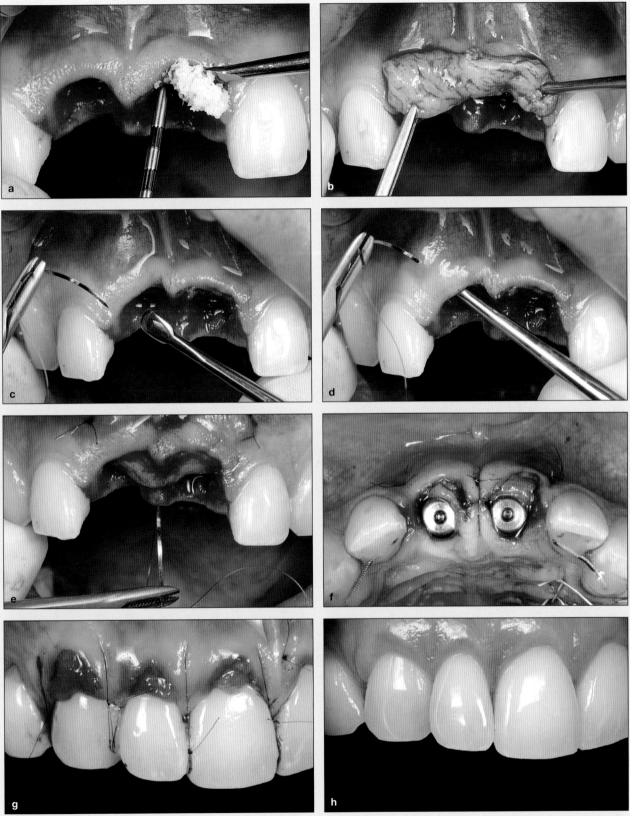

Fig 3-22 / Augmentation for immediate implant placement in the maxillary central incisor sites using microsurgical techniques. *(a)* With the aid of the titanium plugger, the xenograft is placed between the implant and the buccal lamella. *(b)* A connective tissue graft is used to thicken the facial mucosa. *(c)* DSM 16 suture and micro raspatory. *(d)* The buccal mucosa is detached from the bone, creating a tunnel that is kept open while the needle enters the tunnel from the buccal aspect. *(e)* The connective tissue graft is pulled under the buccal mucosa and fixed with vertical mattress sutures. *(f)* Microsurgical approximation of the connective tissue graft buccal to the gingiva former. *(g)* Tunneling technique in plastic-periodontal microsurgery according to Zuhr and Hürzeler.[9] *(h)* Outcome after healing of recession coverage (for recession coverage treatment of this case, see Fig 4-10 in chapter 4).

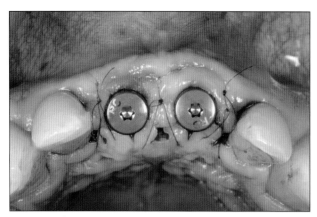

Fig 3-23 / Delicate techniques for soft tissue management, such as the split-finger technique, can only be performed by microsurgery.

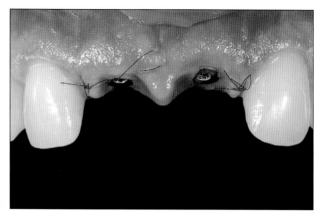

Fig 3-24 / Perfect wound conditions of a patient 1 week after papilla reconstruction thanks to monofilament atraumatic suture material and a microsurgical technique.

Acknowledgments

The authors wish to thank Dr Eva Nadenau for her assistance in creating this chapter.

References

1. Cortellini P, Tonetti MS. Microsurgical approach to periodontal regeneration. Initial evaluation in a case cohort. J Periodontol 2001;72:559–569.
2. Wachtel H, Schenk G, Böhm S, Weng D, Zuhr O, Hürzeler MB. Microsurgical access flap and enamel matrix derivative for the treatment of periodontal intrabony defects: A controlled clinical study. J Clin Periodontol 2003;30:496–504.
3. Zadeh HH, Daftary F. Minimally invasive surgery: An alternative approach for periodontal and implant reconstruction. J Calif Dent Assoc 2004;32:1022–1030.
4. Shanelec DA. Anterior esthetic implants: Microsurgical placement in extraction sockets with immediate provisionals. J Calif Dent Assoc 2005;33:233–240.
5. Burkhardt R, Lang NP. Coverage of localized gingival recessions: Comparison of micro- and macrosurgical techniques. J Clin Periodontol 2005;32:287–293.
6. Happe A, Khoury F. Complications and risk factors in bone grafting procedures. In: Khoury F, Antoun H, Missika P (eds). Bone Augmentation in Oral Implantology. Chicago: Quintessence, 2007:405–429.
7. Tabanella G. Oral tissue reactions to suture materials: A review. J West Soc Periodontol Periodontal Abstr 2004;52:37–44.
8. Lilly GE, Cutcher JL, Jones JC, Armstrong JH. Reaction of oral tissues to suture materials. IV. Oral Surg Oral Med Oral Pathol 1972;33:152–157.
9. Zuhr O, Hürzeler M. Plastic-Esthetic Periodontal and Implant Surgery: A Microsurgical Approach. London: Quintessence, 2011.

"Lost time is never found again."

BENJAMIN FRANKLIN

4

Immediate Implant Placement in the Esthetic Zone

/ Arndt Happe, Gerd Körner

Socket Healing

Loss of a tooth is inevitably accompanied by loss of hard and soft tissue. Reconstruction of dentofacial harmony in the esthetic zone is currently one of the greatest challenges facing modern implantology. After removal of a tooth, the alveolar bone undergoes powerful remodeling processes that usually result in three-dimensional (3D) alveolar ridge defects.

Dynamic changes occur in the socket after dental extraction. Cardaropoli et al[1] studied this change in detail in an animal model. If the periodontal ligament is still present, a blood clot forms immediately after extraction. If the ligament is lost, the clot develops into a temporary matrix due to the migration of fibroblasts; over the course of weeks, this matrix is transformed into a delicate network of bone. After about 180 days, this network of bone is largely remodeled into medullary space and fatty tissue. By this stage, the hard tissue portion in the socket makes up only around 15%. Histologic examination has shown that cortical bone coverage (ie, coronal bridging) predictably results in closure of the alveolus. Although the transferability of data from an animal model to human situations—especially the precise timescales—is obviously limited, the study does provide valuable indicators of possible changes to the composition of the tooth socket in humans.[1] The highest level of mineralization of the alveolus in humans usually occurs between 12 and 16 weeks postextraction.[2,3]

Araújo et al[4,5] discovered that bundle bone plays a crucial role in the resorption processes. *Bundle bone* is the part of the alveolar bone that contains the collagen fibrils of Sharpey fibers. Bundle bone, like the cementum and periodontal ligament, originates phylogenetically from the dental follicle and—unlike the rest of the jawbone—it is not of periosteal origin. Extraction is therefore inevitably followed by bone resorption in the area of bundle bone because the physiologic function of bundle bone (ie, to anchor the tooth) is no longer required. The nature and extent of the resorption depend on the bony composition of the buccal lamella.[4] If the lamella predominantly consists of bundle bone, a bony deficit is unavoidable; however, if a cortical portion is still present, there is a relatively high probability of the lamella being retained even after immediate implant placement. In practice, the composition of the buccal lamella can be subjectively assessed by measuring its thickness. Clinical trials have shown that the extent of volume loss after extraction is inversely proportional to the thickness of the buccal lamella.[6] In a radiologic study, Nevins et al[7] showed that the buccal lamella was clearly visible on a radiograph immediately after extraction but could no longer be detected in some patients after 37 to 42 days, and even well-trained clinicians could not foresee which patients were prone to buccal lamella resorption. A study on nearly 500 teeth using cone beam computed tomography (CBCT) diagnostics concluded that the thickness of the buccal lamella is less than 1 mm in over 90% of teeth, particularly in the esthetic zone.[8]

Schropp et al[9] studied the change to the horizontal crestal width after extraction of molars or premolars in 46 patients and found that resorption mainly happens on the buccal aspect of the alveolar ridge. After 12 months, approximately 50% of the buccolingual crest width had been lost, the majority of the resorption (ie, around 60%) having happened within the first 3 months following extraction.

Timing of Implant Placement

Considering the physiologic changes that occur after extraction, the following strategically significant times postextraction have been defined or classified, and any of these could be suitable for implant placement depending on the patient's specific circumstances[2]:

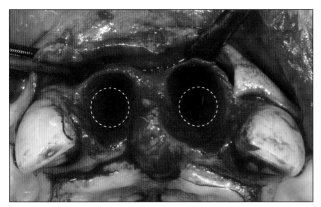

Fig 4-1 / The socket is intact at the time of extraction, so immediate implant placement is possible. (However, the flap formation in this case was completed for a different reason and is not desirable for performing immediate implant placement.)

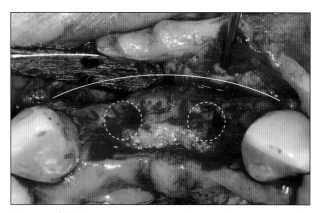

Fig 4-2 / Findings are comparable to those in Fig 4-1, but this shows the condition 6 weeks after extraction. Resorption of the buccal lamella and therefore a 3D alveolar ridge defect have already occurred.

- Immediately after extraction (Fig 4-1)
- When soft tissue healing of the socket is completed, so it is covered with mucosa (about 4 to 8 weeks after extraction; Fig 4-2)
- Distinct clinical or radiologic bone regeneration (about 12 to 16 weeks after extraction)
- Socket fully healed (longer than 16 weeks after extraction)

These timings can vary depending on the clinical situation and degree of inflammation of the tissue. Depending on the treatment plan for the patient, implant-related interventions may be useful at different points in time. If the socket is intact, immediate implant placement may be considered, provided an appropriate risk analysis has been performed. However, it is important to bear in mind that there might be a tissue deficit around the socket opening. At this stage, no resorption processes have yet begun.

If the socket is damaged and requires augmentation, it might be better to wait for complete soft tissue healing of the alveolus to ensure that there is mature mucosa to work with. This facilitates soft tissue management and adequate coverage of the hard tissue augmentation material. If bony healing is desirable (eg, because socket geometry or anatomy do not allow for adequate implant anchorage), implant placement should occur at a suitably later stage. This may be advisable in the posterior dentition, for teeth with multiple roots, or if the fundus of the socket is located in close proximity to important anatomical structures (eg, nasal floor, maxillary sinus, nerve canal). In these cases, advanced resorption is to be expected, which means augmentation techniques will nearly always be required.

Immediate Implant Placement

In an animal model, Botticelli et al[10] and Araújo et al[5] concluded that the immediate placement of implants into extraction sockets does not lead to preservation of bony structures but still results in the remodeling process. Therefore, the therapeutic concept of immediate implant placement was reevaluated, and the range of indications became limited. Furthermore, the previously described classification regarding timing of implant placement was proposed (see the previous section).

Additional studies in dogs showed that the surgical protocol as well as the position of the implant can have an influence on the resorption process of the buccal lamella. For instance, Araújo et al[11] repeated their dog study using smaller-diameter implants that were placed in the lingual area of the socket, and the resulting gap was augmented with xenogeneic substitute material. The results showed that buccal resorption could be greatly reduced.[11] Covani et al[12] conducted a similar animal study and showed that simply using reduced-diameter implants in the lingual area of the socket leads to minimal buccal resorption.

In a clinical trial by Chen et al[13] involving 30 patients who underwent immediate implant placement, the horizontal resorption without augmentation of the gap between implant and buccal lamella was nearly 50%—just as much as that observed by Schropp et al[9] after extraction without implant placement. The authors of the study managed to reduce horizontal resorption to 17% to 20% in patients in whom the gap was augmented with bovine substitute material. However, these procedures involved the formation of a mucoperiosteal flap. For less bone resorption and better esthetic results, current approaches forgo the formation of a flap.[14,15]

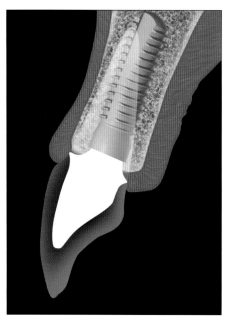

Fig 4-3 / Illustration of the 3D position of an implant in an extraction socket.

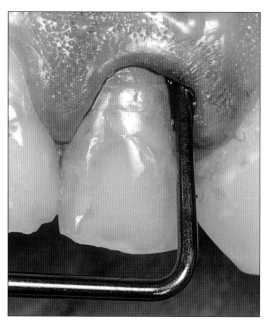

Fig 4-4 / The lack of buccal lamella can frequently be diagnosed using a periodontal probe, as seen here in the case of longitudinal fracture of a maxillary lateral incisor.

The 3D positioning of the implant is another fundamentally important factor in the esthetic outcome (Fig 4-3). This must be guided by the planned restoration.[16] Chen et al[13] studied the influence of the implant position on the degree of buccal recession on 42 immediate implants. They concluded that too buccal of an implant position causes significantly more recession at immediate implants. Clinically, this means that the implant should be placed slightly palatally, and an angulation in the buccal direction must be avoided.

Another significant influencing factor is the individual tissue biotype (also known as *phenotype* or *morphotype*), which describes tissue thickness.[17] A literature review from 2011 regarding the influence of the tissue biotype reached the conclusion that the biotype is a very important factor in the esthetic outcome of immediate implants as well as a prognostic factor for the occurrence of recession at immediate implants in the longer term.[18]

Literature review articles that reviewed and analyzed all of the available studies on immediate implant placement recognized typical pros and cons and identified risk factors. In 2009, Chen and Buser reported in a literature review[19] that augmentation methods are more successful in conjunction with immediate and delayed immediate implant placement than with late placement. However, recession was common in immediate implant placement.

A thin periodontal biotype, a buccal implant position, and a thin or damaged buccal lamella were identified as risk factors (Fig 4-4). A systematic Cochrane review[20] found a rather higher rate of complications and loss for immediate implants and delayed immediate implants than for late implants. However, the authors concluded that the esthetic outcome is best with immediate implants.

The best results with immediate implants can therefore be expected in patients with thick periodontal biotypes and an intact buccal lamella. The diameter of these implants should be smaller than that of the socket, and the implant should be placed palatally in the alveolus. The resulting space between implant and buccal lamella should be at least 2 mm wide and augmented with a suitable slowly resorbable or minimumly resorbable bone substitute material.

Because implant placement occurs in the extraction socket, primary stability becoms a concern. Primary stability can only be achieved if enough bone is available apical to the socket to ensure stabilization. Furthermore, the implant design must permit apical or palatal anchorage. This means that the macro design of the implant must be suitable for this purpose (eg, apically conical or with a good cutting thread). The implant is also usually placed without formation of a flap, allowing for transmucosal healing. Clinical studies have shown that submerged

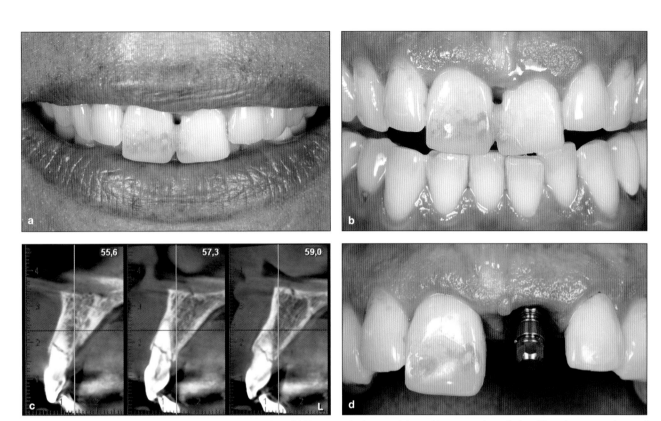

Fig 4-5 / (a) Smile a few weeks after anterior tooth injury. (b) Preoperative intraoral view with composite splinting. There is excess tissue of approximately 1 mm at the left central incisor. The right central incisor had sustained an extra-alveolar crown fracture; the left an intra-alveolar root fracture. (c) CBCT clearly shows the root fracture; the buccal lamella is retained. (d) A bone-level implant 4.1 mm in diameter is placed 4 mm apical to the soft tissue margin. The superstructure will be used to displace the soft tissue apically. Therefore, the implant shoulder lies 3 mm below the intended soft tissue margin.

and transmucosal healing lead to similar clinical results for single-tooth implants, even when a small amount of peri-implant augmentation is needed.[21,22]

As early as 1993, Salama and Salama[23] proposed orthodontic extrusion of teeth to improve the anatomical situation prior to immediate implant placement. As a consequence, socket diameter is diminished, and socket size is simultaneously reduced vertically. This produces better anchorage of the implant. In addition, tissue is gained vertically, and extraction is simplified.

Immediate Implant Placement with Immediate Restoration

Immediate provisional restorations on temporary abutments can be used to avoid collapse of the periodontal tissue and to close the orifice of the socket. The provisional crowns are adjusted so that they have no contact with the opposing arch in static and dynamic occlusion. The immediate attachment of a provisional restoration produces better esthetic results than immediate implant placement without a provisional restoration[24] (Fig 4-5).

The primary stability of the implant does not always permit restoration with a provisional crown. In these cases, a customized anatomical gingiva former can be used to seal the socket and support the tissue. Tarnow et al[25] compared four different therapeutic approaches for immediate implant placement:

1. Without augmentation of the gap between implant and buccal lamella and without provisional restoration but with a narrow prefabricated gingiva former
2. Without augmentation of the gap but with a provisional crown
3. With augmentation of the gap and a wide anatomical gingiva former
4. With augmentation of the gap and with a provisional abutment and provisional crown

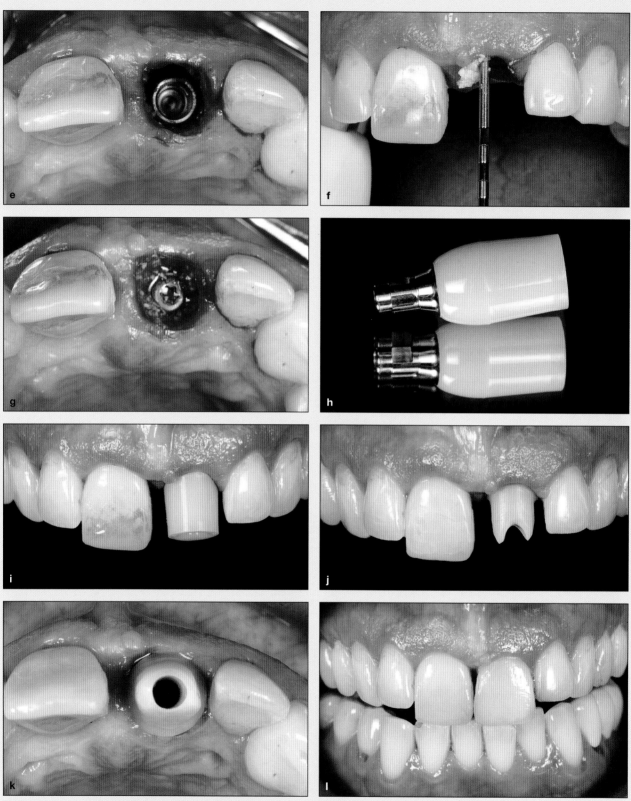

Fig 4-5 *cont.* / *(e)* Palatal position of the implant. A gap of 2 to 3 mm from the buccal lamella remains. *(f)* Bone substitute material is introduced with a titanium plugger. *(g)* The spaces between the implant and the bony socket are filled with substitute material. *(h)* A temporary abutment with a titanium base and acrylic material. The emergence profile needs to be adapted buccally because it is still too convex. *(i)* The abutment fits well into the soft tissue socket. *(j)* Prepared abutment in situ. *(k)* The customized abutment seals the socket. Further reduction is required palatally. *(l)* Provisional acrylic resin restoration in situ.

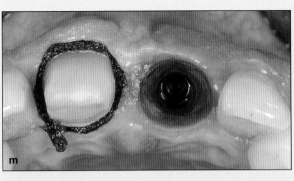

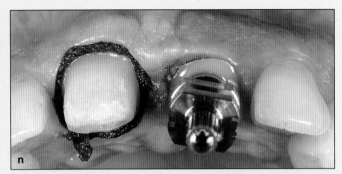

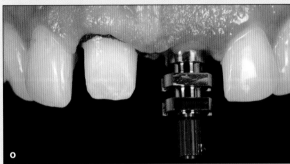

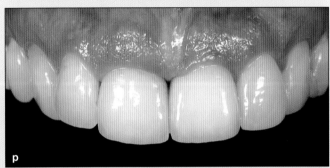

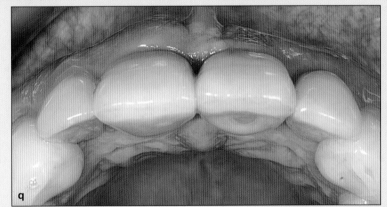

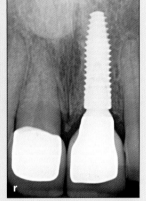

Fig 4-5 *cont.* / *(m)* The adjacent right central incisor is prepared for a crown. *(n and o)* The contoured emergence profile is transferred using a customized impression post. *(p)* Definitive restoration with crown on the right central incisor, implant crown on the left central incisor, and nonprep veneer on the left lateral incisor 1 year postoperatively. The patient wanted the central incisors to be shorter than before treatment. *(q)* Buccal volume after 1 year. *(r)* Radiograph of the restorations after 1 year. *(s)* Patient's smile.

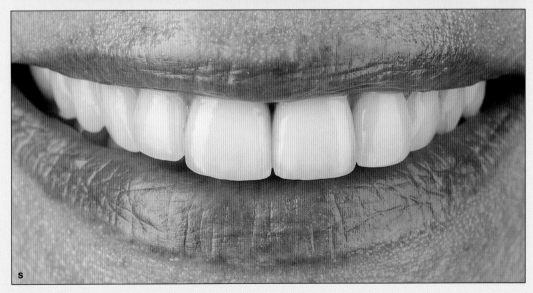

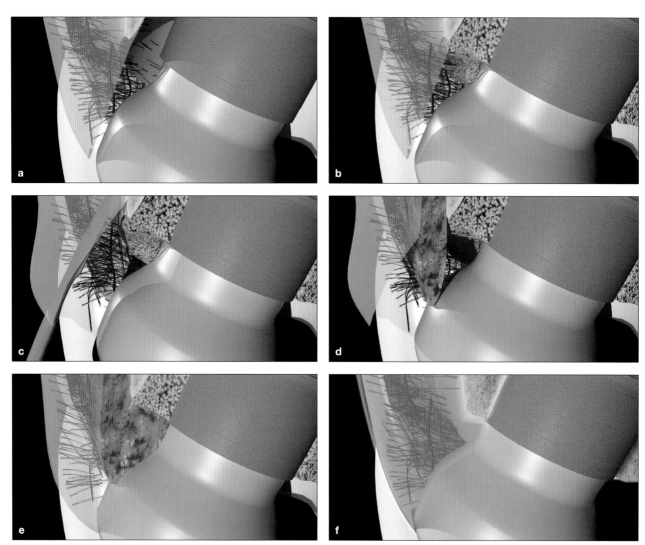

Fig 4-6 / Illustration of the technique. *(a)* Place the implant 2 to 3 mm palatal to the buccal lamella and 3 to 4 mm below the planned soft tissue margin. *(b)* Fill the space with bone substitute material. *(c)* Prepare a supraperiosteal pocket buccal to the buccal lamella; this merges into the mucogingival junction. *(d)* Introduce a subepithelial CTG into the pocket. *(e)* Adapt the mucosa to the gingiva former with sutures. *(f)* Ideally, the volume of the alveolar process is preserved after healing.

Over an observation period of up to 4 years, the smallest contour changes were observed in groups 3 and 4: the two groups in which the gap was filled with bone substitute material and in which the orifice of the socket was supported and closed with either a provisional crown or an anatomical gingiva former.[25]

There are contrasting statements in the literature about long-term results of immediate implant placement with immediate provisional restoration. While Barone et al[26] reported good esthetic results and stable soft tissue conditions after 7 years, other authors observed continuous soft tissue recession and loss of contour after 5 and 8 years, respectively.[27,28]

Immediate Implant Placement with a Connective Tissue Graft

To avoid the problems of soft tissue recession and loss of contour, connective tissue grafts (CTGs) are frequently used to thicken the facial soft tissue. This technique has been described by several authors and tested in clinical trials.[29–31]

In 2011, Grunder[31] published a comparative case series with 24 patients who received immediate implants in the esthetic zone. He divided the patients into two groups of 12; one group received a CTG via the tunneling technique at the same time as implant placement, while the other group did not. The results after 6 months showed a mean horizontal loss of 1.063 mm in the group without

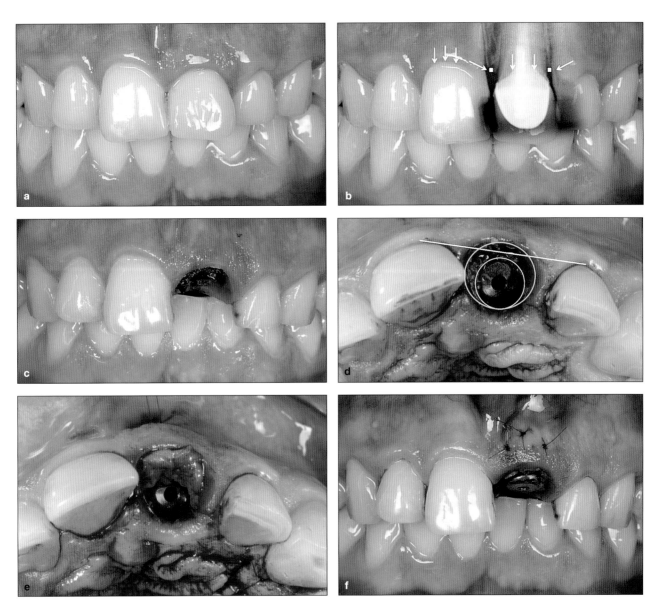

Fig 4-7 / (a) The maxillary left central incisor is not worth preserving, and it exhibits an excess of tissue buccally. (b) The adjacent teeth show no loss of attachment. (c) The root remnant is no longer usable for prosthodontic purposes. (d) An implant 4.3 mm in diameter is placed in the palatal area of the socket. The diameter of the implant (inner circle) is significantly smaller than that of the socket (outer circle). (e) A CTG is introduced into the supraperiosteal pocket buccal to the buccal lamella. (f) The procedure is completed. The socket is closed with the gingiva former and the CTG.

47

the CTG and a mean gain of 0.34 mm in the group that received the CTG.

In a prospective case series of 10 patients in 2011, Tsuda et al[30] reported 1-year results showing a similar trend. They demonstrated that the combination of augmentation of the gap buccal to the implant with a xenograft and additional augmentation of the soft tissue with connective tissue leads to retention of volume and avoids soft tissue recession during this period.

The graft essentially has three functions in this process. First, it is intended to thicken the facial soft tissue and

thereby compensate for loss of volume. Second, it is meant to close the orifice of the socket at the buccal aspect and thereby cover the substitute material once it has been introduced. In addition, together with the gingiva former, it supports the marginal soft tissue (including papillae) and thereby prevents collapse of the periodontal soft tissue (Figs 4-6 and 4-7). The last two functions of the graft might alternatively be performed by the provisional restoration, as has already been described (Fig 4-8).

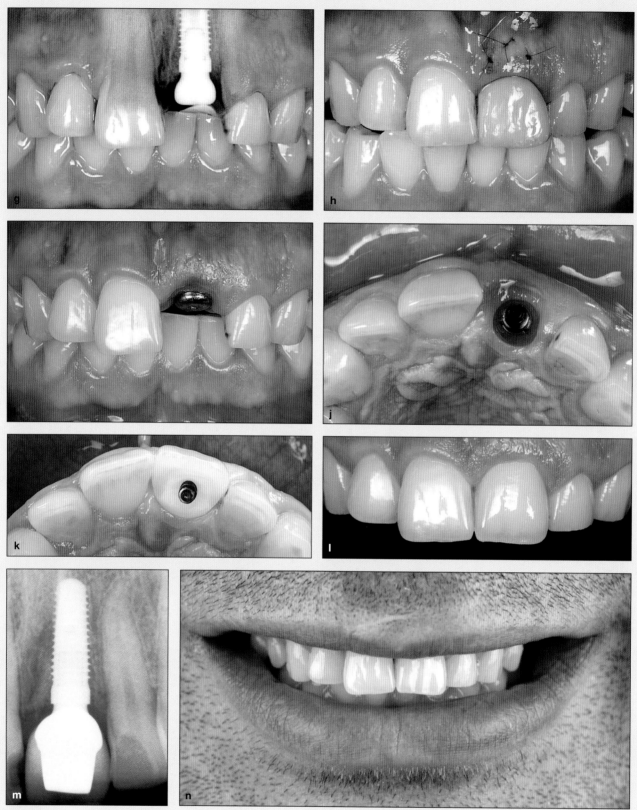

Fig 4-7 *cont.* / *(g)* Superimposed postoperative radiograph. *(h)* The soft tissue is supported by a bonded provisional restoration immediately after surgery. *(i)* Frontal view 3 months postoperatively. *(j)* Occlusal view 3 months postoperatively. *(k)* Screw-retained restoration. *(l)* Final image 6 months after crown placement. *(m)* Radiograph 6 months after placement. *(n)* Smile. (Surgery and prosthodontics performed by A. Happe; laboratory work performed by A. Nolte.)

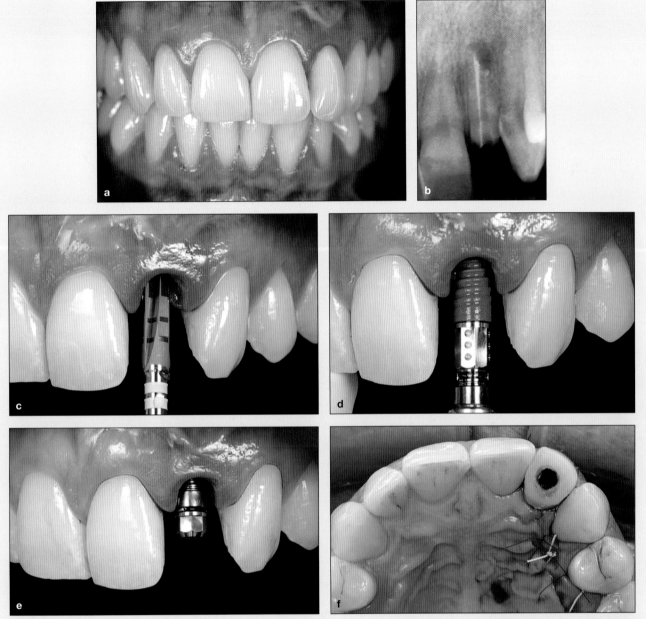

Fig 4-8 / *(a)* The maxillary left lateral incisor is not worth preserving. *(b)* Radiograph of the lateral incisor. *(c)* Preparation for implant without flap formation; the buccal lamella is preserved. *(d)* Implant placement. *(e)* The 4.1-mm-diameter implant in situ. *(f)* A temporary titanium abutment is placed on the implant, and a provisional veneer is suitably adapted. The harvest site for the CTG can be seen in the region of the premolars and first molar. *(g)* Radiograph with provisional restoration immediately after surgery.

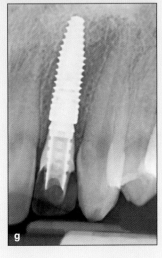

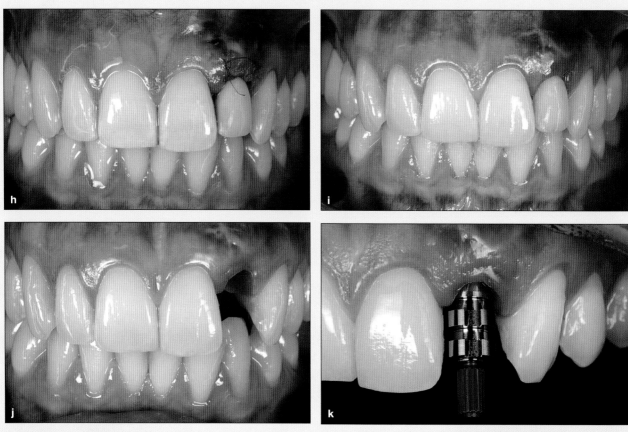

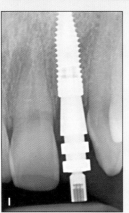

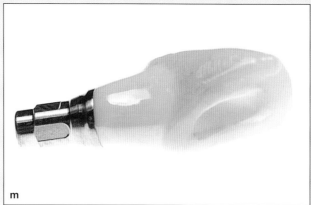

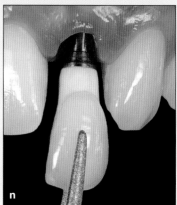

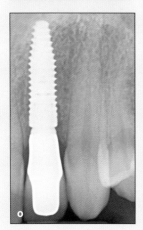

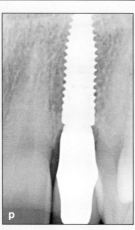

Fig 4-8 *cont.* / *(h)* Finished provisional for the lateral incisor screwed in place. *(i)* Final postoperative image. With the provisional in situ, a CTG was placed buccally. *(j)* Healing 3 weeks postoperatively. *(k)* Implant impression-taking. *(l)* Radiograph with impression post in situ. *(m)* Fully screw-retained superstructure with titanium base. *(n)* Insertion of the superstructure. *(o)* Radiograph of the superstructure 3 months after placement. *(p)* Periapical radiograph at 5 year follow-up. →

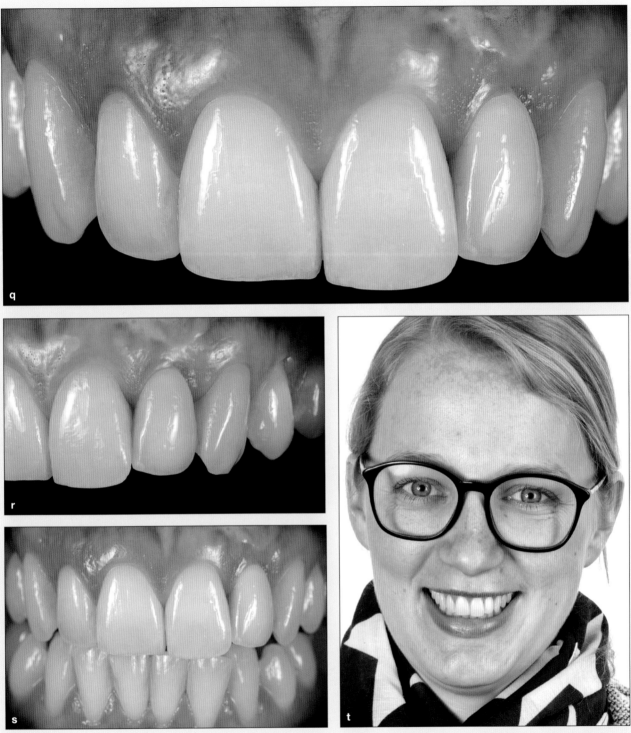

Fig 4-8 *cont.* / *(q to s)* Clinical photographs 5 years after treatment. *(t)* Final portrait. (Surgery and prosthodontics performed by A. Happe; laboratory work performed by P. Holthaus.)

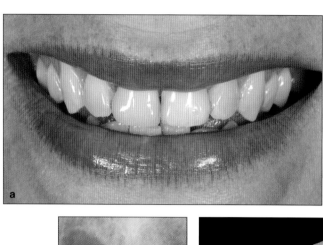
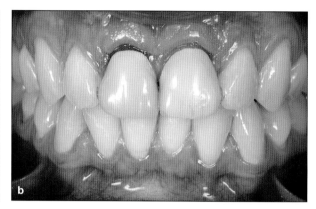
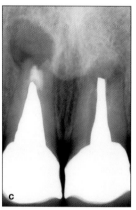
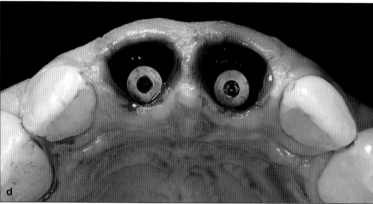
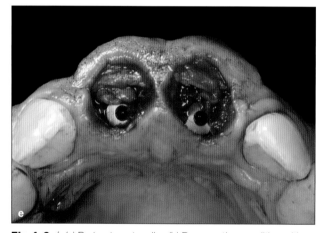
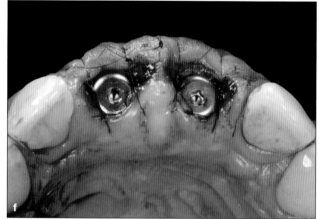

Fig 4-9 / *(a)* Pretreatment smile. *(b)* Preoperative condition with provisional crowns in situ. *(c)* Radiograph of central incisors. Neither tooth is worth preserving. *(d)* Two implants (3.8 mm in diameter) were placed in the palatal area of the sockets with primary stability. *(e)* A tunnel was created in the buccal tissue, and a CTG was placed. *(f)* Gingiva formers in situ and microsurgical adaptation of the soft tissue.

Impressive results can be achieved with this technique even if the preoperative situation itself is difficult, involving two adjacent teeth that need to be replaced by implants (Fig 4-9). The technique can also be combined with other periodontal plastic surgery methods. For instance, a CTG used to cover recession may also serve the purpose of thickening the soft tissue for immediate implant placement (Fig 4-10).

The authors' own results with substitute materials for connective tissue, which were collected as part of a prospective study, also show very good outcomes (Figs 4-11 to 4-13), although adequate long-term results were not yet available at the time of printing. The cases involved the use of an acellular porcine matrix obtained from the dermis of pigs (Mucoderm, Botiss).

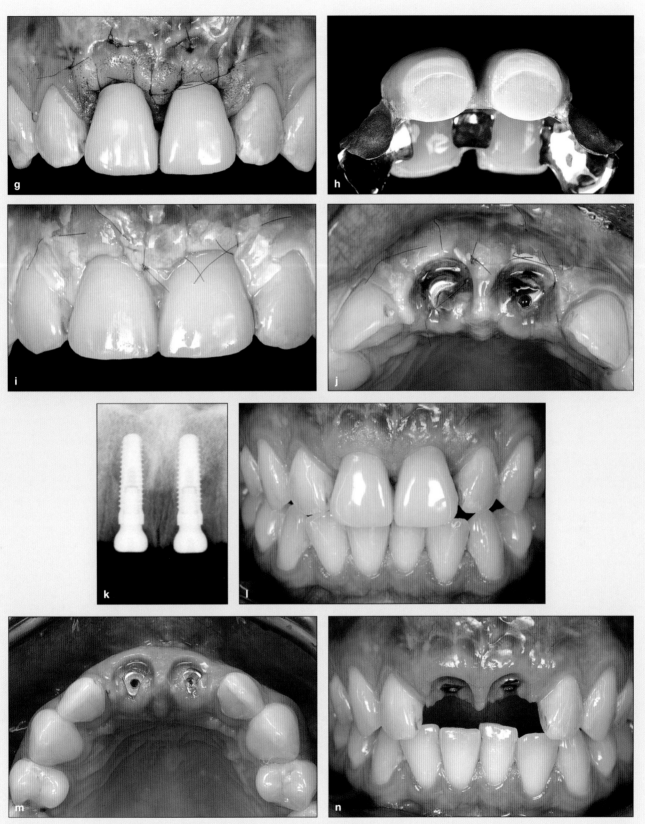

Fig 4-9 *cont.* / *(g)* Postoperative condition with bonded partial denture. *(h)* The bonded partial denture was reduced palatally for the gingiva former. Buccally, the pontics support the cervical tissue. *(i and j)* One week postoperatively with and without provisional restoration. *(k to m)* Radiograph and clinical situation 3 months postoperatively. *(n)* There is almost excessive soft tissue formation and good contouring as a result of the bonded partial denture 3 months postoperatively.

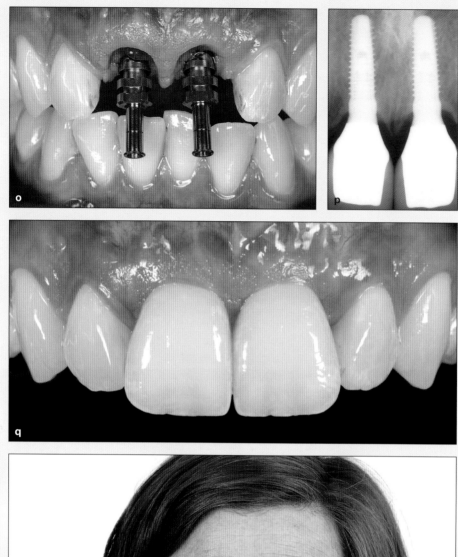

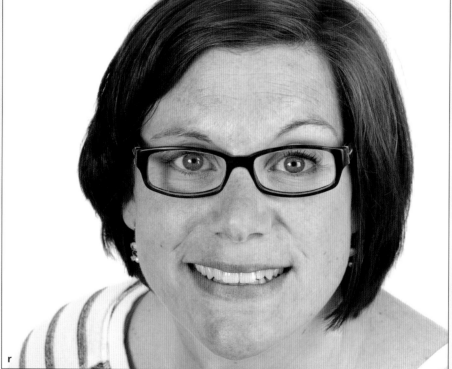

54

Fig 4-9 *cont.* / *(o)* Taking impressions of the implants. *(p)* Radiograph of the superstructure 1 year after implant placement. Note the height of the interimplant bone, which is very important for supporting the papillae. *(q)* All-ceramic crowns 1 year after implant placement. *(r)* Portrait after completion of the treatment. (Surgery performed by A. Happe; prosthodontics performed by B. van den Bosch; laboratory work performed by A. Nolte.)

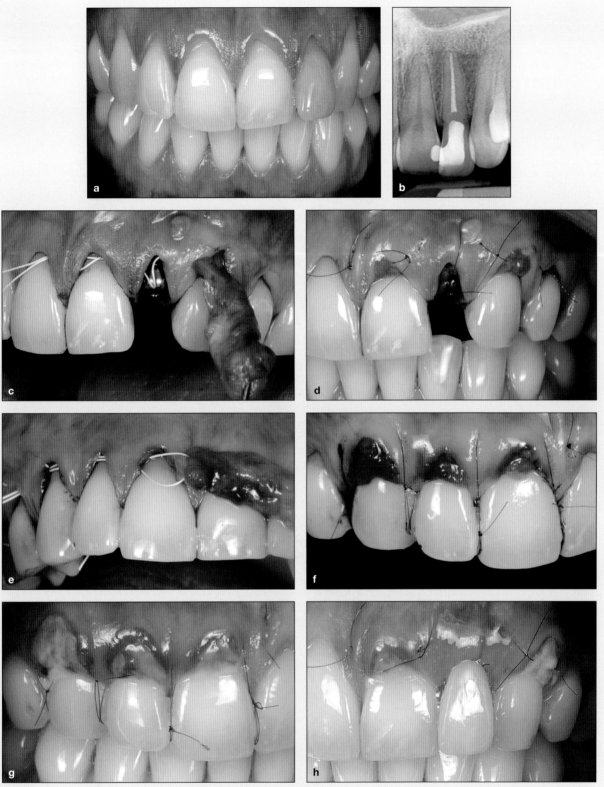

Fig 4-10 / *(a)* Preoperative view with pronounced recession in the maxillary anterior dentition and a left lateral incisor not worth preserving. *(b)* Radiograph of the lateral incisor with a horizontal crown fracture at the height of the limbus alveolaris. *(c)* After extraction, an implant 3.3 mm in diameter was placed along with a gingiva former. In the same session, a CTG was placed via the tunneling technique in the region of the left incisors and canine to cover the recession and thicken the mucosa of the lateral incisor buccally following immediate implant placement. *(d)* Completed immediate implant and CTG placement. *(e)* A few weeks after treatment on the left side, recession coverage was performed using the tunneling technique at the maxillary right central incisor to canine. *(f)* Final view of the procedure on the right with suspended sutures for coronal displacement of the soft tissue. *(g)* Condition of the first quadrant 1 week postoperatively. *(h)* Condition of the second quadrant 1 week postoperatively with bonded partial denture at the lateral incisor in situ.

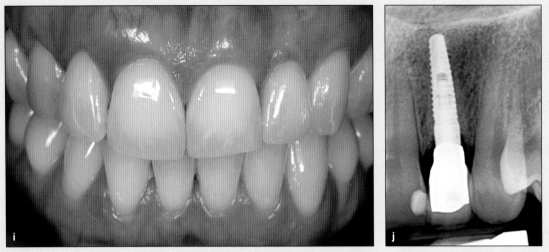

Fig 4-10 *cont.* / *(i)* Condition 12 months after immediate implant placement and recession coverage. *(j)* Radiograph at 12 months.

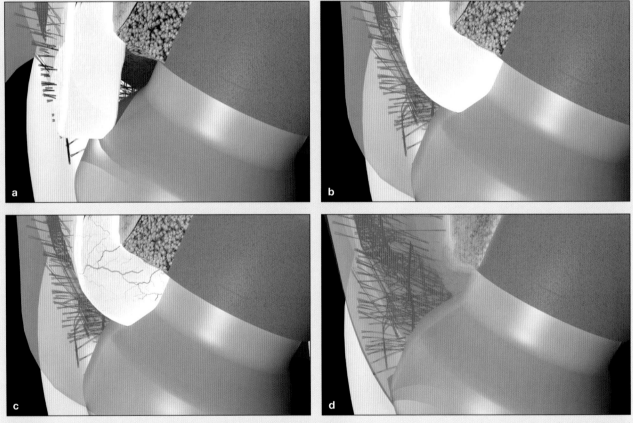

Fig 4-11 / Immediate implant placement with substitute material for CTG. *(a)* A substitute material for connective tissue (acellular dermal matrix) is placed buccal to the bony lamella. *(b)* Adaptation to the gingiva former. *(c)* Tissue integration of the substitute material. *(d)* Complete healing of the area with volume retained.

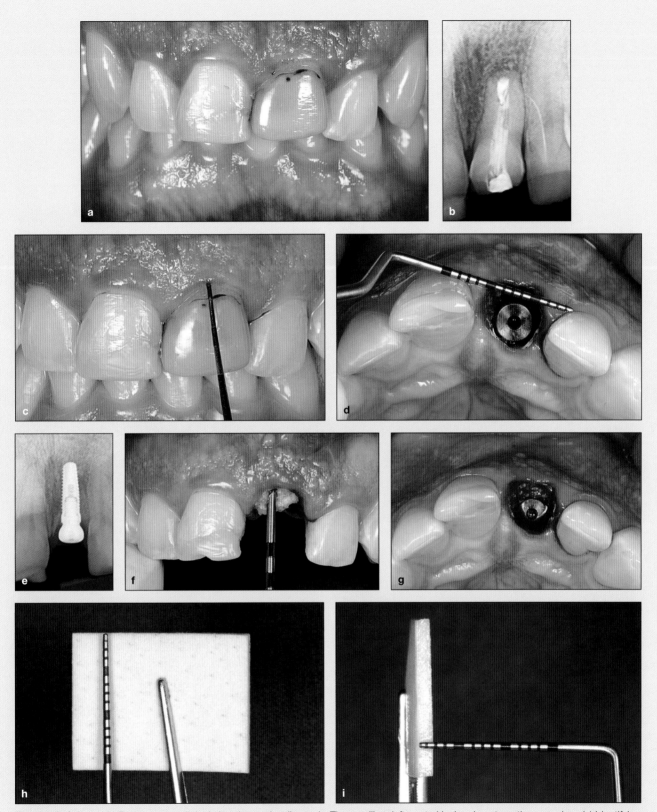

Fig 4-12 / *(a and b)* Pretreatment clinical situation and radiograph. The maxillary left central incisor is not worth preserving. *(c)* Identifying the biotype with a periodontal probe. *(d and e)* An implant 4.3 mm in diameter is placed in the correct 3D position. *(f)* The bone substitute material is introduced with a titanium plugger. *(g)* Implant in situ; the gap is augmented. *(h)* The acellular dermal matrix after rehydration. *(i)* Thickness of the matrix.

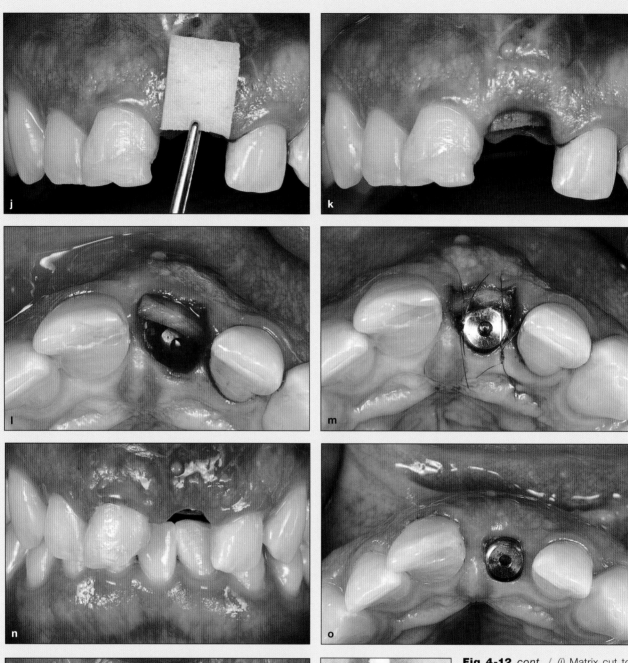

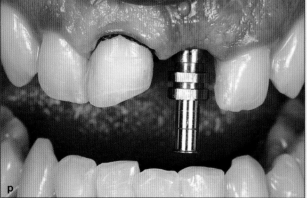

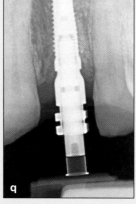

Fig 4-12 *cont.* / *(j)* Matrix cut to size. *(k)* The matrix was introduced buccally as a substitute material for connective tissue. *(l)* Occlusal view. *(m)* Gingiva former in situ and adaptation of the soft tissue. *(n and o)* Healing 2 weeks postoperatively. *(p and q)* Three months after implant placement, before impression-taking: preparation of the right central incisor for veneer and the left central incisor with impression post for a crown. →

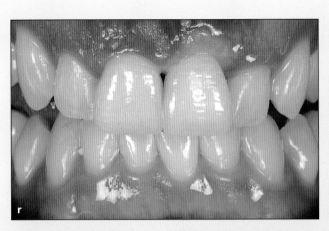

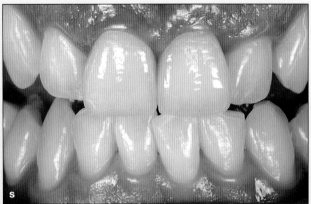

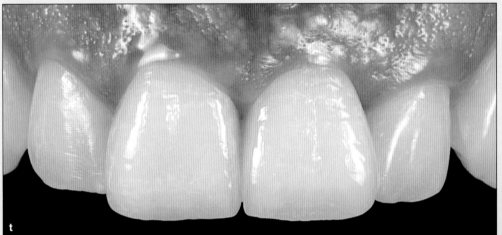

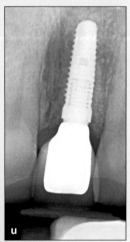

59

Fig 4-12 *cont.* / *(r to v)* Final images and portrait after placement of veneer and implant crown. (Surgery and prosthodontics performed by A. Happe; laboratory work performed by P. Holthaus.)

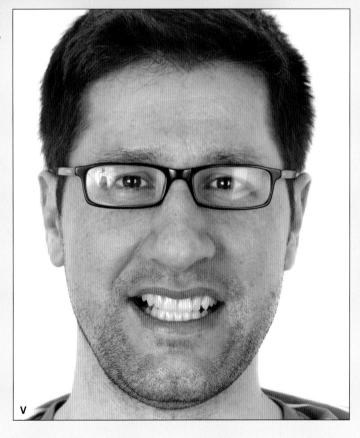

60

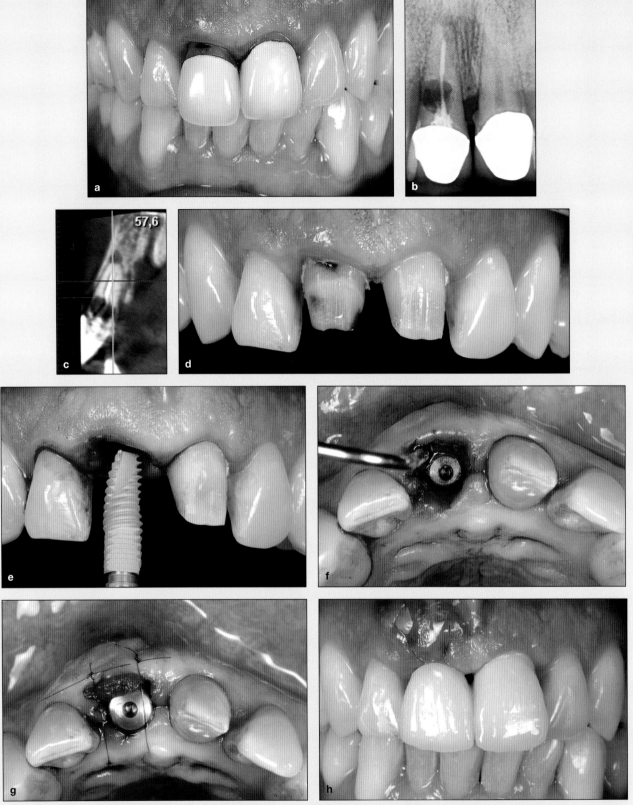

Fig 4-13 / *(a)* Preoperative view with old porcelain-fused-to-metal crowns on the maxillary central incisors. *(b)* The radiograph shows resorption at the right incisor. *(c)* CBCT shows that a buccal lamella is present. *(d)* Condition after removal of the crowns, before extraction of the right incisor. The crown on the left incisor was removed to guarantee a fixed provisional restoration. *(e)* Insertion of an implant with an innovative macro design (ie, triangular cross-section in the crestal part). *(f)* Augmentation of the space between implant and buccal lamella. *(g)* Gingiva former in situ and buccal augmentation of the soft tissue with an acellular dermal matrix. *(h)* Immediate postoperative condition with fixed provisional restoration that is cemented to the left central incisor and has a shear distributor palatal to the right lateral incisor.

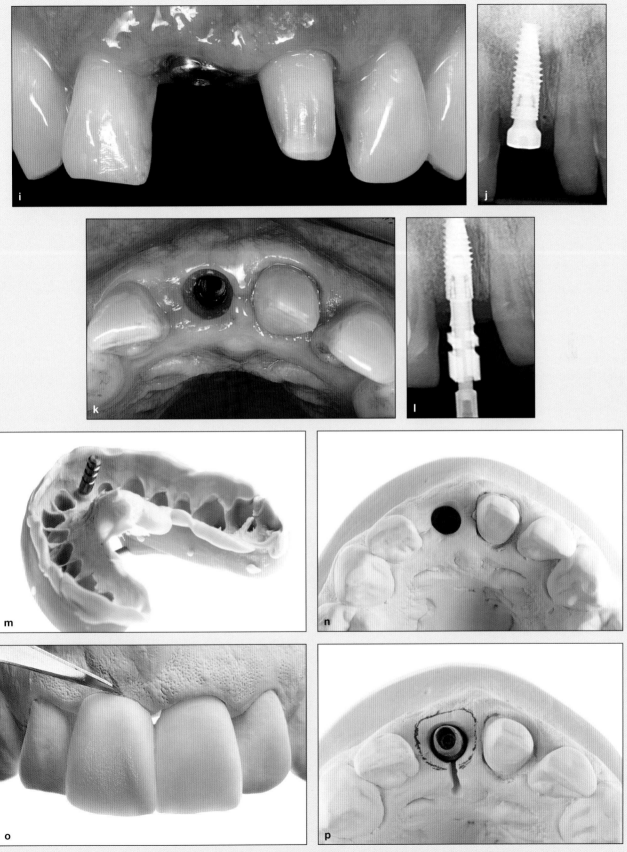

Fig 4-13 *cont.* / *(i)* After 12 weeks, the area is fully healed, and the definitive restoration can be created. *(j)* Radiograph of the implant with the gingiva former. *(k)* The contour of the alveolar ridge was largely preserved with the surgical protocol. *(l)* Radiograph with impression post in situ. *(m)* Impression of right incisor implant and left incisor die with customized tray and silicone impression material. *(n)* With the impression post, the circular soft tissue profile was transferred to the plaster cast. *(o)* Transferring the emergence profile to the cast with a wax-up. *(p)* Contour of the emergence profile marked in pencil, and titanium base fitted. ⟶

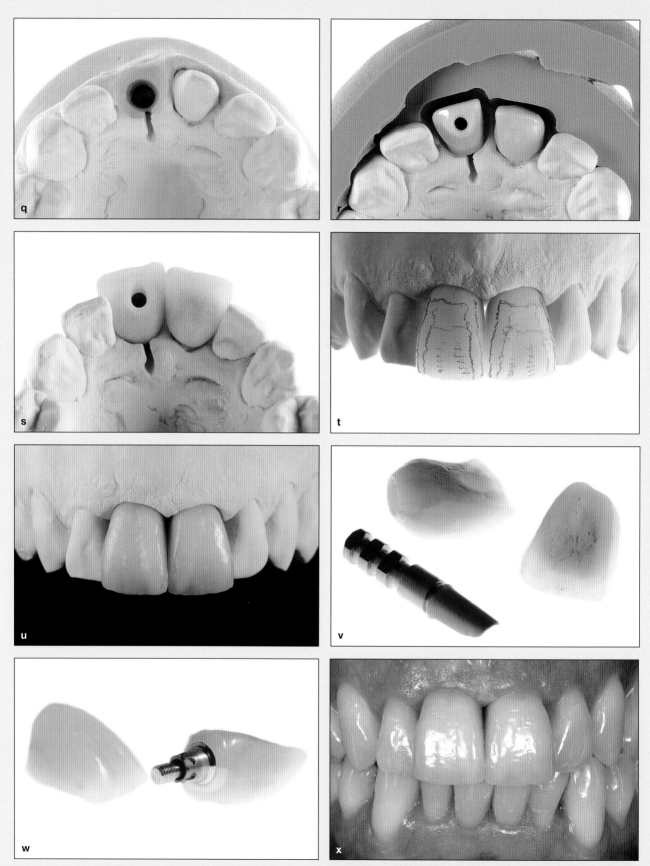

Fig 4-13 *cont.* / *(q)* Emergence profile ground in the cast. *(r)* Zirconia copings with silicone indexes. This shows that the coping design represents the reduced tooth form. *(s)* Veneered copings on the cast. *(t)* The surface characteristics are planned and marked. *(u)* The restorations before mechanical polishing. *(v)* Titanium base and the all-ceramic restorations before assembly. *(w)* The implant crown of the right central incisor was bonded to the titanium base; all-ceramic single crown for the left central incisor. *(x)* Restorations inserted in the mouth.

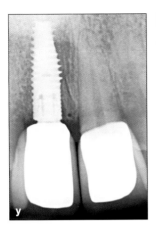
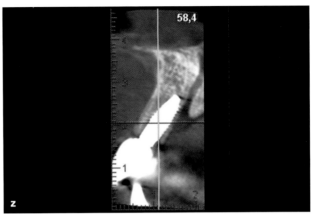

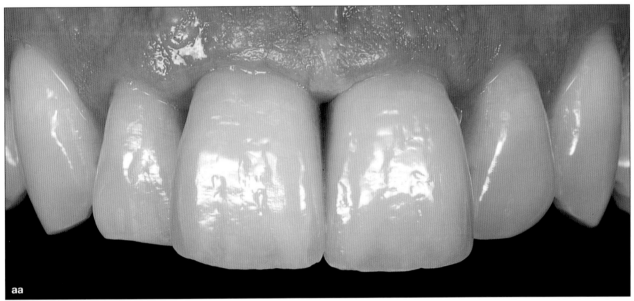

Fig 4-13 *cont.* / *(y)* Radiograph of the definitive screw-retained implant crown and the cemented crown. *(z)* CBCT 4 months after immediate implant placement shows that the surgical protocol managed to retain the buccal lamella at the right incisor. *(aa)* Symmetric soft tissue contour at the implant and the natural abutment. (Surgery and prosthodontics performed by A. Happe; laboratory work performed by P. Holthaus.)

White zirconia implants have been chosen with more frequency, particularly in the maxillary anterior dentition. The more favorable color and good biocompatibility of this material make it an alternative to titanium, especially in the anterior region because there is likely to be less biomechanical loading than in the posterior dentition (Fig 4-14). The two-part system depicted (White Implants) comprises a transgingival implant and a fiberglass abutment that can be cemented to the implant. The implant can be loaded immediately after placement or after a healing period depending on whether primary stability has been achieved.

In relation to immediate implants, however, the question that constantly arises is whether the presence of chronic apical periodontitis at extraction is a contraindication to immediate implant placement or whether it should be rated as a risk factor. No significant differences were found in an animal study with a split-mouth design.[32] Two prospective clinical trials on the subject, each involving about 30 patients and an observation period of 2 to 3 years, also revealed no clinical or radiologic differences and reported 100% survival rates for the implants.[33,34] Similarly, no statistically significant differences were found in a retrospective study with 665 patients and 992 implants (285 test and 637 control implants). However, the presence of an apical lesion affecting the adjacent tooth was identified as a risk factor.[35]

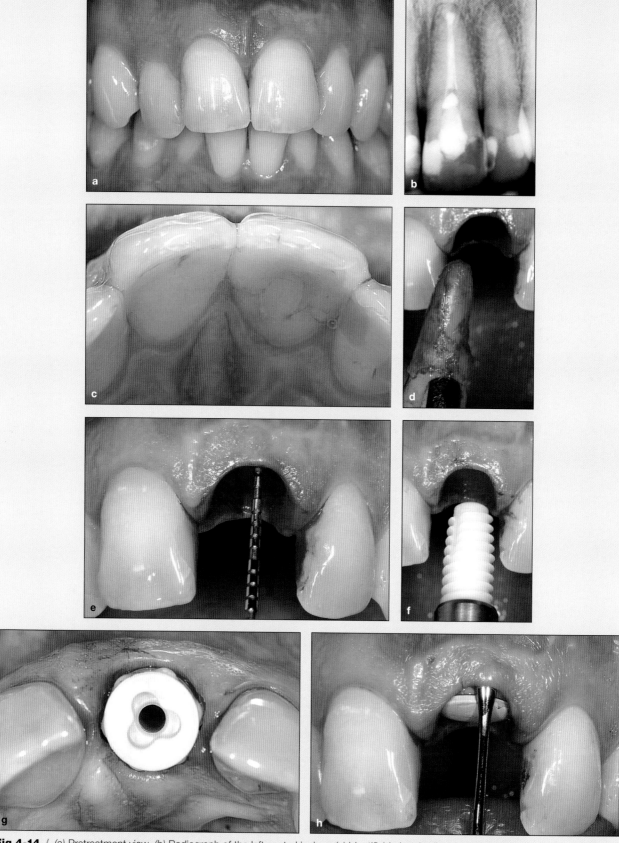

Fig 4-14 / *(a)* Pretreatment view. *(b)* Radiograph of the left central incisor. *(c)* Identifiable longitudinal fracture palatal to the central incisor; the tooth is not worth preserving. *(d)* Extraction of the tooth. *(e)* Buccal lamella is intact. *(f)* Insertion of a zirconia implant (White Implants). *(g)* Implant in situ. *(h)* Dissection of a buccal pocket for placement of a CTG.

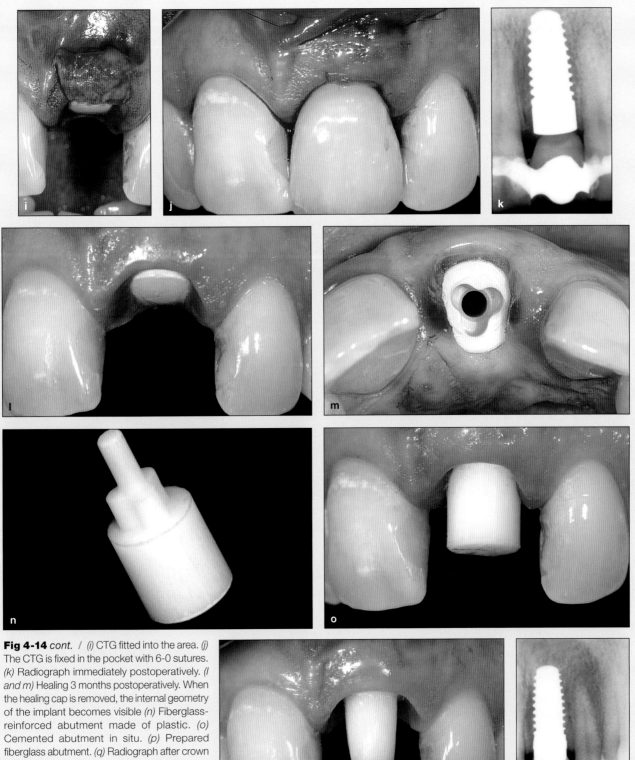

Fig 4-14 *cont.* / *(i)* CTG fitted into the area. *(j)* The CTG is fixed in the pocket with 6-0 sutures. *(k)* Radiograph immediately postoperatively. *(l and m)* Healing 3 months postoperatively. When the healing cap is removed, the internal geometry of the implant becomes visible *(n)* Fiberglass-reinforced abutment made of plastic. *(o)* Cemented abutment in situ. *(p)* Prepared fiberglass abutment. *(q)* Radiograph after crown placement.

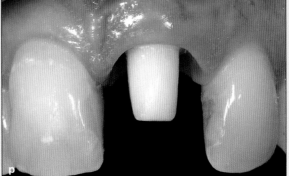

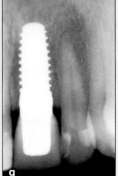

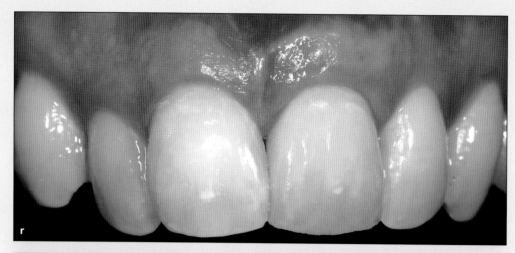

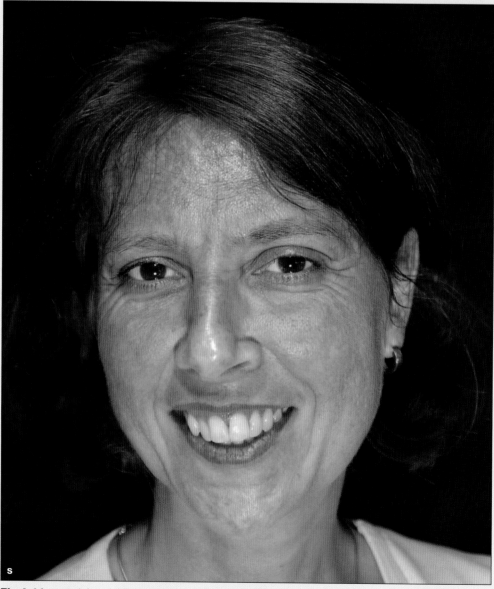

Fig 4-14 *cont.* / *(r and s)* Final clinical image and portrait with all-ceramic crown. (Surgery and prosthodontics performed by G. Körner; laboratory work performed by K. Müterthies.)

Conclusion

The success of immediate implant placement in the esthetic zone is highly dependent on the patient selection and the surgical protocol. Even before extraction, the situation should be assessed, and the correct timing of implant placement should be selected based on the criteria described in this chapter. Primarily, the anatomical situation—and more specifically, the nature of the socket and the tissue biotype—are significant prognostic factors. If the selection criteria for immediate implant placement are met and the correct surgical protocol is adhered to, highly esthetic outcomes can occur with this method. The consensus and recommendation of the European Association for Osseointegration (2014) is that immediate implant placement is a demanding form of treatment and should only be performed by experienced practitioners in specific situations.[36] After extraction, a thick buccal lamella should be available (ie, > 1 mm). A thick periodontal biotype should also be present. There should be no acute inflammation, and there must be enough bone available apically and palatally for an implant to be placed in the correct 3D position.

References

1. Cardaropoli G, Araújo M, Lindhe J. Dynamics of bone tissue formation in tooth extraction sites. An experimental study in dogs. J Clin Periodontol 2003;30:809–818.
2. Hämmerle CH, Chen ST, Wilson TG Jr. Consensus statements and recommended clinical procedures regarding the placement of implants in extraction sockets. Int J Oral Maxillofac Implants 2004;19(suppl):26–28.
3. Amler MH, Johnson PL, Salman I. Histological and histochemical investigation of human alveolar socket in undisturbed extraction wounds. J Am Dent Assoc 1960;61:32–44.
4. Araújo MG, Lindhe J. Dimensional ridge alterations following tooth extraction. An experimental study in the dog. J Clin Periodontol 2005;32:212–218.
5. Araújo MG, Sukekava F, Wennström JL, Lindhe J. Ridge alterations following implant placement in fresh extraction sockets: An experimental study in the dog. J Clin Periodontol 2005;32:645–652.
6. Cardaropoli D, Tamagnone L, Roffredo A, Gaveglio L. Relationship between the buccal bone plate thickness and the healing of postextraction sockets with/without ridge preservation. Int J Periodontics Restorative Dent 2014;34:211–217.
7. Nevins M, Camelo M, De Paoli S, et al. A study of the fate of the buccal wall of extraction sockets of teeth with prominent roots. Int J Periodontics Restorative Dent 2006;26:19–29.
8. Braut V, Bornstein MM, Belser U, Buser D. Thickness of the anterior maxillary facial bone wall: A retrospective radiographic study using cone beam computed tomography. Int J Periodontics Restorative Dent 2011;31:125–131.
9. Schropp L, Wenzel A, Kostopoulos L, Karring T. Bone healing and soft tissue contour changes following single-tooth extraction: A clinical and radiographic 12-month prospective study. Int J Periodontics Restorative Dent 2003;23:313–323.
10. Botticelli D, Berglundh T, Lindhe J. Hard-tissue alterations following immediate implant placement in extraction sites. J Clin Periodontol 2004;31:820–828.
11. Araújo MG, Linder E, Lindhe J. Bio-Oss collagen in the buccal gap at immediate implants: A 6-month study in the dog. Clin Oral Implants Res 2011;22:1–8.
12. Covani U, Marconcini S, Santini S, Cornelini R, Barone A. Immediate restoration of single implants placed immediately after implant removal. A case report. Int J Periodontics Restorative Dent 2010;30:639–645.
13. Chen ST, Darby IB, Reynolds EC. A prospective clinical study of non-submerged immediate implants: Clinical outcomes and esthetic results. Clin Oral Implants Res 2007;18:552–562.
14. Boardman N, Darby I, Chen S. A retrospective evaluation of aesthetic outcomes for single-tooth implants in the anterior maxilla. Clin Oral Implants Res 2016;27:443–451.
15. Merheb J, Vercruyssen M, Coucke W, Beckers L, Teughels W, Quirynen M. The fate of buccal bone around dental implants. A 12-month postloading follow-up study. Clin Oral Implants Res 2017;28:103–108.
16. Garber DA. The esthetic dental implant: Letting restoration be the guide. J Oral Implantol 1996;22:45–50.
17. Müller HP, Heinecke A, Schaller N, Eger T. Masticatory mucosa in subjects with different periodontal phenotypes. J Clin Periodontol 2000;27:621–626.
18. Lee A, Fu JH, Wang HL. Soft tissue biotype affects implant success. Implant Dent 2011;20:e38–e47.
19. Chen ST, Buser D. Clinical and esthetic outcomes of implants placed in postextraction sites. Int J Oral Maxillofac Implants 2009;24(suppl):186–217.
20. Esposito M, Grusovin MG, Polyzos IP, Felice P, Worthington HV. Timing of implant placement after tooth extraction: Immediate, immediate-delayed or delayed implants? A Cochrane systematic review. Eur J Oral Implantol 2010;3:189–205.
21. Cordaro L, Torsello F, Chen S, Ganeles J, Brägger U, Hämmerle C. Implant-supported single tooth restoration in the aesthetic zone: Transmucosal and submerged healing provide similar outcome when simultaneous bone augmentation is needed. Clin Oral Implants Res 2013;24:1130–1136.
22. Sanz M, Ivanoff CJ, Weingart D, et al. Clinical and radiologic outcomes after submerged and transmucosal implant placement with two-piece implants in the anterior maxilla and mandible: 3 years results of a randomized controlled clinical trial. Clin Implant Dent Relat Res 2015;17:234–246.
23. Salama H, Salama M. The role of orthodontic extrusive remodeling in the enhancement of soft and hard tissue profiles prior to implant placement: A systematic approach to the management of extraction site defects. Int J Periodontics Restorative Dent 1993;13:312–333.
24. De Rouck T, Collys K, Wyn I, Cosyn J. Instant provisionalization of immediate single-tooth implants is essential to optimize esthetic treatment outcome. Clin Oral Implants Res 2009;20:566–570.

67

25. Tarnow DP, Chu SJ, Salama MA, et al. Flapless postextraction socket implant placement in the esthetic zone: Part 1. The effect of bone grafting and/or provisional restoration on facial-palatal ridge dimensional change—A retrospective cohort study. Int J Periodontics Restorative Dent 2014;34:323–331.

26. Barone A, Marconcini S, Giammarinaro E, Mijiritsky E, Gelpi F, Covani U. Clinical outcomes of implants placed in extraction sockets and immediately restored: A 7-year single-cohort prospective study. Clin Implant Dent Relat Res 2016;18:1103–112.

27. Cosyn J, Eghbali A, Hermans A, Vervaeke S, De Bruyn H, Cleymaet R. A 5-year prospective study on single immediate implants in the aesthetic zone. J Clin Periodontol 2016;43:702–709.

28. Kan JY, Rungcharassaeng K, Lozada JL, Zimmerman G. Facial gingival tissue stability following immediate placement and provisionalization of maxillary anterior single implants: A 2- to 8-year follow-up. Int J Oral Maxillofac Implants 2011;26:179–187.

29. Mankoo T. Single-tooth implant restorations in the esthetic zone—Contemporary concepts for optimization and maintenance of soft tissue esthetics in the replacement of failing teeth in compromised sites. Eur J Esthet Dent 2007;2:274–295.

30. Tsuda H, Rungcharassaeng K, Kan JY, Roe P, Lozada JL, Zimmerman G. Peri-implant tissue response following connective tissue and bone grafting in conjunction with immediate single-tooth replacement in the esthetic zone: A case series. Int J Oral Maxillofac Implants 2011;26:427–436.

31. Grunder U. Crestal ridge width changes when placing implants at the time of tooth extraction with and without soft tissue augmentation after a healing period of 6 months: Report of 24 consecutive cases. Int J Periodontics Restorative Dent 2011;31:9–17.

32. Novaes AB Jr, Vidigal Júnior GM, Novaes AB, Grisi MF, Polloni S, Rosa A. Immediate implants placed into infected sites: A histomorphometric study in dogs. Int J Oral Maxillofac Implants 1998;13:422–427.

33. Crespi R, Capparè P, Gherlone E. Immediate loading of dental implants placed in periodontally infected and non-infected sites: A 4-year follow-up clinical study. J Periodontol 2010;81:1140–1146.

34. Truninger TC, Philipp AO, Siegenthaler DW, Roos M, Hämmerle CH, Jung RE. A prospective, controlled clinical trial evaluating the clinical and radiological outcome after 3 years of immediately placed implants in sockets exhibiting periapical pathology. Clin Oral Implants Res 2011;22:20–27.

35. Bell CL, Diehl D, Bell BM, Bell RE. The immediate placement of dental implants into extraction sites with periapical lesions: A retrospective chart review. J Oral Maxillofac Surg 2011;69:1623–1627.

36. Morton D, Chen ST, Martin WC, Levine RA, Buser D. Consensus statements and recommended clinical procedures regarding optimizing esthetic outcomes in implant dentistry. Int J Oral Maxillofac Implants 2014;29(suppl):216–220.

"A goal without a plan is just a wish."

ANTOINE DE SAINT-EXUPÉRY

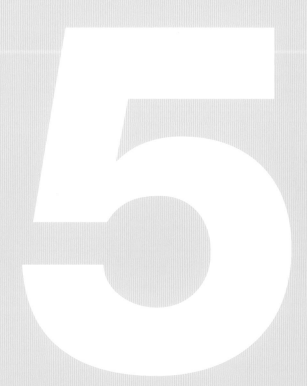

Implant Position, Planning, and Esthetic Analysis

/ Arndt Happe, Christian Coachman, Tal Morr,
Vincent Fehmer, Irena Sailer

As discussed in chapter 1, the correct three-dimensional (3D) positioning of an implant plays a crucial role in the outcome of implant restorations in partially edentulous patients. The 3D implant position is obviously a major determinant of esthetic outcome, but an incorrect 3D position can also lead to biologic and functional complications. The Consensus Conference of the 11th European Workshop on Periodontology therefore issued a consensus statement on the primary prevention of peri-implantitis, which includes the following recommendations[1]:

- Implant placement must allow for proper cleaning.
- The superstructure must allow for good hygiene, ie, it must be free of recesses and flaws that may result in tissue trauma.

These factors are largely influenced by the 3D position of the implant because this is what determines whether the superstructure can be screw-retained via its palatal surface or whether it must be cement-retained. Literature reviews have shown that the different forms of superstructure attachment (cement- versus screw-retained) are associated with different rates of functional and biologic complications, and cement-retained restorations carry specific risks that play a role in the etiology and pathogenesis of peri-implantitis.[2–5] In this regard, the 3D implant position indirectly acts as a prognostic factor because screw-retained restorations cannot be used with certain implant positions.

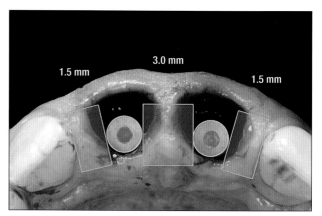

Fig 5-1 / Recommended minimum distances.

Implant Position

Horizontal position

To prevent interproximal tissue loss, the distance between an implant and the adjacent tooth should be at least 1.5 mm. This will ensure that the resorptive processes caused by postrestorative remodeling (see chapter 1) do not influence the attachment of the adjacent teeth. The distance between adjacent implants should be at least 3 mm, and there should be at least 2 to 4 mm of bone buccal to the implant[6] (Fig 5-1). Depending on the nature of the implant-abutment connection (eg, conical connections), smaller distances are possible in individual cases.[7]

If the implant is placed too far facially, soft tissue recession usually results because the implant is positioned outside the geometry of the alveolar ridge (Fig 5-2). An imagined tangent between the facial curvature of the adjacent teeth can be used as a guide (Fig 5-3). If there are no adjacent teeth, a setup or wax-up is required beforehand to plan the correct position.

Vertical position

The biologic width around implants consists of a 2-mm junctional epithelium and a 1- to 1.5-mm connective tissue

Fig 5-2 / Soft tissue recession has occurred at the left central incisor because the implant was positioned too buccally.

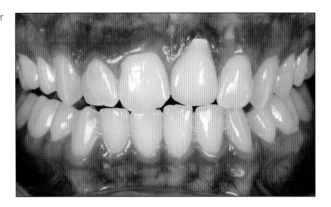

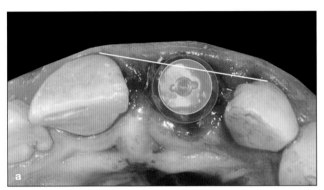

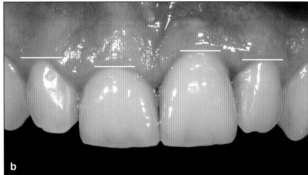

Fig 5-3 / (a) The implant is positioned too far buccally. The implant should be positioned palatal to the tangent *(white line)*. (b) Soft tissue recession caused by malpositioning.

zone, for a total of 3.0 to 3.5 mm.[8] Therefore, in a sense, this dimension (ie, the biologic width) determines the vertical position of the implant from the biologic perspective. From the prosthetic perspective, a certain vertical distance between the implant shoulder and the superstructure is required so that the abutment can be expanded from the circular implant diameter to the far more anatomical emergence profile.

If the implant is not positioned deeply enough, it may become difficult or even impossible to contour the peri-implant soft tissue to result in a natural look and ensure that the abutment is accessible for oral hygiene (see chapter 11).

If the implant is positioned too deeply, there is actually a lot of distance available to develop the abutment toward the emergence profile. However, the interface—including the contaminated microgap—is so far below the tissue that the resorptive effects can lead to tissue loss. This can subsequently result in vertical recession of the mucosa.

Between these two extremes, however, there is room for a functional abutment design. It is important to understand that the macro design of the abutment is determined by the anatomical crown of the tooth being replaced and the position of the implant shoulder.

For a maxillary central incisor, the rule of thumb is that the implant shoulder should be located 3 to 4 mm apical to the planned soft tissue margin (Figs 5-4 and 5-5). Furthermore, the larger the difference between the diameter of the implant and the diameter of the superstructure, the more vertical distance is required by the technician to develop the emergence profile.

As early as 1996, David Garber[9] stipulated, "let the restoration be the guide." This means that the superstructure should determine the implant position. This old stipulation is reflected in modern 3D diagnostics using cone beam computed tomography (CBCT) and template techniques. Yet the first step is still analysis of the situation to identify the correct position of the superstructure.

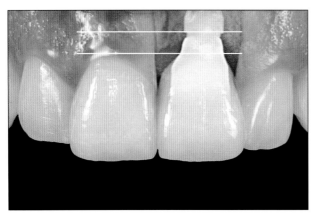

Fig 5-4 / Superimposed radiograph illustrating the ideal vertical situation.

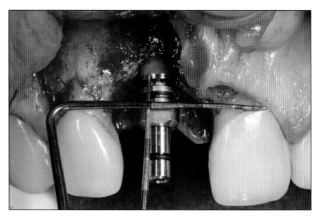

Fig 5-5 / Intraoperative check of the vertical implant position.

Planning and Esthetic Analysis

The literature has described quantifiable criteria for achieving dental esthetics, primarily focusing on the following[10–12]:

* Midline
* Relationship of occlusal plane to bipupillary line
* Position of the incisal edges of the central incisors in the maxilla
* Proportions of the maxillary anterior teeth
* Relationship of the incisal edges of the maxillary anterior teeth to the lips
* Buccal corridor
* Relationship of maxillary anterior dentition to mandibular anterior dentition

Various methods have been described for treatment planning and esthetic analysis, all working with casts, models, photographs, or the patients themselves.[13–15]

When planning in the esthetic zone, it is advisable to create anatomical casts that can both establish the preoperative situation and be used for planning (Fig 5-6). Spatial conditions and occlusal relationships can be assessed very effectively using casts. They can also be used to communicate with patients. If a wax-up is created, it can be transferred to the mouth with the aid of a mock-up produced with silicone indices (Fig 5-7). The silicone indices can also serve as preparation keys to assess the spatial conditions (Fig 5-8). In some cases, it may be necessary to plan with mounted casts. Especially when there is loss of vertical dimension or in patients with impaired function, it is advisable to perform a functional analysis and perhaps do a full wax-up (ie, a complete wax simulation of the new occlusion; Fig 5-9). In addition, dental

photographs are often appropriate. As well as complete intraoral photographs, extraoral images are helpful for the esthetic analysis.

The following clinical cases use the Digital Smile Design (DSD) system developed by Coachman.[14] This is a method of using photographs and technology to easily illustrate and visualize the treatment plan.

Case 1: Single-tooth replacement of right central incisor in a patient with considerable loss of substance due to erosion

As well as the standard intraoral photographic records, the DSD method requires a frontal, centered portrait of the patient smiling with a slightly open mouth and a photograph of the maxillary anterior dentition against a black background (Figs 5-10a to 5-10h). The images are imported into presentation software such as Keynote (Apple) or PowerPoint (Microsoft). Reference lines can then be generated and proportions analyzed via pixel dimensions. To do this, the pictures have to be taken from a standardized perspective to avoid distortion phenomena caused by different recording axes. Even if optical phenomena lead to slight discrepancies, this systematic procedure can still serve as a means of approaching the case, and the analysis can be used to communicate with patients and team partners, such as orthodontists or dental technicians.

Facial reference lines (eg, the midline and bipupillary line) and the smile line are first projected onto the mouth and then onto the intraoral situation (Figs 5-10i to 5-10l). This demonstrates the intraoral situation in relation to the patient's face. The contour of the marginal gingiva is

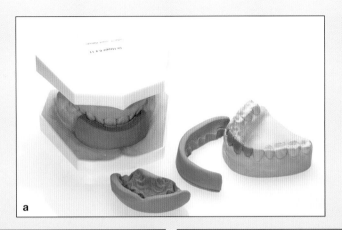

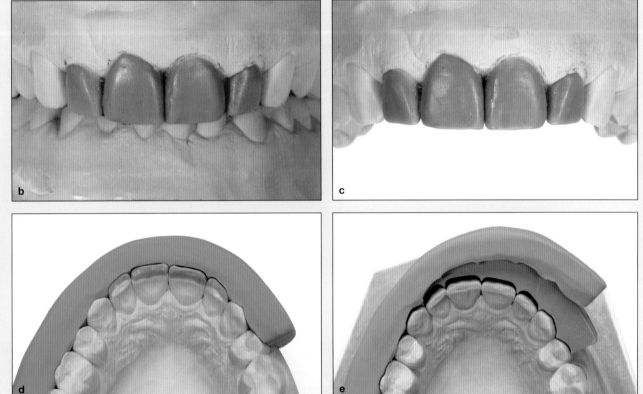

Fig 5-6 / *(a to e)* Cast with wax-up and silicone index for mock-up and preparation key.

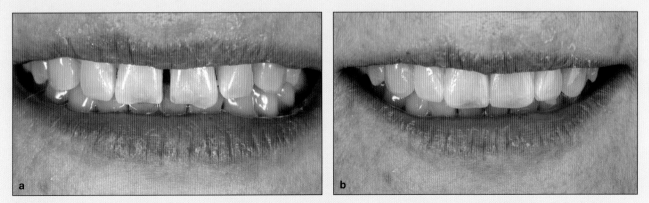

Fig 5-7 / *(a)* Spaced maxillary anterior dentition. *(b)* Mock-up: transferring the wax-up to the mouth with the aid of a silicone index.

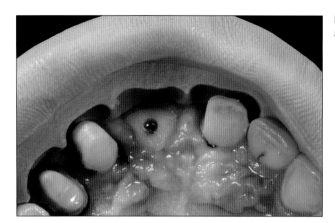

Fig 5-8 / Preparation key in situ for both the natural abutments and the implant.

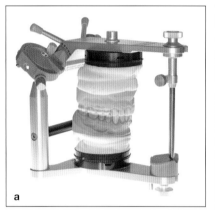

a

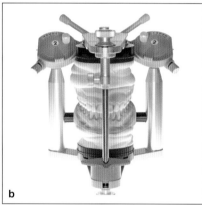

b

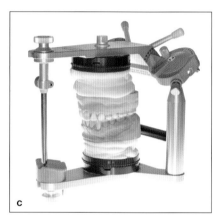

c

Fig 5-9 / *(a to c)* Mounted planning casts with functional wax-up (waxing up the new occlusion).

analyzed. The width-to-length ratio of the teeth can be determined by placing a rectangle in the software congruently over the dental crown and calculating the pixel dimensions. In this case, the ratio of width to length is 99% (Fig 5-10m), which means that the crown of the tooth is almost square. The anatomical shape of the crown of a central incisor generally has a width-to-length ratio of between 75% and 85%.[13] Based on these values, a new contour for the teeth can be developed (Figs 5-10n and 5-10o). This involves checking width ratios visually perceptible from the front according to the golden ratio (Fig 5-10p). This natural proportion, which was espoused by the ancient Greeks in their architecture and art, is reflected in the ratio of the tooth widths of a harmonious maxillary anterior dentition. The visually perceived widths should be in a ratio of roughly 2:3 (lateral incisors to central incisors); and 1:3 (canines to central incisors).[12] Canines appear narrower than lateral incisors because the distal aspect is not visible from a frontal view.

After development of the new contour in this clinical case, it becomes clear that both central incisors need to be elongated and there is an excess of soft tissue (Fig 5-10q). If the teeth were to be lengthened only incisally, this would lead to an incorrect position of the incisal edges of the teeth, which would be esthetically and phonetically problematic. The position of the incisal edge of the central incisors in the maxilla is a significant key to overall planning.[16]

The dental technician can transfer the resulting analysis to a functional wax-up (Fig 5-10r). In this case, the result of the described analysis was surgical crown lengthening of the left central incisor and appropriate adaptation of the right central incisor socket prior to implant placement (Figs 5-10s to 5-10z). Without the analysis, the implant would have been placed solely based on local reference points, such as crestal bone and marginal soft tissue. This in turn would have compromised the width-to-length ratio of the restoration.

As a result of the vertical positioning of the implant shoulder 3.5 mm apical to the preplanned soft tissue margin, the final images shows a harmonious and symmetric soft tissue contour (Figs 5-10aa to 5-10ff). This case shows how DSD can assist decision making, particularly in complex situations, and it is also valuable as an educational tool.

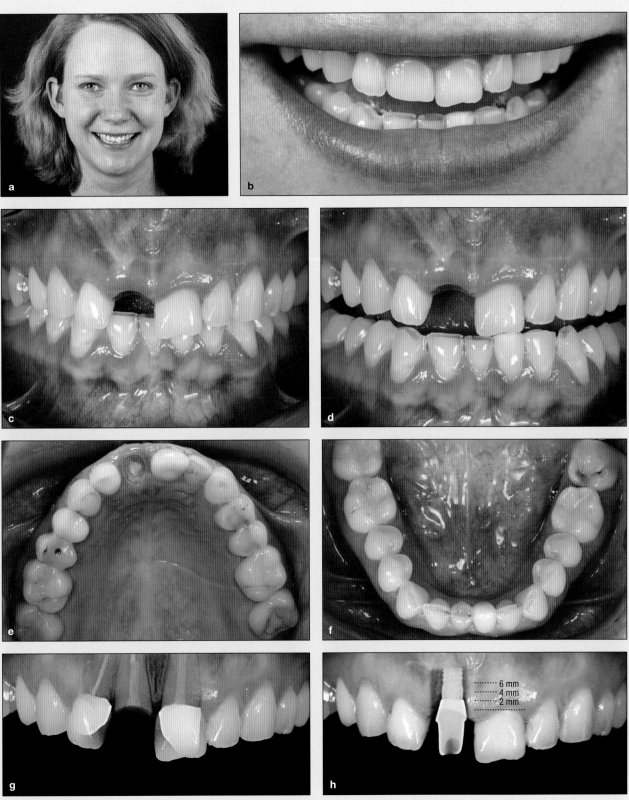

Fig 5-10 / 30-year-old patient. *(a)* Portrait before treatment. *(b)* Smile. *(c)* The maxillary right central incisor is fractured. The root remnant has a longitudinal fracture and is not worth preserving. *(d)* Protrusion. Discernible loss of substance at the incisal edges of the anterior teeth. *(e)* Occlusal view of the maxilla. There is moderate generalized erosion and partially inadequate restorations. *(f)* Occlusal view of the mandible. There is moderate generalized erosion and partially inadequate restorations. *(g)* Radiograph superimposed over the clinical situation. *(h)* It must be decided how deep to place the implant.

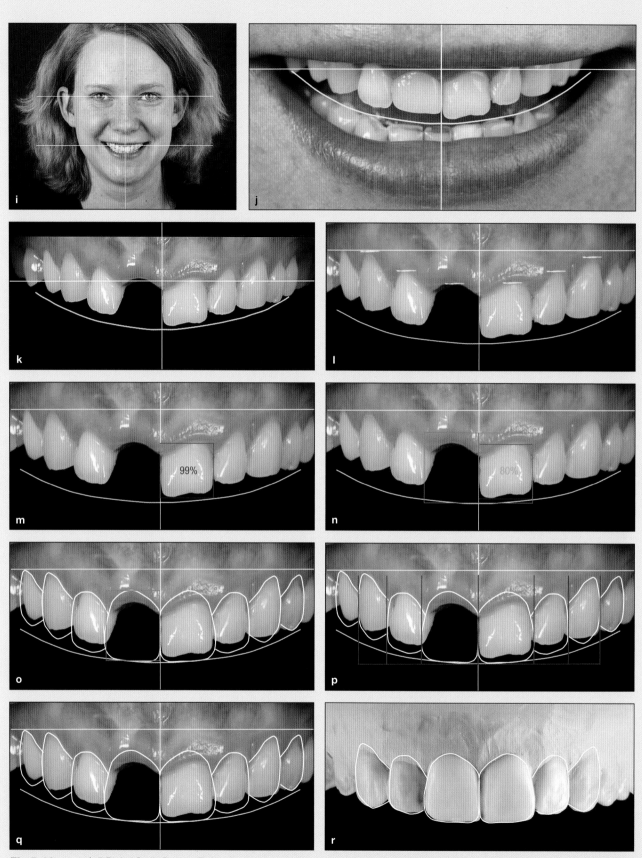

Fig 5-10 *cont.* / *(i)* Digital Smile Design. Reference lines are projected onto the portrait. *(j)* Magnification of the mouth section. *(k)* Reference lines are transferred to the intraoral situation. *(l)* Analysis of the soft tissue contour. *(m)* Analysis of the width-to-length ratio. The crown is almost square. *(n)* Simulation of a correct width-to-length ratio. *(o)* Development of a new tooth shape. *(p)* The dimensions and width ratios are checked with a template, simulating the golden ratio. *(q)* New contour of the maxillary anterior dentition. It becomes clear that there is an excess of tissue at the central incisors. *(r)* Transfer of the tooth shapes to a wax-up.

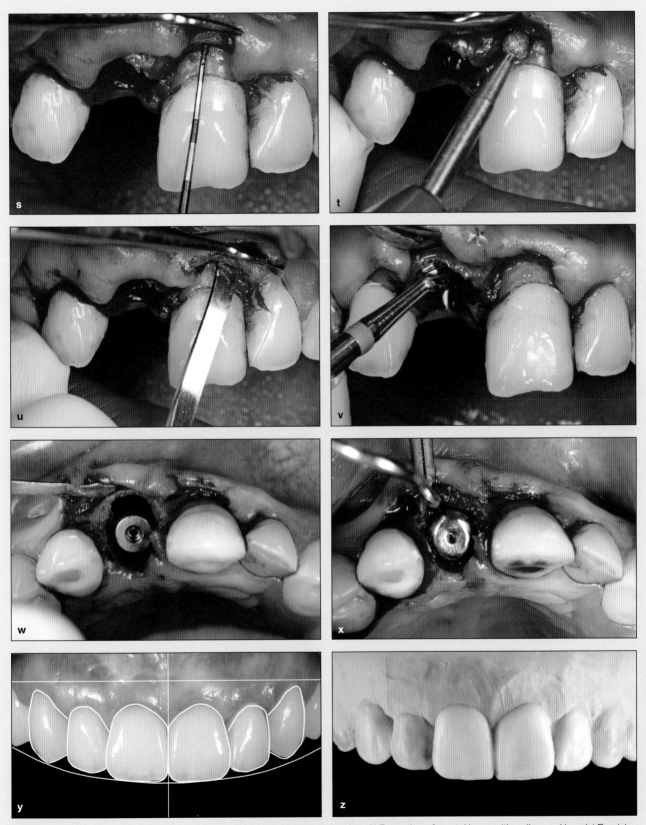

Fig 5-10 *cont.* / *(s)* Measuring the biologic width prior to crown lengthening. *(t)* Resection of crestal bone with a diamond bur. *(u)* Precision adjustment with periodontal chisel. *(v)* Adapting the socket at the right central incisor. *(w)* An immediate implant (3.8-mm diameter) is placed in the site of the right central incisor. *(x)* With a gingiva former in place, the space between implant and buccal lamella is filled with xenograft. *(y)* The end result matches the digital simulation. *(z)* The wax-up for comparison.

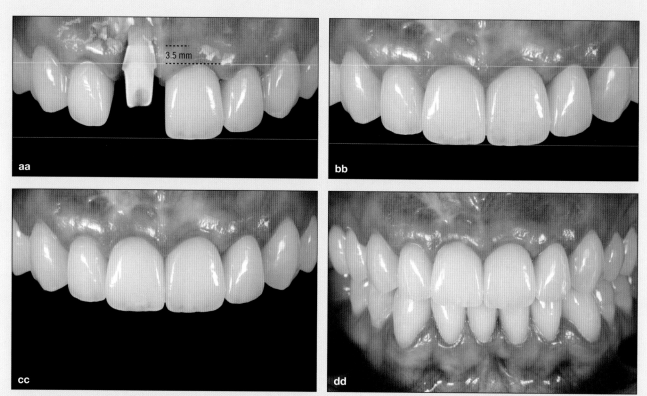

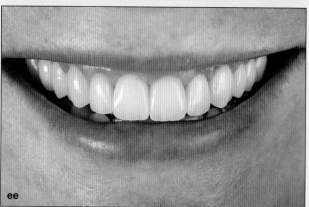

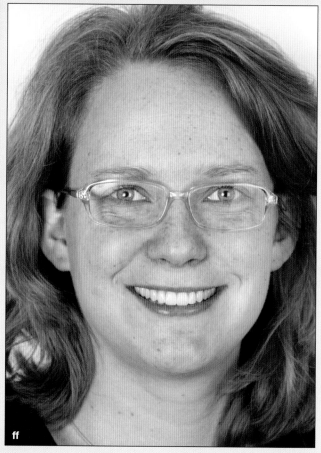

Fig 5-10 *cont.* / *(aa)* The vertical implant position was guided by the soft tissue contour planned for the future. In this case, the implant shoulder lies 3.5 mm apical to the marginal mucosal edge. *(bb)* Symmetric soft tissue contour at the central incisors. *(cc)* Final image of the maxillary anterior dentition. *(dd)* Final image of the intraoral situation. *(ee)* Smile after completion of the treatment. *(ff)* Portrait of the patient after completion of the treatment. (Surgery and prosthodontics performed by A. Happe; laboratory work performed by D. Meyer.)

Case 2: Redesigning the maxillary anterior dentition

The patient in this case had already undergone orthodontic treatment as a child. This resulted in root resorption at the maxillary incisors (Figs 5-11a to 5-11i). Although these four anterior teeth were already splinted with a wire, they exhibited grade III mobility. The patient had extreme difficulty with eating because she was afraid of losing her teeth. The right central incisor had an existing retrograde root filling after apicoectomy. An implant had already been placed in the site of the left canine, which led to esthetic impairment because of its incorrect 3D position and the poor quality of the tissue. The plan was to remove all incisors and place implants in the right lateral and left central incisor sites to allow an implant-supported fixed partial denture from the right lateral incisor to the left canine via the left central incisor. The right central incisor was maintained to preserve the existing anatomy of the ridge. This involved cutting the tooth and root to 0.5 to 1 mm above the bone to preserve the supracrestal fiber attachment and the periodontal ligament attachment. This technique is called *root banking*. This method involves waiting until the mucosa has fully closed over the root remnant so that a pontic rest can be created at that site. The root remains permanently in the alveolar bone in the sense of a *radix relicta* (ie, retained root).

The patient wanted to use the upcoming implant treatment as an opportunity to improve the overall condition of her anterior dentition. The existing situation was analyzed with the aid of DSD, and a proposal was worked out to redesign the maxillary anterior dentition. To do this, the portrait is first aligned horizontally so that the interpupillary plane coincides with the horizontal line of the software. The reference lines (ie, interpupillary plane, base of the nose, midline, smile line) are then drawn (Figs 5-11j and 5-11k) and transferred to the photograph of the intraoral situation (Fig 5-11l).

Figures 5-11m and 5-11n show how a digital ruler can be used to gain metric values for the analysis. The digital ruler is calibrated by means of the real length of the teeth measured in the mouth, and the metric values are then transferred to the model (see Figs 5-11r and 5-11s). This involves taking the real length of the central incisor (8 mm in this case), and adjusting the ruler accordingly. After this process, the ruler can be duplicated, but the size must not be altered any further in the software. Nevertheless, optical distortions have to be taken into account, and the measurements on the model or patient still have to be

checked for plausibility. Deviation of the midline by less than 1 mm is not esthetically problematic and does not necessarily require any correction, but it was corrected in this case because it could be accomplished easily.[17]

It is possible to separate different areas of the photograph and distinguish them with different colors. This can be a helpful way to concentrate on specific parts of the situation individually. In this case, the color of the mucosa was removed in one view to make the tooth shapes easier to assess (Fig 5-11o), and the color of the teeth was removed in another view to reveal the contour of the soft tissue more clearly (Fig 5-11p). Figure 5-11q shows analysis of the width-to-length ratios of the right central and left lateral incisors. Both of these teeth deviate markedly from the ideal ratio of 75:100 to 85:100, where 100 is the tooth length. It can also be expressed in percentages (eg, 80% for 80:100). In this case, the right central incisor is almost square (nearly 100%), and the left lateral incisor is far too narrow or too long (well below 75%).

The soft tissue contour is highly irregular in this case. Figures 5-11r and 5-11s show the difference in level between different papillae. This difference is most pronounced between the reference papilla distal to the right central incisor and the papilla distal to the left lateral incisor. Unilateral papillary deficits are commonly perceived as nonesthetic; they are regarded as problematic above a difference of 1 to 1.5 mm.[18] To develop the new maxillary anterior dentition, a rectangle with a width-to-length ratio of 75% to 85% (to fit the individual anatomical situation) is first aligned with the reference lines (ie, midline and smile line). This rectangle is also created on the left central incisor, and then the new tooth shape is drawn. Templates from the database may be helpful in doing this. Drawing of the lateral incisors and canines is further guided by the smile line and general fundamental esthetic rules. This produces an initial design of the new situation, which the dental technician can transfer to a wax-up (Figs 5-11t to 5-11w). In this case, both lateral incisors and the left central incisor were extracted, and implants were placed in the regions of the right lateral and left central incisors. The teeth to be extracted were first extruded by orthodontic methods to grow excess tissue (Fig 5-11x). This equalized the level of soft tissue and avoided the need for augmentation. The left lateral incisor, in particular, was markedly extruded, and the vertical tissue deficiency was thereby leveled. The root of the right central incisor remained for ridge preservation (Figs 5-11y to 5-11bb).

After osseointegration, a provisional restoration was placed to contour the soft tissue (Figs 5-11cc and 5-11dd).

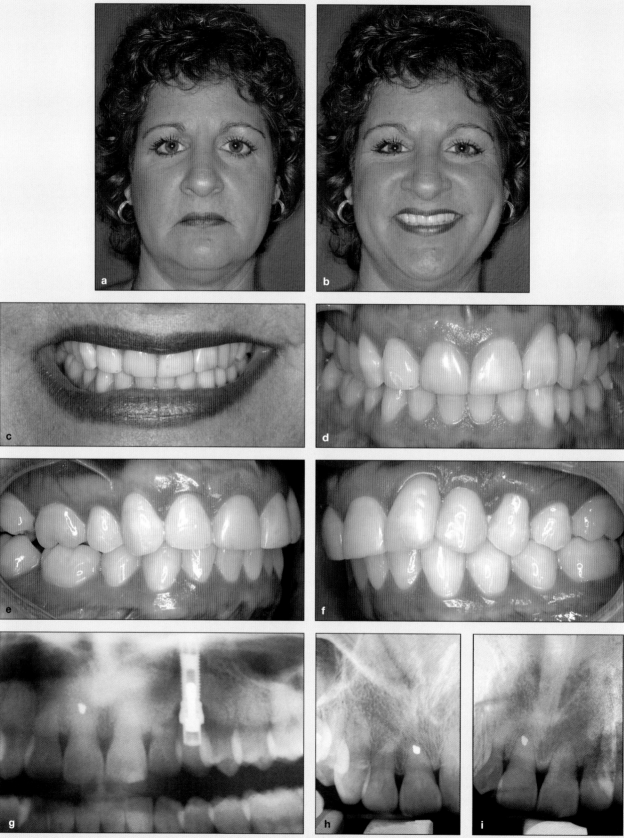

Fig 5-11 / *(a)* Portrait of the patient with mouth in relaxed closed position. *(b)* Portrait of the patient smiling. *(c)* Close-up of smile. *(d)* Intraoral situation with an implant at the maxillary left canine and recession at the left lateral incisor. *(e and f)* Intraoral photographs from the right and left lateral views. *(g)* Radiograph of the entire esthetic zone. *(h)* Periapical radiograph from the right central incisor to the canine. *(i)* Periapical radiograph from the right central incisor to the left lateral incisor.

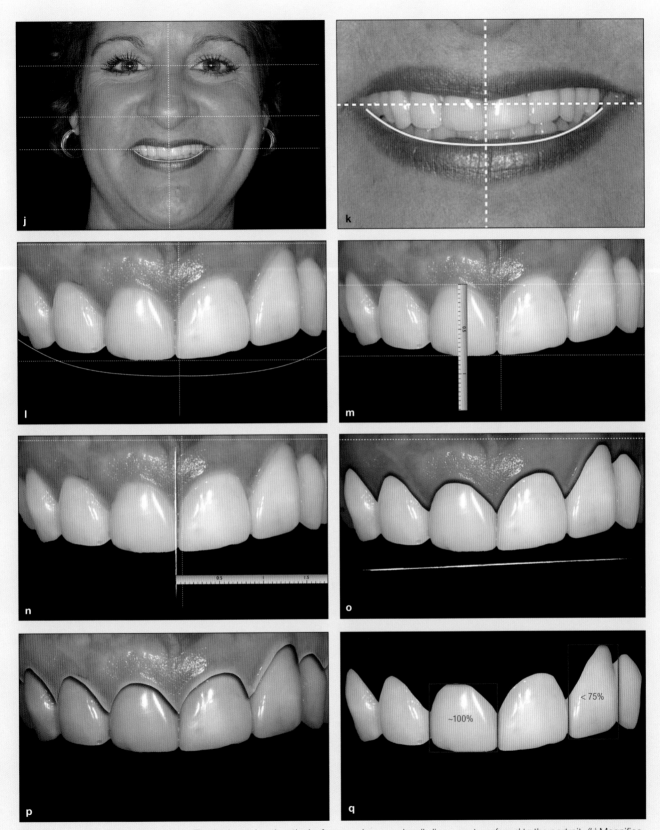

Fig 5-11 *cont.* / *(j)* Esthetic analysis: The horizontal and vertical reference planes and smile line were transferred to the portrait. *(k)* Magnification of the mouth area. *(l)* The key reference planes were transferred to the intraoral situation. *(m)* The digital ruler is calibrated to the real crown length of the right central incisor. *(n)* Once calibrated, the ruler can be used for approximate measurement of dimensions on the image. *(o)* The mucosa was depicted in black and white so that the tooth shapes could be assessed more efficiently. *(p)* The teeth were depicted in black and white to help assess the soft tissue contour. *(q)* Visualization of the width-to-length ratios of the right central incisor and left lateral incisor. →

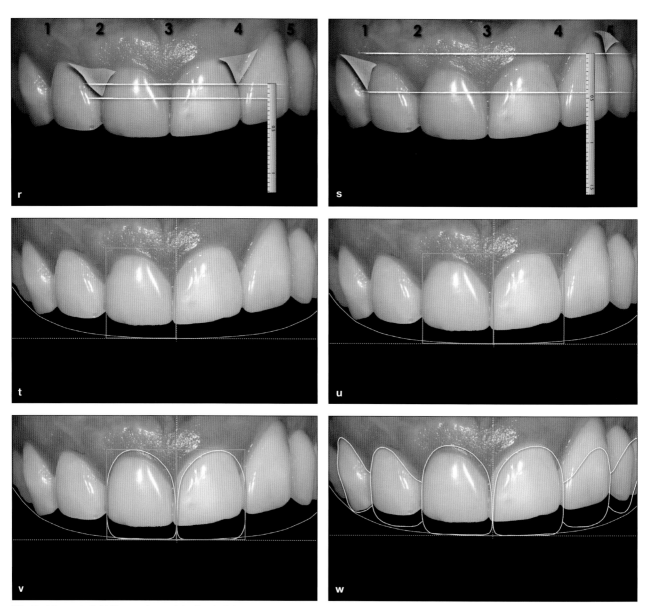

Fig 5-11 *cont.* / *(r)* Comparison of the level of the papilla distal to the left lateral incisor with the reference papilla distal to the right central incisor. *(s)* Pronounced discrepancy between the reference papilla and the papilla distal to the left lateral incisor. *(t)* The planned proportions are transferred to the right central incisor via a rectangle with the ratio of 75% to 85%. *(u)* Alignment of the second rectangle with the left central incisor according to midline and smile line. *(v)* Drawing the tooth shape inside the rectangle. *(w)* Completion of the anterior dentition based on smile line and general esthetic guidelines. ⟶

After the soft tissue had matured, covering the root of the central incisor (a minimum of 3 months postoperatively), the impression was taken for the definitive restoration with transfer of the emergence profile that had been developed (Figs 5-11ee to 5-11hh). Customized zirconia abutments were fabricated, and the emergence profile was further optimized for the definitive restoration (Figs 5-11ii to 5-11kk). After the definitive restoration was placed, the radiographs clearly show the differences in the peri-implant bone con-

figuration between the right lateral incisor and left central incisor implants with a conical connection versus the left canine implant with the classic non-platform-switched connection (Figs 5-11ll to 5-11nn). The final photographs show the redesigned anterior dentition. Unlike the preoperative view, the postoperative result exhibits a far more regular soft tissue contour and much more harmonious form of the teeth. The photograph of the smile shows the natural interaction with the lips (Figs 5-11oo to 5-11rr).

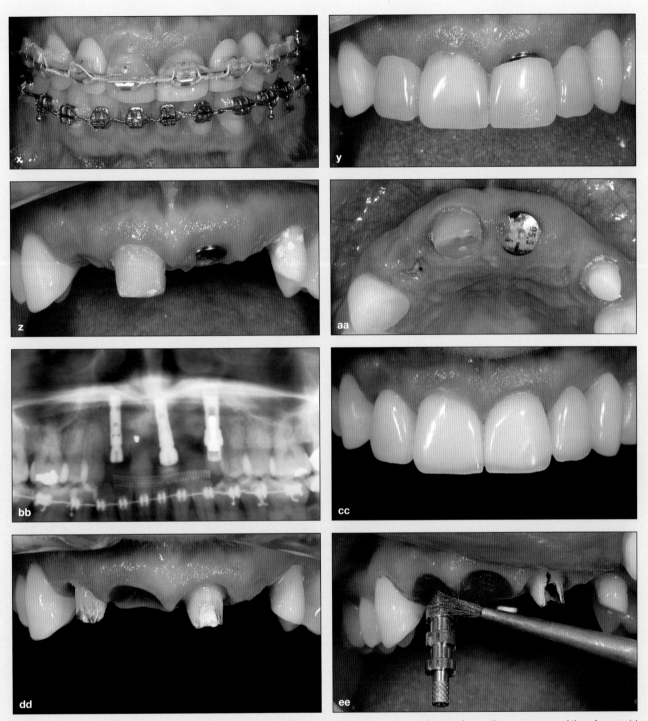

Fig 5-11 *cont.* / *(x)* Extrusion of both left incisors and the right lateral incisor to be extracted to produce a tissue excess and therefore avoid any augmentation. Extrusion of the left lateral incisor was particularly pronounced. *(y)* Chairside provisional restoration over the right central incisor and left canine during the implant incorporation phase. *(z)* Situation after successful osseointegration. *(aa)* Occlusal view with implants in the sites of the right lateral and left central incisors. *(bb)* Detail from panoramic radiograph with an older implant at the left canine (Bråne-mark-type) and newer implants (Astra, Dentsply) in the incisor sites. *(cc)* Implant-supported long-term provisional restoration for contouring the soft tissue. *(dd)* Contoured pontic area of the right central incisor with natural papillary morphology. *(ee)* Transferring the emergence profile of the implants and the pontic area to the impression posts with acrylic resin (Pattern Resin, GC).

84

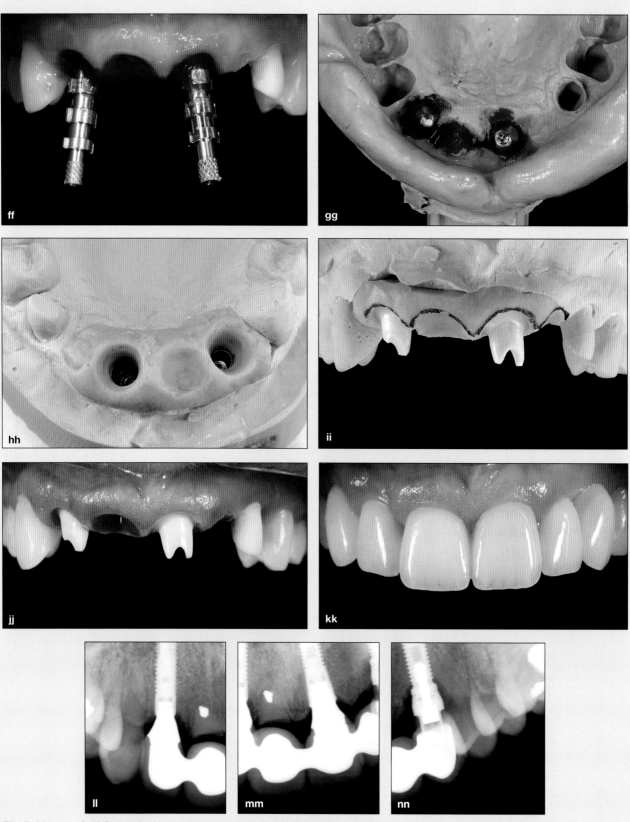

Fig 5-11 *cont.* / *(ff)* Customized impression posts with visualization of the pontic region. *(gg)* Silicone impression with open tray. *(hh)* Cast situation with mucosal mask showing the transferred emergence profile. *(ii)* Drawing the mucosal scalloping with all-ceramic zirconia abutments. *(jj)* The zirconia abutments fit perfectly into the ready-contoured tissue. *(kk)* All-ceramic veneered zirconia anterior partial denture. *(ll to nn)* Radiographs of the old and new implants supporting the fixed partial denture.

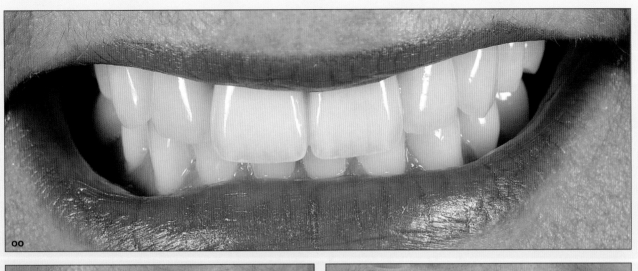

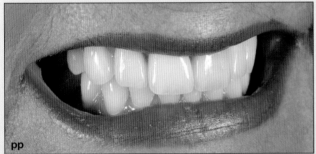

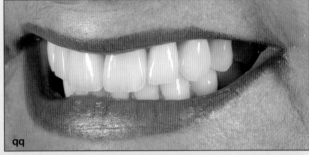

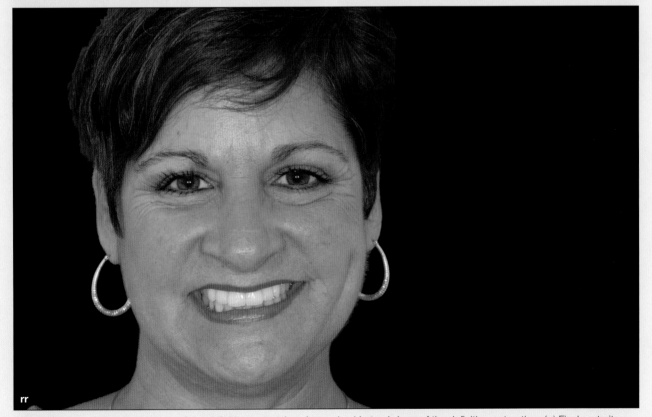

Fig 5-11 *cont.* / *(oo)* Frontal view of the definitive restoration. *(pp and qq)* Lateral views of the definitive restoration. *(rr)* Final portrait.

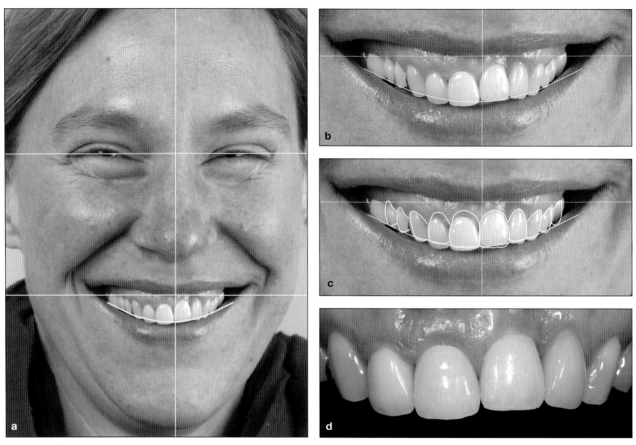

Fig 5-12 / *(a)* Portrait of the patient with DSD reference lines. *(b)* Reference lines transferred to the maxillary anterior dentition. *(c)* Digital planning of the new tooth shapes. *(d)* Intraoral photograph, frontal view.

Case 3: Preexisting implant at left central incisor, new implant for right central incisor

The patient was unsatisfied with the appearance of her maxillary anterior dentition. In addition, she was aware of a considerable degree of abrasion on the occlusal and palatal surfaces of her anterior teeth (Figs 5-12a to 5-12d). After an accident involving anterior tooth trauma about 4 or 5 years previously, her left central incisor was lost and endodontic treatment of the right central incisor became necessary (Fig 5-12e). During implant restoration treatment in the region of the left central incisor, significant complications arose in connection with augmentation, causing structural deficits in that region and additional recession at the left lateral incisor. Over subsequent years, diffuse problems persisted in the region of the right central incisor, the tooth that had undergone endodontic treatment. Endosurgical correction failed to remedy this problem.

Various treatment options were discussed with the patient, including orthognathic surgery. However, the patient was only willing to permit a surgical procedure to correct the maxillary anterior dentition. In view of the existing diffuse problems affecting the right central incisor and the unsightly asymmetric overall situation in the maxilla, the following procedure was therefore proposed and eventually carried out:

1. The right central incisor was extracted atraumatically, and an immediate implant was placed in the site without any soft tissue correction to permit posttreatment recession of 0.5 to 1.0 mm (Figs 5-12f and 5-12g).
2. A minimally invasive clinical crown lengthening of the right lateral incisor was performed concurrently (Fig 5-12h).
3. The superstructure of the left central incisor was reduced at the same time, and surgical tunneling was performed at both left incisors for integration of a subepithelial connective tissue graft. This was done to correct the recessions and thereby reduce the pronounced asymmetry (Figs 5-12i to 5-12k).

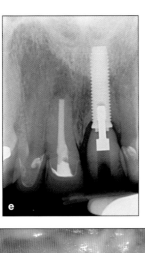

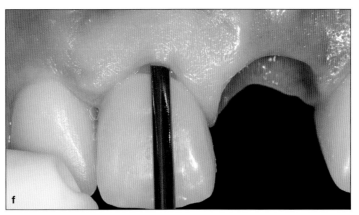

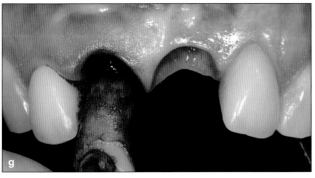

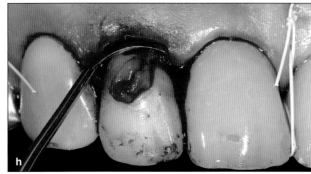

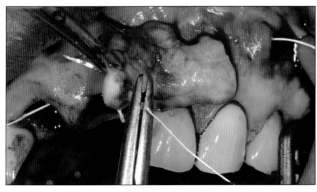

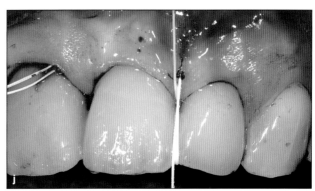

87

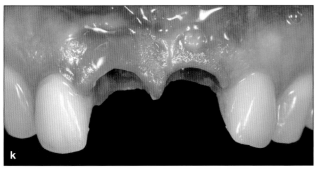

Fig 5-12 *cont.* / *(e)* Radiograph of central incisors. *(f)* Before extraction of the right central incisor, the periodontal tissue is cautiously detached with a periotome. *(g)* Extraction of the right central incisor. *(h)* Crown lengthening of the right lateral incisor. *(i)* A connective tissue graft is introduced through the access incision in the region of the left lateral incisor and canine into the area of the left incisors. *(j)* Coronal displacement of the tissue with suspended suture between the left incisors. *(k)* Healed area of the central incisors contoured with a provisional restoration. ⟶

4. A provisional restoration was immediately placed.
5. The sites of the implants, soft tissue augmentation, and crown lengthening were left to heal for 3 months. Impressions were taken at both central incisors, and the provisional restoration on the definitive zirconia abutments was adjusted for both central incisors.
6. After another 2 to 3 months, the definitive all-ceramic restoration was delivered with the prepared leveled soft tissue margins and incisal edges (Figs 5-12l to 5-12o).

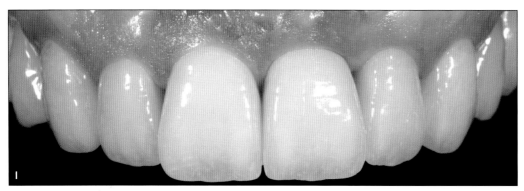

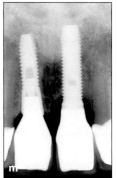

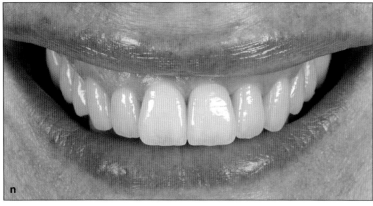

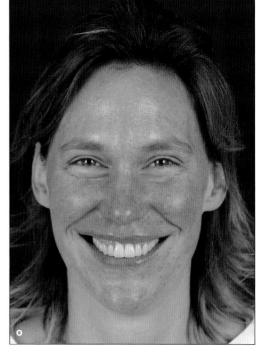

88

Fig 5-12 cont. / (l) Definitive all-ceramic restoration. (m) Radiograph of central incisors. (n) Smile after completion of the treatment. (o) Portrait after completion of the treatment. (Surgery and prosthodontics performed by G. Körner; laboratory work performed by P. Holthaus and K. Müterthies.)

Case 4: Complex implant rehabilitation in a patient with advanced periodontitis

The patient presented for rehabilitation and complained primarily of her long maxillary anterior teeth. She was wearing inadequate removable dentures in both arches. The residual anterior dentition was no longer worth preserving, and the patient wanted a fixed prosthetic solution (Figs 5-13a to 5-13c).

Cases such as this raise the question of how strong the patient's lip dynamics are and how much of the alveolar process or the maxilla they expose. Is it possible to work with fixed restorations? Where should the incisal edges of the teeth lie? Do papillae need to be reconstructed with pink material? It is only with the aid of suitable analysis

and planning that a predictably good esthetic outcome can be achieved and the decision can be made whether a fixed restoration is possible.

In the same manner as cases 1 to 3, the reference lines and the smile line were projected onto the photographs of the lips and the intraoral situation (Figs 5-13d to 5-13g). In this case, additional projection of the upper lip contour onto the intraoral situation is particularly important. This enables the clinician to assess the eventual exposure—and therefore the visibility—of the planned restoration. After analysis of the length-to-width ratio and development of an anatomical tooth shape (Figs 5-13h to 5-13l), it becomes clear how substantial the vertical loss of tissue is. Figure 5-13l illustrates how the upper lip would not conceal the black triangles in the interproximal spaces of the anterior teeth. Because of the biologic limitations of bone and soft tissue grafting, papillae need to be reconstructed with pink

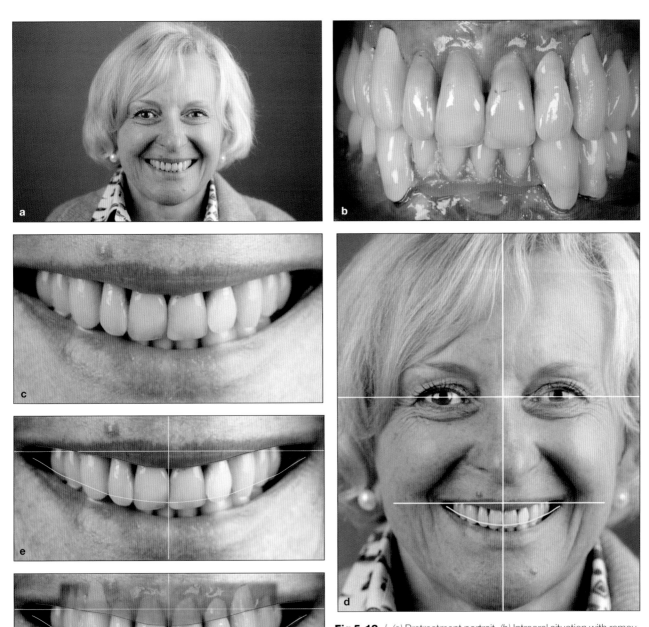

Fig 5-13 / *(a)* Pretreatment portrait. *(b)* Intraoral situation with removable denture; residual dentition has preexisting periodontal damage. *(c)* Smile with elongated anterior teeth. *(d)* Drawing the reference lines in DSD. *(e)* Mouth detail with maximum upper lip retraction marked *(red line)*. *(f)* Intraoral situation superimposed. This makes it clear what proportion is concealed by the upper lip. ⟶

ceramic or acrylic resin. Nevertheless, there is still enough distance from the alveolar process for a fixed restoration to be achievable and for the interface between pink dental material and mucosa not to be exposed. Analysis makes it easier to decide on a fixed restoration.

The patient eventually received fixed treatment with eight implants in the maxilla and six implants in the mandible, and the vertical tissue loss was compensated with pink ceramic[19] (Figs 5-13m to 5-13u). In the interim, the patient wore a fixed provisional restoration on the implants for a year so that function and oral hygiene could be evaluated and monitored. These restorations require very good care and patient compliance. The final extraoral photographs show the natural dentofacial esthetics of the definitive restoration.

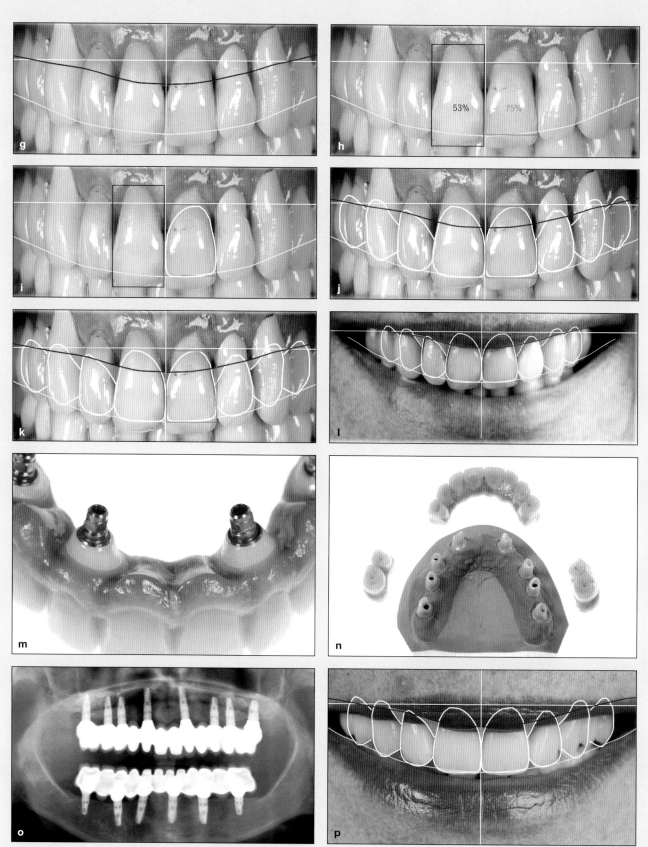

Fig 5-13 *cont.* / *(g)* Reference lines of the portrait, including top lip contour on maximum retraction, transferred to the intraoral situation. *(h)* Analysis of the correct width-to-length ratio of the anterior teeth. *(i)* Development of a new contour. Establishing the position of the incisal edge of the incisors. *(j)* Newly developed contour of maxillary anterior dentition. *(k)* Coloring the resulting interdental triangles. There is a need for papillary reconstruction with pink material. *(l)* Projection of the design onto the extraoral smile. *(m)* The superstructure was created with skillful reconstruction of the vertical defect in pink ceramic; the base is accessible for proper oral hygiene. *(n)* Segmented prostheses with cast. There are three zirconia partial dentures with zirconia abutments. *(o)* Panoramic radiograph after completion of treatment. *(p)* Smile after completion of treatment with planning superimposed.

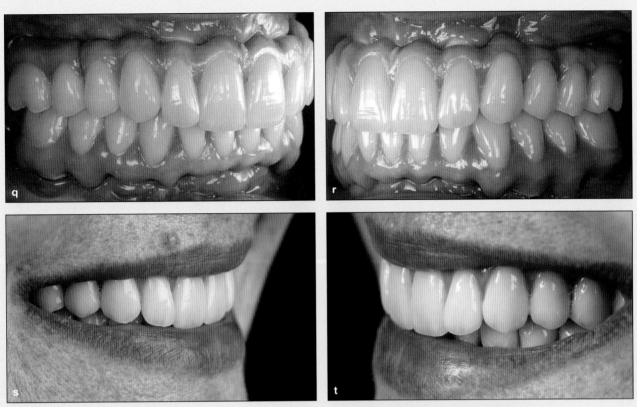

Fig 5-13 *cont.* / *(q and r)* Intraoral situation from left and right after completion of treatment. *(s and t)* Lateral views of smile after completion of treatment. *(u)* Final portrait. (Surgery and prosthodontics performed by A. Happe; laboratory work performed by A. Kunz.)

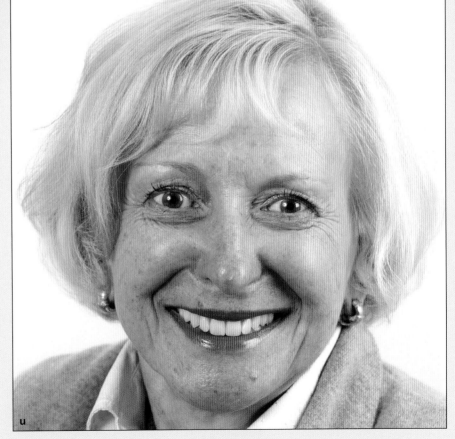

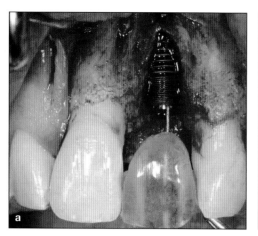
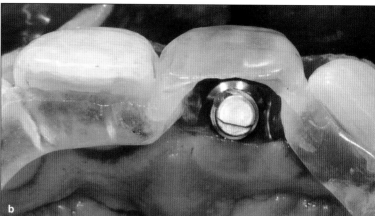
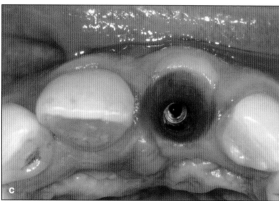
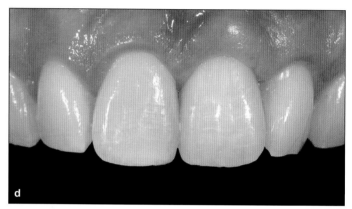

Fig 5-14 / *(a)* With the conventional guide in place, the clinician can perform a 3D position assessment based on the adjacent anatomical structures and the shape of the planned superstructure on the model. In this example, the depth of implant placement is being assessed. *(b)* The guide leaves space for drilling on the palatal aspect and facilitates controlled implant positioning. *(c)* Implant position after osseointegration and exposure. *(d)* An esthetic outcome was achieved after the crown was placed and soft tissue had matured.

Templates

Portions of this section have been adapted with permission from Happe et al.[20]

As described in the first section of this chapter, it is necessary to have the best 3D position of the implant for an optimal functional and esthetic outcome. Templates are intended to aid orientation during implant placement and therefore achieve this ideal position.

Simple surgical orientation templates

In the past, diagnostics and planning for implant placement were often based on models and two-dimensional radiographs. Clinical structures such as the crowns of adjacent teeth, soft tissue margins, and tooth axes were used as orientation landmarks, and a template with composite resin simulating the planned crown served as a surgical guide as well as a means of assessing the 3D implant position (Fig 5-14). These templates did not allow for transfer of information from the radiograph to the clinical situation.

Surgical templates with radiopaque components

Now available are plastic templates that have additional radiopaque components. For example, metallic spheres can be used to provide information about the magnification factor of the 2D radiograph (Fig 5-15a). Radiopaque teeth can also be used (Fig 5-15b). Radiopaque templates represent a considerable gain in information for 3D planning by means of CBCT. They allow for a relatively simple transfer of information from diagnostic radiographs.

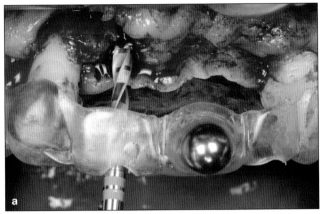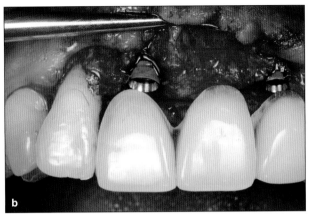

Fig 5-15 / *(a)* Plastic template with radiopaque spheres. *(b)* Template with radiopaque teeth. This template also contains the information about the cervical limit of the clinical crown for vertical positioning of the implant shoulder.

Guided surgery templates

Today, 3D digital imaging technologies such as CBCT make it possible to plan the positioning of dental implants using appropriate 3D positioning software and to transfer the information from the 3D imaging data sets to the surgical guides to help perform the surgery. These technologic advances have increased the accuracy of implant positioning, which also makes implant placement safer, especially in locations such as narrow spaces or in close proximity to vulnerable anatomical structures.[21]

In general, the restorative team has the following three options for the implementation and transfer of prosthetic reference points to a surgical guide:

1. Transferring information from a conventional diagnostic wax-up to a radiographic template
2. Using planning software to match CBCT and surface scan data of the wax-up
3. Using planning software to directly create a digital wax-up

Conventional diagnostic wax-up to radiographic template

This option represents the oldest conventional fabrication process associated with guided implant surgery. Before the CBCT scan is acquired, the laboratory technician must fabricate a radiographic template with radiopaque reference structures (eg, titanium pins or gutta-percha markers) or a radiopaque duplicate of the provisional restoration

made of acrylic resin (Fig 5-16a). The reference structures are placed in the template as specified by the planning software. CBCT scans are taken with the radiographic template correctly placed in the patient's mouth. Exact spatial positioning of the prosthetic reference in the dental arch can therefore be achieved (Fig 5-16b). The reference structures also serve as an interface to the planning software afterward. The CBCT scan with the clearly visible radiographic template is then uploaded into the planning software and aligned and calibrated based on the reference structures (Fig 5-16c). It is important to note that in situations such as this, legally the person who uploads the CBCT data into the software has sovereignty over the data. In this example, the software used was DWOS coDiagnostiX (Dental Wings) with three titanium pins.

The radiopaque prosthetic references can then be used for implant planning, but the lack of a surface scan of the actual intraoral conditions makes it difficult to identify important parameters (eg, soft tissue thickness) that are relevant and useful for planning. With most commercially available implant planning systems, the radiographic template must be sent back to the dental laboratory at this stage. The laboratory will then fabricate the drilling guides for guided surgery by using drilling tables specifically developed for the planning system. Exact fabrication is achieved by fixing the radiographic template in the correct position with plaster, followed by precise preparation of the sleeve bed for the respective implant position (Figs 5-16d and 5-16e). Take caution because this step of the fabrication process can be very prone to error, even for experienced dental technicians.

93

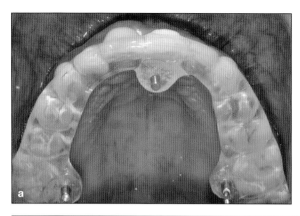
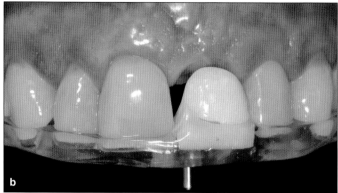
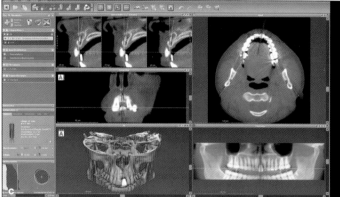
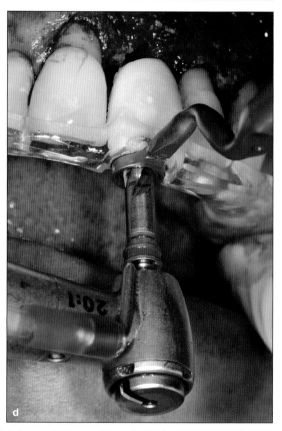
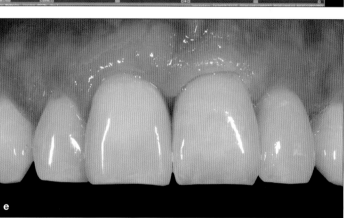

Fig 5-16 / *(a)* View of the radiographic template in place for CBCT with metal pins serving as markers. *(b)* Radiopaque composite represents the shape of the planned superstructure (in this case, a single crown). *(c)* View of the CBCT data set for guided surgery in the planning software. *(d)* Implant site preparation is performed using the sleeve inserted into the surgical guide according to the planning. *(e)* View of the single implant restoration (maxillary left central incisor) after completion of treatment. Correct positioning of the implant ensured a predictable esthetic outcome.

A second option is to send the planning data and stone cast of the current conditions to an industrial laboratory, where a surgical guide will be fabricated via a mostly additive process based on aligning these data and the planning data. The industrialized process step has the advantage of excluding many laboratory processing errors, but it also has certain disadvantages for the clinician, such as longer delivery times, higher costs, and a loss of control over the design process of the surgical guide.

Matching CBCT and surface scan data

With this option, it is possible to upload and align the surface scan data of the current intraoral situation with the CBCT data as well as with data from a scan of the wax-up (Fig 5-17). The data are uploaded in stereolithography (STL) format. The available software solutions allow for a decentralized workflow: The use of cloud-based software enables each member of the restorative team

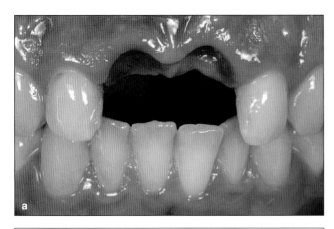

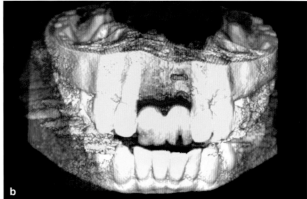

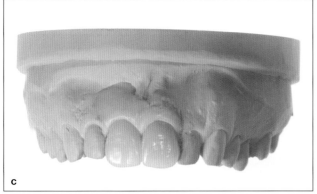

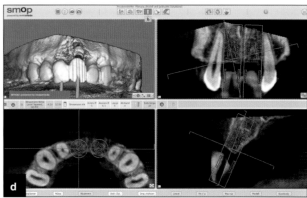

Fig 5-17 / *(a)* Clinical view of 3D alveolar ridge defects before treatment. *(b)* CBCT data set. *(c)* Wax-up of the central incisors simulating the tissue defects. *(d)* CBCT data set in the planning software. *(e)* Matching the CBCT data with the surface scan of the wax-up.

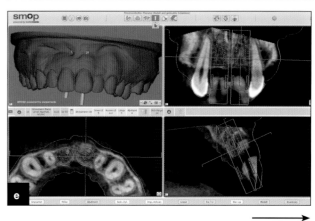

95

to independently upload the data sets and perform surgical planning with all of the prosthetic references. This approach allows for maximum freedom of software selection; the only requirement is that the system must be able to read the data in the standard STL format. These cloud-based systems also have the advantage of enabling different practitioners to work on a case simultaneously, thus greatly simplifying coordination with the referring clinician.

After all thorough examinations have been completed and the results and options discussed with the patient, the clinician can take a CBCT scan and upload the data into the planning software without any preliminary work

by a dental technician (see Fig 5-17d). After an initial review of the findings, the clinician can share the planning data and discuss the case with colleagues and/or dental technicians via cloud-based technology. With the corresponding alginate impression or intraoral impression, the dental technician can then produce any type of setup or wax-up needed. This may require an intraoral try-in as an intermediate step, or it may be generated by the software directly as STL data via a scan. To start the matching process, the user must first upload and open the files containing the surface scan data of the current intraoral situation and the planning data for the future restoration (wax-up or setup) (see Fig 5-17e). As with the

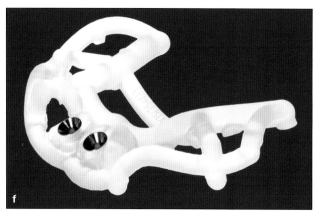

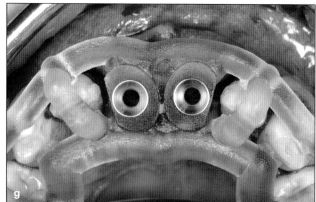

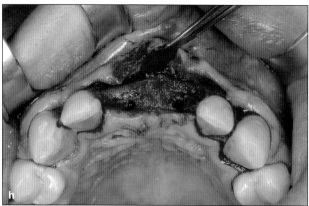

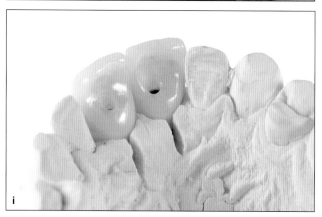

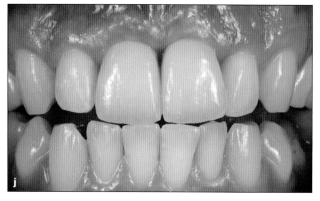

Fig 5-17 *cont.* / *(f)* 3D printed surgical guide with sleeves for the pilot holes. *(g)* View of the 3D guide in place. *(h)* Drilling the pilot hole is the cornerstone of 3D positioning. *(i)* Computer-assisted implant planning made it possible to use palatally screw-retained superstructures, which have several advantages over cemented crowns. *(j)* Final view of implant-supported crowns for the maxillary central incisors.

DWOS coDiagnostiX software described in the previous section, this is accomplished by marking identical areas and later making fine adjustments as needed.[22] Correct matching of the STL surface scan data with the CBCT data (as determined by gray level differences) is crucial, and the accuracy of implant planning and placement rises and falls with it. Consequently, this option may be contraindicated under various conditions. For example, the presence of an insufficient number or distribution of remaining teeth or large metal or zirconia restorations in the arch to be treated can make it difficult or impossible to achieve accurate data matching. In these cases, the conventional diagnostic wax-up option is the only way to proceed, and radiographic templates with reference structures must be used during CBCT scanning.

Once the clinician has gathered all of the necessary information, the actual process of prosthetic-driven implant planning can begin. It is possible to plan and save

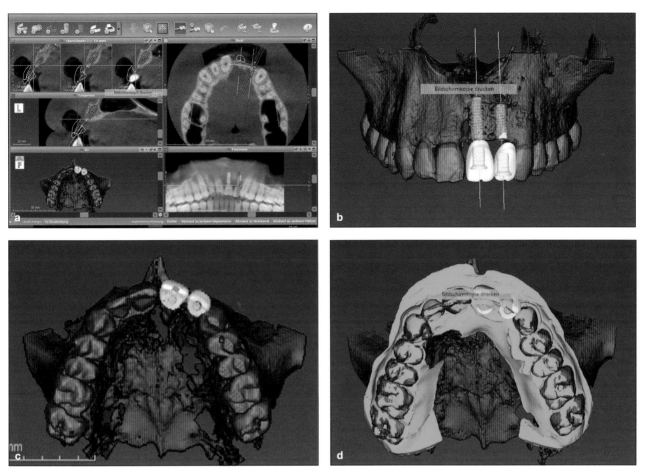

Fig 5-18 / *(a)* Overview of the different planning software views. *(b)* Digital wax-up of the maxillary left incisors. *(c)* Occlusal view of the digital wax-up: palatal screw retention is planned. *(d)* Surface scanned data matched with the CBCT data.

several versions of the surgical guide without reimporting the data, which means different treatment options can be presented to the team and the patient.[23] Once the final planning version of the surgical guide has been approved, the guide can be fabricated directly in the dental laboratory or ordered from the software manufacturer, if applicable (see Figs 5-17f and 5-17g). The splint module of the SMOP software package (SwissMeda) used to design the drill guide also produces STL data sets. Like all other systems currently available, this software contains details about all the relevant implant systems and the drill sleeves that accompany them. The SMOP workflow also has another interesting feature: Depending on which implant system is used, it may be possible to save the metal sleeve, which simplifies the manufacturing process and reduces costs, and also minimizes another source of error (eg, fitting the sleeves, luting the sleeves).[24,25] Unfortunately, this software only supports the implant-planning program and cannot be used in the restorative phase.

Creating a digital wax-up directly with the planning software

With this option, it is not only possible to upload and match the surface scan data of the current intraoral situation with the 3D CBCT data (as with the previously described options), but a digital wax-up can be created directly with the planning software (Figs 5-18a to 5-18d). Performing the workflow in this manner is highly efficient because the steps involved in displaying and then scaling and correctly positioning the virtual wax-up in the software can be completed very quickly.[26,27] Most guided surgery systems available today, however, are intended for planning purposes only. They are equipped with rather rudimentary tooth libraries and design software tools. These are sufficient for single-tooth implant planning if there are enough prosthetic references, including those on the adjacent teeth; however, if they are used for cantilever and partial denture restorations that span multiple teeth, proper adaptation and positioning of the

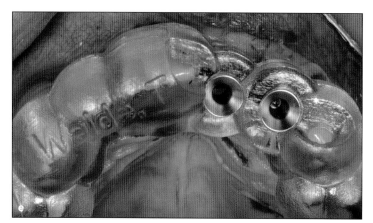

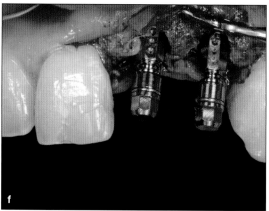

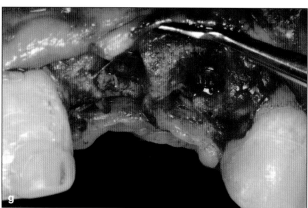

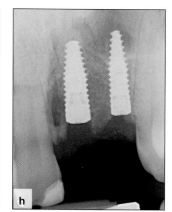

Fig 5-18 *cont.* / *(e)* Surgical guide in place. *(f)* The implants in the planned positions. *(g)* Correct vertical position with interimplant bone to support the papilla. *(h)* Postoperative radiograph of the implants.

virtual teeth can be very difficult. There is great potential for the new generations of computer-assisted design/computer-assisted manufacturing (CAD/CAM) software to fill this gap. Through the merging or modular docking of implant planning software with the manufacturing software used in the dental laboratory, digital implant planning can now be completed in the virtual articulator with modern design tools, taking all the relevant information (eg, the exact course of the soft tissue margins) into consideration. The data can then be visualized in the implant planning software in real time, eg, by creating a Straumann DWOS Synergy connection. This allows the dental technician to continuously adapt the wax-up, but only the clinician has the capability to change the implant position in the software module.

After the implant planning proposal has been finalized and approved, the dental technician designs the surgical guide using the software elements intended for dental laboratory use. The planned guide can be milled or 3D printed either in-house or by an external provider who is sent the corresponding data sets (Figs 5-18e to 5-18h). This blending of software solutions also opens up new possibilities. For example, it is possible to design and manufacture provisional restorations or abutments directly using the planned implant positions without the need to laboriously export them from the planning software and then reimport them into the design software.

In principle, the positioning of splints can be used to guide all or part of the implant site preparation process. Some splints allow for implant placement via the guide. Ultimately, it is up to clinicians to decide how much autonomous control they want over the entire process, ie, how much they want to rely on the planning software and surgical guide (Fig 5-19).

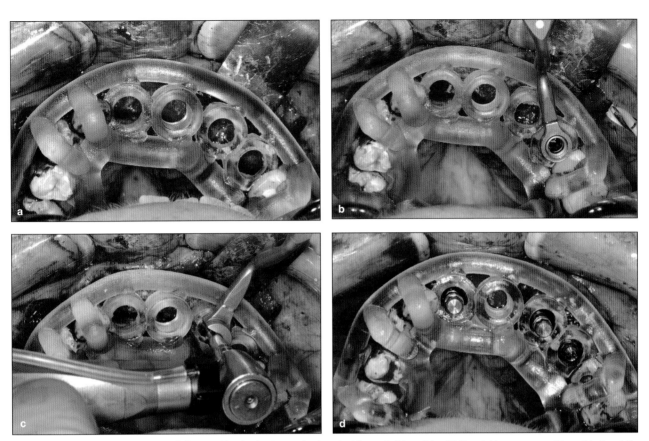

Fig 5-19 / *(a)* Guide without metal sleeves. The implants can be inserted through this guide. *(b)* Special keys are used to guide the drills into the plastic guide. *(c)* Drilling through the key inserted in the guide. *(d)* Implants inserted through the guide.

References

1. Jepsen S, Berglundh T, Genco R, et al. Primary prevention of peri-implantitis: Managing peri-implant mucositis. J Clin Periodontol 2015;42(suppl 16):S152–S157.
2. Sailer I, Mühlemann S, Zwahlen M, Hämmerle C, Schneider D. Cemented and scew-retained implant reconstructions: A systematic review of the survival and complication rates. Clin Oral Implants Res 2012;23(suppl 6):163–201.
3. Wilson TG Jr. The positive relationship between excess cement and peri-implant disease: A prospective clinical endoscopic study. J Periodontol 2009;80:1388–1392.
4. Linkevičius T, Vindašiūtė E, Puišys A, Linkevičienė L, Maslova N, Puriene A. The influence of the cementation margin position on the amount of undetected cement. A prospective clinical study. Clin Oral Implants Res 2013;24:71–76.
5. Linkevičius T, Puišys A, Vindašiūtė E, Linkevičienė L, Apse P. Does residual cement around implant-supported restorations cause peri-implant disease? A retrospective case analysis. Clin Oral Implants Res 2013;24:1179–1184.
6. Grunder U, Gracis S, Capelli M. Influence of the 3-D bone-to-implant relationship on esthetics. Int J Periodontics Restorative Dent 2005;25:113–119.

7. Vela X, Méndez V, Rodríguez X, Segalá M, Tarnow DP. Crestal bone changes on platform-switched implants and adjacent teeth when the tooth-implant distance is less than 1.5 mm. Int J Periodontics Restorative Dent 2012;32:149–155.
8. Berglundh T, Lindhe J. Dimension of the periimplant mucosa. Biological width revisited. J Clin Periodontol 1996;23:971–973.
9. Garber DA. The esthetic dental implant: Letting restoration be the guide. J Oral Implantol 1996;22:45–50.
10. Goldstein RE. Esthetics in Dentistry: Principles, Communication, Treatment Methods, ed 2. Ontario: BC Decker; 1998.
11. Rufenacht CR. Fundamentals of Esthetics. Chicago: Quintessence, 1990.
12. Magne P, Belser U. Bonded Porcelain Restorations in the Anterior Dentition: A Biomimetic Approach. Chicago: Quintessence, 2002.
13. Fradeani M. Esthetic Rehabilitation in Fixed Prosthodontics. Vol 1: Esthetic Analysis: A Systematic Approach to Prosthetic Treatment. Chicago: Quintessence, 2004.
14. Coachman C, Van Dooren E, Gürel G, Landsberg CJ, Calamita MA, Bichacho N. Smile design: From digital treatment planning to clinical reality. In: Cohen M. Interdisciplinary Treatment Planning. Vol 2: Comprehensive Case Studies. Chicago: Quintessence, 2012:119–174.
15. Kois JC. Diagnostically driven interdisciplinary treatment planning. Seattle Study Club J 2002;6:28–34.

16. Spear FM. The maxillary central incisor edge: A key to esthetic and functional treatment planning. Compend Contin Educ Dent 1999;20:512–516.

17. Kokich VO Jr, Kiyak HA, Shapiro PA. Comparing the perception of dentists and lay people to altered dental esthetics. J Esthet Dent 1999;11:311–324.

18. Kokich VO, Kokich VG, Kiyak HA. Perceptions of dental professionals and laypersons to altered dental esthetics: Asymmetric and symmetric situations. Am J Orthod Dentofacial Orthop 2006;130:141–151.

19. Happe A, Kunz A. Complex fixed implant-supported restoration in a site compromised by periodontitis: A case report. Int J Esthet Dent 2016;11:186–202.

20. Happe A, Fehmer V, Herklotz I, Nickenig HJ, Sailer I. Possiblities and limitations of computer-assisted implant planning and guided surgery in the anterior region. Int J Comp Dent 2018;21(2):1–16.

21. Nickenig HJ, Wichmann M, Hamel J, Schlegel KA, Eitner S. Evaluation of the difference in accuracy between implant placement by virtual planning data and surgical guide templates versus the conventional free-hand method: A combined in vivo - in vitro technique using cone-beam CT (Part II). J Craniomaxillofac Surg 2010;38:488–493.

22. Flügge T, Derksen W, Te Poel J, Hassan B, Nelson K, Wismeijer D. Registration of cone beam computed tomography data and intraoral surface scans: A prerequisite for guided implant surgery with CAD/CAM drilling guides. Clin Oral Implants Res 2017;28:1113–1118.

23. Sancho-Puchades M, Fehmer V, Hämmerle C, Sailer I. Advanced smile diagnostics using CAD/CAM mock-ups. Int J Esthet Dent 2015;10:374–391.

24. Van Assche N, Quirynen M. Tolerance within a surgical guide. Clin Oral Implants Res 2010;21:455–458.

25. Schneider D, Schober F, Grohmann P, Hämmerle CH, Jung RE. In-vitro evaluation of the tolerance of surgical instruments in templates for computer-assisted guided implantology produced by 3-D printing. Clin Oral Implants Res 2015;26:320–325.

26. Benic GI, Mühlemann S, Fehmer V, Hämmerle CH, Sailer I. Randomized controlled within-subject evaluation of digital and conventional workflows for the fabrication of lithium disilicate single crowns. Part I: Digital versus conventional unilateral impressions. J Prosthet Dent 2016;116:777–782.

27. Sailer I, Benic GI, Fehmer V, Hämmerle CHF, Mühlemann S. Randomized controlled within-subject evaluation of digital and conventional workflows for the fabrication of lithium disilicate single crowns. Part II: CAD-CAM versus conventional laboratory procedures. J Prosthet Dent 2017;118:43–48.

"'Experience' is the name we give
to our mistakes."

OSCAR WILDE

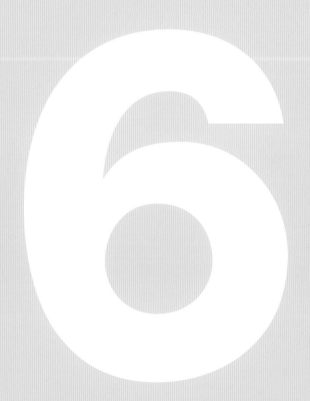

Tooth Preservation Versus Extraction and Implant Placement

/ Gerd Körner, Arndt Happe

102

T he goal of the dental practitioner is to select treatment measures that will satisfy patients and prove successful in the long term. This decision will depend on an appropriate indication and a critical evaluation of the various options. Assessment of the influencing factors separately or in combination plays a crucial strategic role, and the factors should be considered at three different levels:

- Patient level
- Dental level (locally and extended)
- Practice level

Patient Level

Strategic assessment of the use of implants addresses a variety of scenarios that may involve an indication in the esthetic zone:

- Tooth agenesis
- Tooth loss following trauma (eg, tooth fracture or avulsion)
- Teeth not worth preserving because of significant loss of substance (eg, carious destruction or traumatic erosion or abrasion)
- Teeth not worth preserving because of periodontal or endoperiodontal lesions

The patient's underlying preferences have a significant effect on the ultimate decision to choose implant treatment. There are few data on this aspect available in the literature.

Many patients seem to be very satisfied with fixed partial dentures, and there is a tendency for implant-supported restorations to be preferred by patients from a high socio-economic background. The esthetic aspects and preservation of substance mainly appeal to younger patients.[1] Generally, the patient's fundamental decision can and must be influenced by the dental practitioner. Because patients are usually more interested in a long-term stable esthetic outcome than in the methods to achieve this outcome, it is incumbent on the dentist to explain the pros and cons as well as the risks involved.

At the patient level, it must be clearly emphasized that marginal infections must be avoided to maintain an esthetic solution. To achieve this, it is essential to integrate the treatment into a rigorous precare and aftercare regimen. In addition, it might become necessary to address negative effects of endogenous diseases (eg, diabetes) and recommend optimal clinical management. In particular, the complication rate of augmentation measures is significantly higher in patients who smoke. Depending on the extent of nicotine abuse and scope of surgical measures, clinicians may advise against an implantology procedure for these patients.[2,3]

It is therefore important to perform a risk and prognostic assessment that is as precise as possible. The assesment should consider systemic factors (especially compliance and smoking) as well as local factors, such as plaque control and the microbiologic makeup of the periodontal microflora. The patient's specific wishes; requirements in terms of esthetics, phonetics, and function; and the cost-benefit relationship against the patient's specific background must be incorporated into the decision-making process (Fig 6-1).[4]

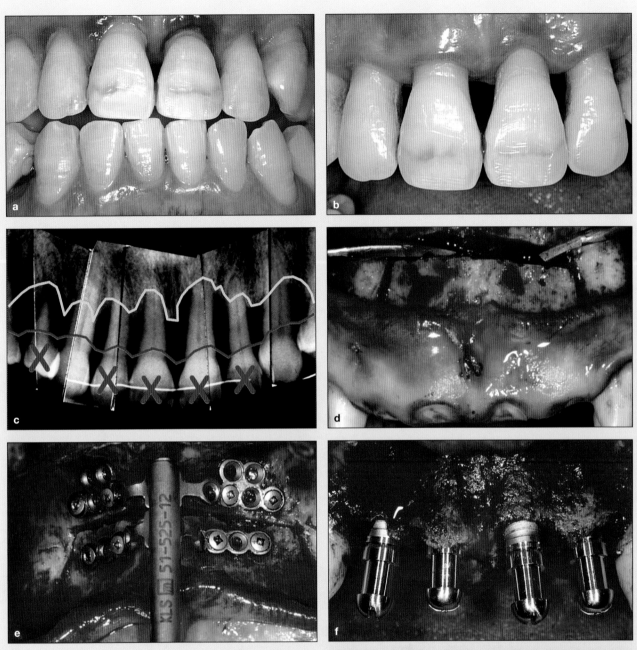

Fig 6-1 / *(a)* This 49-year-old patient has aggressive periodontitis, and microbiologic testing was positive for *Aggregatibacter actinomycetemcomitans*. *(b)* Condition of maxillary anterior dentition after extensive hygiene treatment, including antibiotic treatment with a van Winkelhoff cocktail (ie, amoxicillin and metronidazole). *(c)* Prognostic assessment of the maxillary anterior dentition based on bone level (*yellow line*, actual status; *blue line*, desired status; *X*, to be extracted). *(d)* Alveolar osteotomy for vertical distraction with root segments left in place for the purpose of socket preservation until immediate implant placement is carried out 4 months later. *(e)* Distractor with basal wings fixed to the local subnasal alveolar process, and screwable wing in the osteotomized bone segment. *(f)* Immediate implant placement with Frialit Synchro (Dentsply) after removal of the four root segments of the maxillary incisors. *(g)* Occlusal view after placement of immediate implants in the ideal restorative positions. Note the buccal bony deficits.

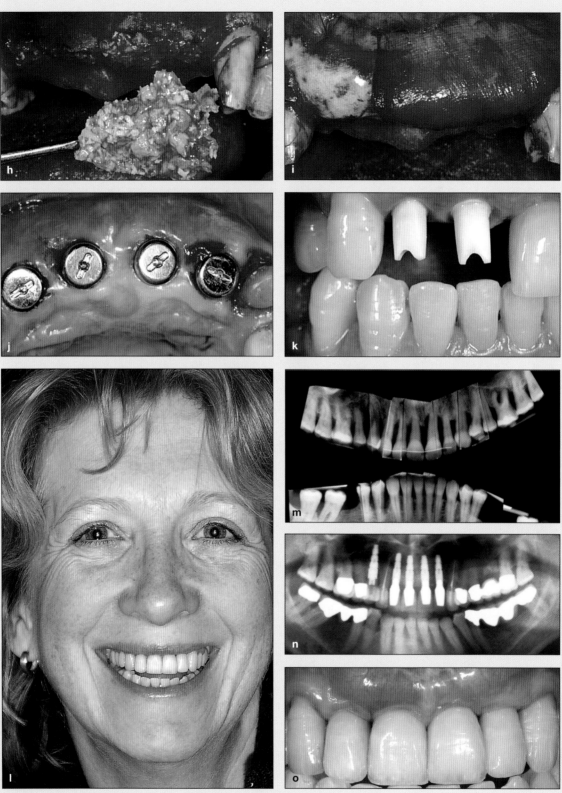

Fig 6-1 *cont.* / *(h)* Bone particulate augmentation in conjunction with plasma rich in growth factors (PRGF) for the horizontal deficits of the incisors. *(i)* Membrane coverage (Bio-Gide, Geistlich) of the mixed autogenous and xenogeneic augmentation material (Bio-Oss, Geistlich). *(j)* Minimally invasive exposure by the keyhole access expansion technique according to Happe et al.[4] *(k)* All-ceramic restorative treatment: implants with zirconia hybrid abutments at maxillary right first premolar and all maxillary incisors. *(l)* Final portrait after combined periodontal, implant, and restorative treatment. *(m)* Pretreatment radiograph. *(n)* Follow-up radiograph 6 years after completion of the treatment. The radiograph also shows socket preservation of the region of the maxillary left first molar and status after guided tissue regeneration (GTR) at the region of the mandibular right canine, first premolar, and second molar. *(o)* Clinical view of the maxillary anterior dentition 6 years after completion of the treatment. (Surgery and prosthodontics performed by G. Körner; laboratory work performed by K. Müterthies.)

Fig 6-2 / Tooth loss or survival rate over 15 to 16 years corresponding to prognostic classification according to McGuire[9] and McGuire and Nunn.[10]

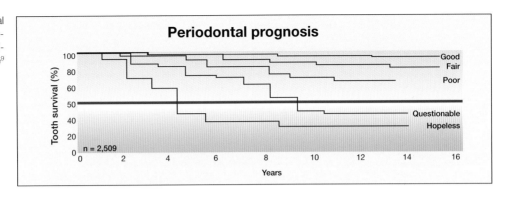

Fig 6-3 / Prognosis classification according to the "traffic light principle" proposed by McGuire and Nunn.[10] Note: Treatment decision requires the most consideration in the yellow group.

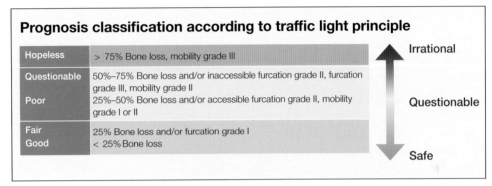

Dental Level

Decision making at the so-called dental level can prove equally complex, as indicated by various long-term studies regarding tooth type and associated loss rates.[5–7] This primarily affects decision making related to periodontal suitability for preservation; it is less relevant to the course of action in cases of agenesis and posttrauma tooth loss and only to a limited extent to excessive loss of substance caused by caries, abrasion, or erosion. The decision to preserve a tooth or use an implant must be guided primarily by the probability of long-term success of the periodontal therapeutic measures.[8] Therefore, the threshold of what is rational or irrational to treat needs to be defined against the background of this probability of long-term success, the requirements for the best possible esthetic solution, and possible alternatives.

Because *therapeutic success* does not have a single agreed-upon definition, data in the literature only provide limited information about the correct timing of the transition from appropriate periodontal treatment to an implant replacement. This can only be approached gradually by examining different parameters. Differentiation of prognostic classes of periodontally damaged teeth and their probability of survival is an important entry point into the decision-making process. The classic studies by McGuire[9] and McGuire and Nunn[10] are useful for this purpose (Fig

Box 6-1 Parameters for determining the prognosis classification (see also determining bone loss, Fig 6-6)

Viable	Questionable	Hopeless
< 50% bone loss	> 50% bone loss	> 75% bone loss
< Furcation grade II	≥ Furcation grade II ≥ Mobility grade I or II	Mobility grade III

6-2). The resulting prognostic classification is based on the parameters listed in Box 6-1 and is typically the basis of the so-called traffic-light principle (Fig 6-3).[10]

The survival rate after 8 years is set as a demarcation point to make a reliable statement that is relevant to dental practice. The classifications that fall below 50% survival rate at this time result in an "irrational to treat" rating. A sufficient margin above that must be the goal for the long-term success of a treatment strategy.

Therefore, further criteria are needed to classify tooth preservability in the transitional range, (ie, when there is 50% loss of bony support, grade II furcation, and grade II mobility). For teeth that are strategically significant specifically from a prosthodontic viewpoint, further probing and a more critical assessment usually have to be completed at the different levels. In practice, a staged approach has proved valuable: A primary assessment is first performed according to the traffic light principle derived from the prognosis classification developed by McGuire and Nunn[10]

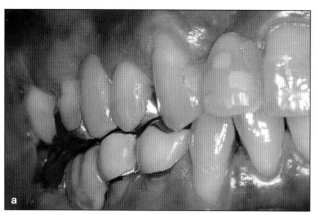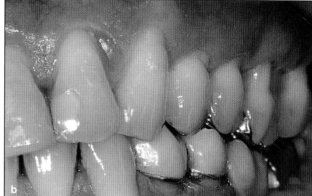

Fig 6-4 / *(a and b)* This patient has aggressive periodontitis, and microbiologic testing is positive for *A actinomycetemcomitans*.

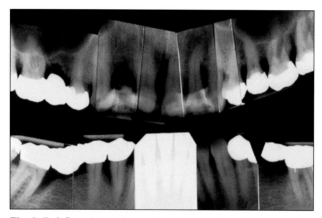

Fig 6-5 / Complete radiographic status for risk assessment of the periodontally impaired situation.

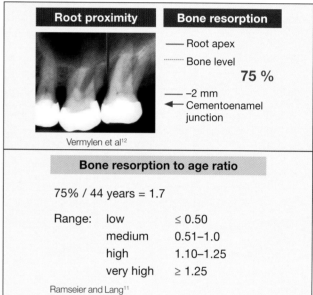

Root proximity	Bone resorption
	— Root apex
	⋯⋯ Bone level
	75 %
	— –2 mm
	← Cementoenamel junction
Vermylen et al[12]	

Bone resorption to age ratio	
75% / 44 years = 1.7	
Range: low	≤ 0.50
medium	0.51–1.0
high	1.10–1.25
very high	≥ 1.25
Ramseier and Lang[11]	

Fig 6-6 / Root proximity according to Vermylen et al[12] and bone resorption/age index according to Ramseier and Lang.[11] Bone resorption is determined as percent of root length (cementoenamel junction minus 2 mm up to root apex). The bone resorption/age index is calculated by dividing the bone resorption by the patient's age (eg, index 1.7 indicates a very high risk).

(Fig 6-4). After this, the other extended local factors are examined, as described in the following paragraphs.

The *bone resorption/age index* according to Ramseier and Lang[11] is an important patient factor when assessing the risk in complex periodontal cases. This measures bone resorption in relation to root length at the most advanced site in the whole dentition using a radiograph, and it should be put into context with the extended local findings at the dental level. This ratio is divided by the patient's age to gain an impression of the severity of the periodontal disease and hence the risk of treating it. If only bitewing radiographs are available without a complete image of the root dimensions,

1 mm loss is equated to 10% bone resorption relative to the entire root length (Figs 6-5 and 6-6).[11,12]

There are several factors that are highly heterogenous and must be viewed as limiting in esthetically demanding situations. These play a significant role at the dental level:

• The extended local examination
• The basic strategic assessment regarding restorative versus nonrestorative treatment
• The influence of multiple risks from the endodontic and conservative perspectives (eg, apical lesions, root discolorations, resorption, posts and cores, residual substance)

Table 6-1 Single-tooth prognosis in overall restorative situation derived from heterogenous factors at the dental level

	Viable	Questionable	Hopeless
Periodontal	0% to 50% bone loss Furcation grade I	50% to 75% bone loss Furcation grade II	> 75% bone loss Furcation grade II to III Mobility grade III
Endodontic	Vital No endodontic issues No restorative issues No apical radiolucency	Incomplete root fracture Apical radiolucency Nonvital without root fracture "Micro-endo" apicectomy Hypersensitivity Perio-endo lesion Instrument fracture	Perforation Fracture Cyst Symptomatically obliterated teeth Root resorption
Defect	Formal design possible Intact biologic width Favorable tooth or root length Reconstruction height > 4 mm	Prior to pin restoration Prior to crown lengthening Circular cervical filling Small root cross-section Tooth position prosthetically unfavorable	Deeply destroyed teeth

Table 6-2 Dental and practice level: survival of molars in patients with periodontal disease in long-term studies overall and in the case of practice-specific endodontic and resective therapy

Study	Survival rate (%)	Duration (years)
Molar risk overall after completed periodontal therapy		
Wasserman et al[5]	68	22
McFall[6]	43	19
Goldmann et al[7]	56	22
Svårdström et al[13]	89	8–12
In the case of endodontic/restorative therapy		
Basten et al[14]	92	12
Carnevale et al[15]	93	10
Svårdström et al[13]	89	8–12
Langer et al[16]	62	10
Bühler[17]	68	10

Beware of the exponential accumulation of risk. Multiple risks in the questionable section change the classification to hopeless (Table 6-1). Underestimated factors, such as orthodontic malpositioning, functional disorders of the stomatognathic system, and root proximity can make a more stringent assessment necessary under certain circumstances.[12] *Root proximity*, especially for molars, is understood to mean limited bony alveolar structure with adverse nutritional circumstances and a small root distance.

These patient-specific factors are significant, above all, to the final direction of decision making in the group that is primarily classified as questionable. Consideration should be given to the numbers in the classic studies regarding tooth loss by Hirschfeld and Wasserman,[5] McFall,[6] and Goldman et al.[7] These illustrate a good prognosis for teeth that have previous periodontal damage, are treated, and receive long-term aftercare (average of 19 to 22 years). This good prognosis applies particularly to the esthetically relevant anterior dentition. However, the slightly increased risks for the premolars and especially molars must be borne in mind (Table 6-2 and Fig 6-7).[5–7,13–17] A more recent study by Svårdström and Wennström[13] shows similar loss rates for the molars as those reported in the previously mentioned classic studies with regard to the duration under optimal conditions.

Practice Level

The influence of the practice level becomes particularly clear when the results of root amputations are viewed in relation to furcations in patients with extremely compromised molars. The 10-year survival rates of 89% to 93% for one group and only 62% to 68% for another group differ markedly and highlight the so-called center effect at the practice level (ie, interdependences of the specific conditions prevailing in an individual practice).[13–17]

The following factors should be taken into consideration when making the final decision against or in favor of retaining the natural tooth:

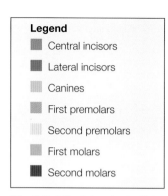

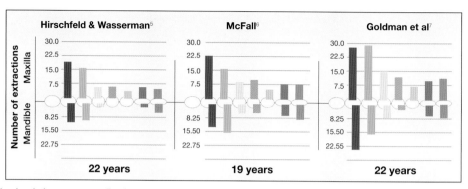

Fig 6-7 / Tooth loss by tooth type in classic long-term studies in patients with periodontal disease.

Box 6-2 Influence of different factors on the target variable of tooth loss*

Patient level
- Age
- Sex
- Average bone loss
- Interleukin genotype
- Relationship of interleukin genotype to bone loss

Dental level
- Tooth mobility
- Prosthetic restoration
- Tooth type
- Intra-alveolar periodontal defect component
- Residual alveolar bone support

*Data from Muzzi et al.[18]

- It is essential to keep a critical eye on the efficacy of endodontic treatment and the effectiveness of the periodontal aftercare regimen, but also the restorative potential of the clinician's own practice (ie, center effect) in avoiding complications, especially root fractures.
- Of relevance to the esthetic zone, all the quoted studies show a far better long-term prognosis for single-rooted teeth than for multiple-rooted teeth, which can be achieved with comparatively minimal therapeutic effort and therefore low economic cost.
- A complete assessment of the factors at the patient and dental levels takes time, and this should be allotted for in the treatment process to ensure a reliable risk assessment. An interim long-term restoration (laboratory-fabricated long-term temporary/therapeutic agent) may prove beneficial for a definitive evaluation of preservability and continuing strategic directions such as tissue conditioning, maintenance of chewing comfort, initial functional therapy and esthetic diagnostics, eg, mock-ups and Digital Smile Design.

- At the practice level, decision making must include the question of whether and how effective an aftercare concept is, which is essential for all patients but especially when treating periodontitis.

Choosing to Keep the Tooth

A 10-year study by Muzzi et al[18] provides valuable assistance in further decision making for or against tooth preservation. This group investigated the influence of various factors on the target variable of tooth loss (Box 6-2).[18] The conclusion reached was that only a few factors—primarily at the dental level—have a decisive impact on tooth loss:

- Molars are generally more susceptible as a tooth type ($P < .001$).
- Residual bone support is inversely proportional to tooth loss.
- The larger the intra-alveolar defect component, the less future tooth loss there is.
- None of the other indicators had a similarly evident influence on the outcome.

With regard to influence on the radiographic bone level, again over 10 years, a similar study by the same group[19] additionally reported that larger pocket depths and greater tooth mobility at initial measurment had the poorest prognoses. The bony intra-alveolar component of the periodontal defect, however, was associated with a relatively good prognosis in terms of remedying the defect, provided appropriate periodontal treatment was performed. The other factors had less significant influence on changes to the bone level.

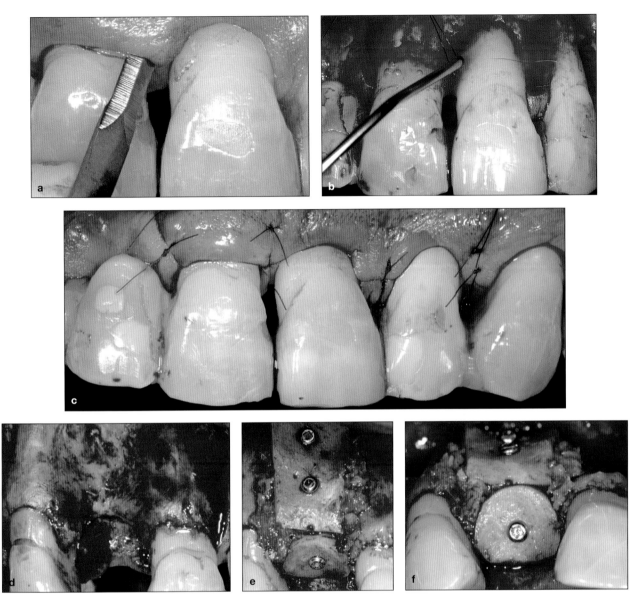

Fig 6-8 / *(a and b)* Minimally invasive regenerative periodontal treatment using the minimally invasive surgical technique (MIST) according to Cortellini and Tonetti[27] with Emdogain (Straumann). *(c)* Multilayer interdental wound closure at completion of periodontal surgery. *(d to f)* Bone augmentation in the region of the right lateral incisor with autogenous blocks harvested from the oblique line of the right mandible using piezoelectric technology and a trephine, packed in multiple layers with autogenous bone chips and xenograft (Bio-Oss), and covered by a collagen membrane (Bio-Gide).

Another concept suggests extracting periodontally damaged teeth at an early stage. The idea is to preserve the alveolar ridge so implants can be placed without regenerative and augmentative therapy, even if implant placement is slightly compromised. However, this results in loss of bundle bone even with immediate implant placement and is not justified; it often leads to excessive implant treatment and inadequate esthetic results.[20–24] Regenerative therapy, on the other hand, has shown positive long-term results.

The results of the study by Cortellini and Tonetti[25] make it clear that the survival rate of teeth more than 10 years after guided tissue regeneration (GTR) is higher than 96%. The clinical attachment level gain was the same or better after 15 years in 92% of cases. As well as the cost-benefit advantages, which emerged when inferring the benefits of regenerative treatment even with seemingly hopeless teeth, the advantages cannot be rated highly enough, especially in the esthetic zone (Fig 6-8).[26–28] This needs to be offset by the significant alveolar bone loss rates due to resorption and remodeling (ie, up to 63% horizontally and 22% vertically) in the case of periodontally undamaged teeth 3 and 6 months after extraction.[29,30]

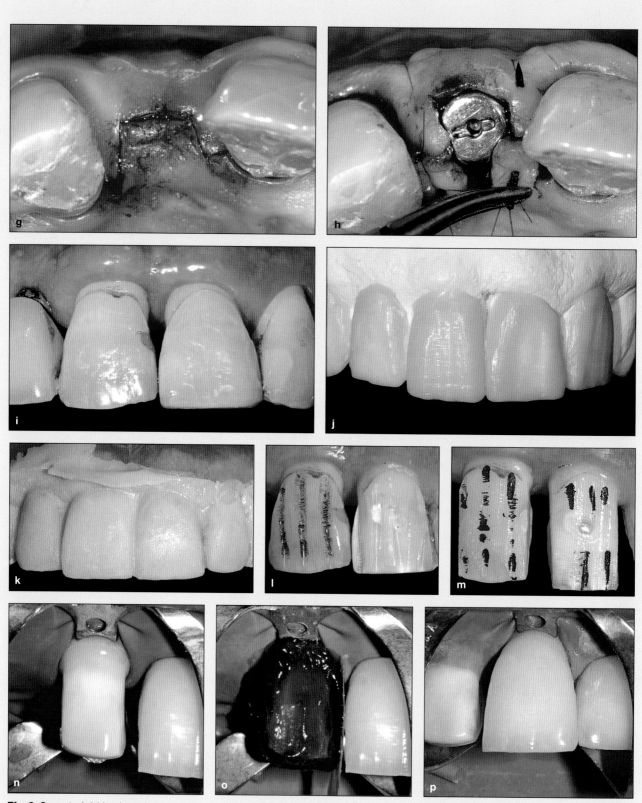

Fig 6-8 *cont.* / *(g)* Implant placement site (Xive 3.8, Dentsply) 4 months after bone augmentation. *(h)* After another 3 months, the implant was exposed based on the split-finger technique according to Misch et al.[28] The volume and extent of the keratinized structures is visualized with Lugol's solution. *(i)* Condition 2 months after implant exposure at the right lateral incisor and 8 months after regenerative treatment from the right central incisor to the left canine. A resin-bonded partial denture is used for long-term provisional restoration at the right lateral incisor. *(j)* Wax-up of the deficient maxillary anterior dentition for esthetic analysis and initiation of the definitive restorative treatment. *(k to m)* Converting the wax-up into a restorative mock-up for a minimally invasive veneer preparation. It must be ensured that there is sufficient interproximal resection for perio-prosthetic recontouring of an esthetic-restorative emergence profile. *(n to p)* Controlled adhesive cementing of incisor veneers under rubber dam.

⟶

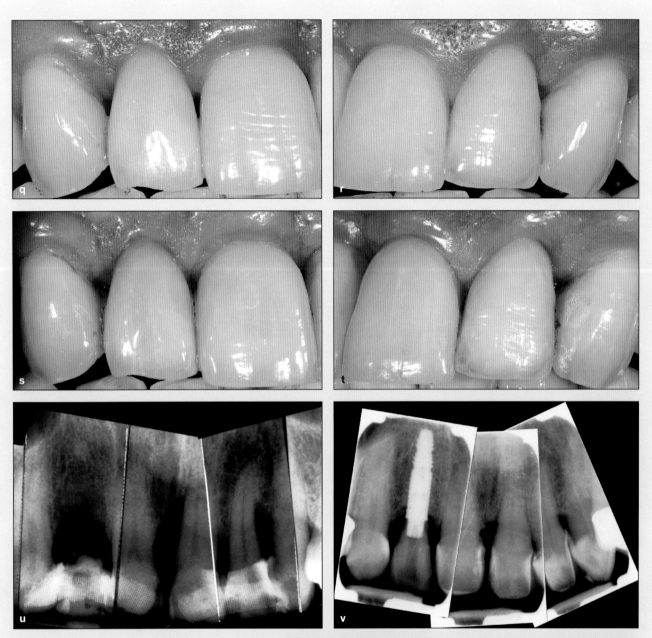

Fig 6-8 *cont.* / *(q and r)* All-ceramic restoration on implant at the right lateral incisor and veneers at the other maxillary incisors after 3 months. *(s and t)* Clinical appearance after 2 years. *(u)* Radiographs of maxillary anterior dentition before treatment. *(v)* Radiographs 10 years after periodontal regeneration, implant restoration, and ceramic restoration. Note the considerable regeneration of intra-alveolar defects. *(w)* Clinical appearance 10 years after combined periodontal, implant, and restorative treatment. (Surgery and prosthodontics performed by G. Körner; laboratory work performed by K. Müterthies.)

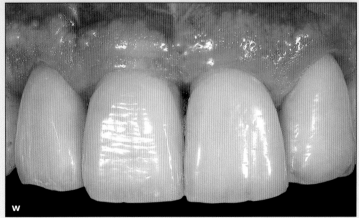

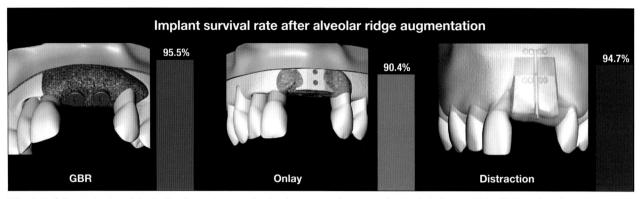

Fig 6-9 / Survival rates of implants after various methods of augmentation according to Aghaloo and Moy.[32] Note that these data come from different time periods of the follow-up examinations (ie, 5 to 74 months).

Table 6-3 Assignment of different patient-specific parameters to different risk profiles with regard to periodontal disease recurrence or tooth loss*

Risk profile	BOP (%)	PD ≥ 5 mm (no. of teeth)	Tooth loss (no. of teeth)	Bone resorption/ age index	Systemic/ generalized	Smoking
Low	≤ 9	≤ 4	≤ 4	< 0.5	No	Nonsmoker (< 10 cigarettes/ day) or former smoker
Medium	10 to 25	5 to 8	5 to 8	0.5 to 1	No	10 to 19 cigarettes/day
High	≥ 26	≥ 9	≥ 9	> 1	Yes	> 20 cigarettes/day

BOP, bleeding on probing; PD, probing depth.
*Data from Matuliene et al.[33]

Interestingly, the essentially high probability of success and long-term stability of regenerative measures correlates with the results of Fiorellini and Nevins[31] with respect to the predictable implant survival rate in cases of guided bone regeneration (GBR) and distraction osteogenesis.[20,21,25,26] The results of augmentative and ridge-preserving or buildup techniques indicate that a high survival rate of implants in previously deficient areas is to be expected (Fig 6-9).[32] These results must be interpreted with the understanding that in some cases the number of follow-up examinations is small (eg, in cases of distraction) and that the time intervals vary. Nevertheless, the results do emphasize the growing predictability of such techniques.

An approach that involves prophylactic extraction of teeth with moderate periodontal damage to permit or improve the success of implants must therefore be rejected in principle. Instead, as predictable an assessment as possible of the future risk of a periodontally diseased tooth should determine the decision making against the background of local and systemic influencing factors. For this purpose, the results of a long-term study by Matuliene et al[33] provide valuable insight into the risk of recurrence of periodontal diseases and tooth loss during periodontal aftercare. The role of patient compliance is specifically highlighted in this context. The study describes a systematic assignment of various factors (Table 6-3).[33] The conclusion was reached that even if only one of the tested parameters was in the high risk profile, the probability of periodontal disease recurrence or tooth loss significantly increased. As the number of parameters in this risk profile increases, the risk increases accordingly. Considering the influencing factors, extraction tends to be required when the value of tooth preservation is questionable and if there is a lack of supportive therapy after periodontal disease treatment. For high-risk patients, there is a chance of recurrence even with supportive therapy. Accordingly, teeth that are severely periodontally compromised should be sacrificed if there is a lack of compliance and extensive restorative measures are planned.

Choosing Implants

If the decision is made to use implants, this raises the question of how to assess treatment success with implants in patients with periodontal disease and how long-term that assessment can be. A basic distinction must be made between survival and success.[34] The survival rate of implants in periodontally diseased or susceptible patients may be high, but the higher incidence of peri-implantitis can greatly limit the sustainable success depending on the criteria applied. Accordingly, even if implant therapy is not entirely contraindicated, it should be made conditional on appropriate infection control and aftercare.

Other Considerations

The results of a prospective long-term study by Karoussis et al[35] reveal marked differences between periodontally healthy patients and those with a previous history of periodontal disease. The main conclusion is that an association between periodontal and peri-implant conditions and the corresponding alterations becomes clear after 10 years of follow-up.

The rate of progression with regard to loss of attachment to teeth and to implants is similar in an individual patient. Smoking has a significant correlation with bone loss around implants: roughly 1 mm greater after 10 years than in nonsmokers. Lindquist et al[36] discovered even greater bone loss than Karoussis et al,[35] although this was in patients with tobacco consumption greater than 10 cigarettes per day.

The differing survival rate associated with a past periodontitis history is made clear in another study by Karoussis et al,[37] and this has been confirmed by other authors. In their meta-analysis, Wen et al[38] conclude that a previous periodontal disease must be assessed as a statistical risk factor for the long-term survival of dental implants (Table 6-4).[39–51] This negative effect is more likely when the influence is more advanced, aggressive, and prolonged.

However, in the review article comparing the longevity of teeth and implants by Holm-Pedersen et al[52] (Fig 6-10), even follow-up examination of implants without identified periodontal impairment shows that the overall implant survival rate after 5 years and estimated after 10 years certainly does not surpass the survival rate of treated teeth, even those that were periodontally compromised.[53–57]

The results reported by Lulic[54] regarding the survival rate of periodontally treated teeth that served as abutments for very wide-span partial dentures represent a relatively small number of cases. However, the trend is still impressive: The survival rate of these abutment teeth, which came nowhere near to following Ante's law[58] (related to periodontal anchorage), was 92.9% after 10 years; this is at least as high as for implants serving a similar function as abutments for shorter-span partial dentures (ie, one or two units) at 92.8%.[59]

Only the results extrapolated to 10 years for single implants (96.3%) came close to those for periodontally compromised but successfully treated teeth.[60] If possible, so-called hybrid partial dentures (ie, units of combined natural teeth and implants) should be avoided because of the lower survival rates.[57]

After careful consideration of all these aspects, the final treatment decision of tooth versus implant—especially when faced with periodontal problems—should focus on removing the "questionable" classification: the yellow in the traffic light system (see Fig 6-3). Insecure teeth that were rated with a question mark in the first prognostic assessment must be reevaluated because the decision to keep or extract is very often strategically important. If these insecure teeth had to be used as abutments, for example, they should no longer be considered because of the increased risk to the overall restorative situation. If a natural tooth can no longer be preserved, an implant can take its place. Therapeutic approaches must strategize by choosing an abutment that produces a synergistic addition to the remaining stock of natural teeth and fully exploits the diverse potential. The neighboring situation of implants and natural teeth plays a key role, especially in the esthetically relevant appearance of the interproximal papilla.[61,62] The overall therapeutic approach must take into account these neighboring relationships as well as the advantage of pontic areas that can be dynamically influenced to optimize the restorative outcome.[63]

In addition to esthetic and functional demands, the need to strive for biologic stabilization of the interface between the involved structures arises from the basic fact that implants only succeed in a sustained, long-term fashion if they are part of a periodontally oriented therapeutic approach.

The varied histologic aspects and the pathologic changes that may result need to be properly addressed by augmentative and preservative structural measures similar to those around compromised natural teeth such as modern periodontal plastic surgery. In addition, it is essential to ensure suitable exposure techniques to optimize the peri-implant environment.[64] In fact, two authoritative Cochrane database systematic reviews in recent years concluded that there is still no robust evidence of advantages arising from an increase in peri-implant keratinized mucosa.[65,66] However, there have recently been a growing number of reports of a positive influence, and achieving

113

Table 6-4 Meta-analysis of the survival rate of implants in patients with a previous history of periodontitis*

Authors	Study type	Implant type	Groups	Patients (n)	Implants (n)	Implant survival rate	Follow-up (months)
Hardt et al[39]	Retrospective	Brånemark	Periodontally healthy	25	92	96.74%	60
			Periodontally diseased	25	100	92%	
Karoussis et al[40]	Prospective	ITI	Periodontally healthy	45	91	96.5%	120
			Chronic periodontitis	8	21	90.5%	
Evian et al[41]	Retrospective	Paragon	Periodontally healthy	72	72	91.67%	118
			Periodontally diseased	77	77	79.22%	
Mengel et al[42]	Prospective	Brånemark	Periodontally healthy	12	30	100%	36
			Chronic periodontitis	12	43	100%	
			Aggressive periodontitis	15	77	97.4%	
De Boever et al[43]	Prospective	ITI	Periodontally healthy	110	261	96.94%	140
			Chronic periodontitis	68	193	96.38%	
			Aggressive periodontitis	16	95	84.75%	
Roccuzzo et al[44]	Prospective	TPS	Periodontally healthy	28	61	96.6%	120
			Moderate periodontitis	37	95	92.8%	
			Severe periodontitis	36	90	90%	
Anner et al[45]	Retrospective	–	Periodontally healthy	164	455	96.5%	114
			Periodontally diseased	311	1,171	94.8%	
García-Bellosta et al[46]	Retrospective	–	Periodontally healthy	–	283	97.8%	132
			Periodontitis	–	697	95.6%	
Matarasso et al[47]	Retrospective	Brånemark	Periodontally healthy	40	40	95%	120
		TPS	Periodontally diseased	40	40	90%	
Aglietta et al[48]	Retrospective	Brånemark	Periodontally healthy	20	20	95%	120
		TPS	Periodontally diseased	20	20	85%	
Levin et al[49]	Prospective	–	Periodontally healthy	283	747	96.9%	144
			Moderate chronic periodontitis	149	447	96.6%	
			Severe chronic periodontitis	285	1,065	94.8%	
Swierkot et al[50]	Prospective	Brånemark	Periodontally healthy	18	30	100%	192
			Aggressive periodontitis	35	149	96%	
Jiang et al[51]	Prospective	–	Periodontally healthy	30	127	97.6%	24
			Chronic periodontitis	30	149	95.97%	

–, not reported; TPS, titanium plasma sprayed.
*Data from Wen et al.[38]

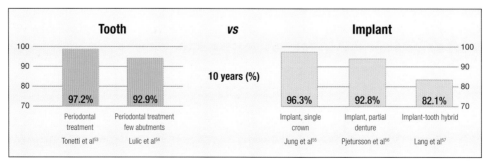

Fig 6-10 / Survival rates of teeth and implants.[52]

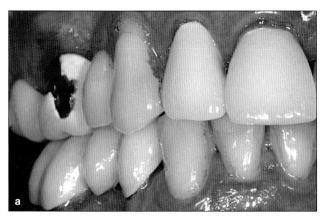 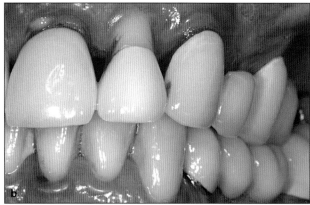

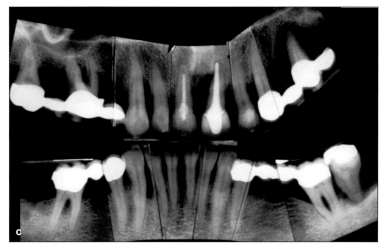

115

Fig 6-11 / *(a and b)* This 52-year-old patient has aggressive periodontitis with microbiologic testing positive for *A actinomycetemcomitans*, restorative deficiencies, and extremely increased mobility with significant impairment of chewing comfort and esthetics. *(c)* Pretreatment radiographs show substantial periodontal bone resorption with multiple vertical fractures, furcation involvement at the both mandibular right first molars and the mandibular left second molar, and an incomplete root filling at the maxillary right central incisor with periapical bone disintegration. This disintegration is even more extensive at the maxillary left second premolar and mandibular left third molar. ⟶

an adequate dimension of keratinized tissue seems to be essential for sustained stability of the peri-implant/restoration interface.[67-78]

Conclusion

In summary, the decision of tooth versus implant must consider the following influencing factors:

- The prognosis of the individual tooth rated according to the traffic light principle
- Critical evaluation of the extended local findings
- Multifactorial influence due to existing treatment situation (eg, endodontic)
- Decision between restorative or nonrestorative therapy
- Integration of the patient and practice level

- Enough time for the definitive evaluation (using provisional restorations)
- Critical evaluation of molars in particular

If the decision is made in favor of implants, the following steps should be taken:

- A chronologic, spatial, and restorative strategy should be established.
- The principles of periodontal plastic surgery should be carefully applied when placing and especially when exposing implants.
- A sufficient volume of keratinized mucosa should be created to ensure long-term esthetic results with implant treatment.

The case study presented in Fig 6-11 illustrates periodontally-oriented decision making for a complex preoperative situation.[79]

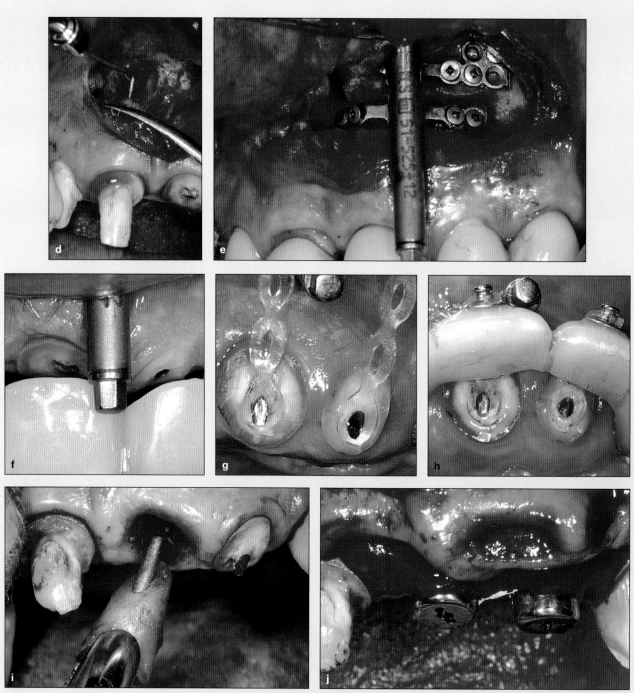

Fig 6-11 *cont.* / *(d and e)* Simultaneous retrograde endosurgical revision at the maxillary right central incisor and a horizontal as well as a vertical osteotomy to initiate distraction with the decapitated root segments of the maxillary left incisors (TRACK distractor, KLS Martin). *(f to h)* Vertical distraction of the maxillary left incisors under the shortened pontic area of the provisional restoration; after completion of vertical distraction, the horizontal position is corrected buccally by elastics mounted on root posts. *(i and j)* Four months after completion of distraction, implants are immediately placed in the sites of the maxillary left incisors with a palatal incision for papilla preservation from the right central incisor to the left canine.

→

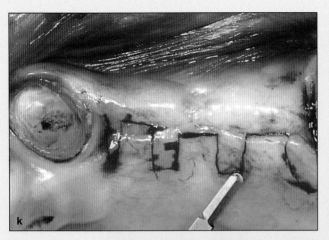
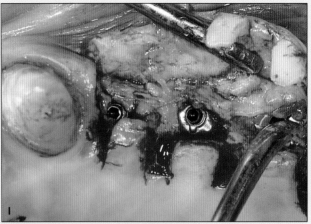

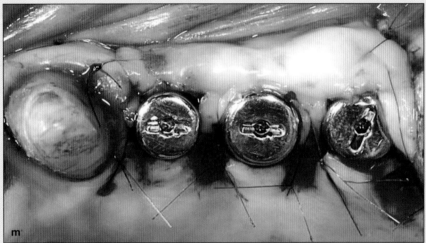

117

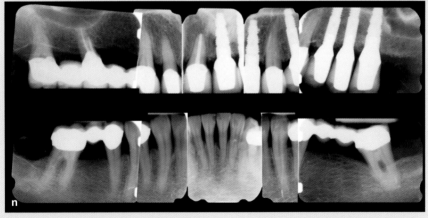

Fig 6-11 *cont.* / *(k)* Exposure of implants from the maxillary left first premolar to first molar by the meander method.[79] Note the displacement of keratinized mucosa for simultaneous widening of the relevant structures buccally and interproximally to the implants and the canine. *(l and m)* Raising a split-thickness flap by the meander method to expose the implants and apical displacement of keratinized mucosa to improve the buccal and interproximal peri-implant situation. *(n)* Radiographs 10 years after completion of the treatment. Note results after GTR of the vertical periodontal defects and furcations at the mandibular left second and right first molars, the root amputation of the maxillary right first molar, the condition after distraction at the region of the maxillary left canines, bone augmentation (onlay graft and sinus elevation at the region of the left premolars and first molar), and appropriate implant restoration.

⟶

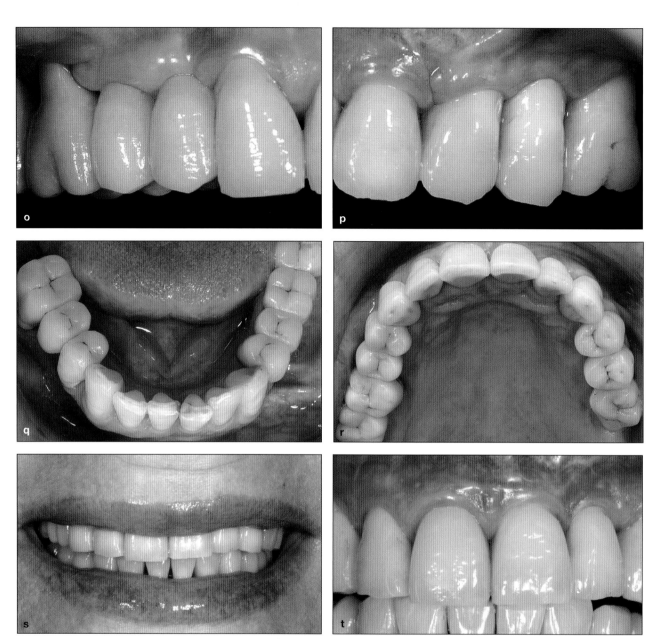

Fig 6-11 *cont.* / *(o to t)* Clinical situation 10 years after completion of the treatment. (Surgery and prosthodontics performed by G. Körner; laboratory work performed by K. Müterthies.)

References

1. Dhingra K. Oral rehabilitation considerations for partially edentulous periodontal patients. J Prosthodont 2012;21:494–513.
2. Strietzel FP, Reichart PA. Oral rehabilitation using Camlog screw-cylinder implants with a particle-blasted and acid-etched microstructured surface. Results from a prospective study with a special consideration of short implants. Clin Oral Implants Res 2007;18:591–600.
3. Sørensen LT. Wound healing and infection in surgery. The clinical impact of smoking and smoking cessation: A systematic review and meta-analysis. Arch Surg 2012;147:373–383.
4. Happe A, Körner G, Nolte A. The keyhole access expansion technique for flapless implant stage-two surgery: Technical note. Int J Periodontics Restorative Dent 2010;30:97–101.
5. Hirschfeld L, Wasserman B. A long-term survey of tooth loss in 600 treated periodontal patients. J Periodontol 1978;49:225–237.
6. McFall WT Jr. Tooth loss in 100 treated patients with periodontal disease. A long-term study. J Periodontol 1982;53:539–549.
7. Goldman MC, Ross IF, Goteiner D. Effect of periodontal therapy on patients maintained for 15 years or longer. A retrospective study. J Periodontol 1986;57:347–353.
8. Beikler T, Flemmig TF. Implantat versus Zahnerhalt aus parodontologischer Sicht. Implantologie 2006;14:9–18.

9. McGuire MK. Prognosis versus actual outcome: A long-term survey of 100 treated periodontal patients under maintenance care. J Periodontol 1991;62:51–58.

10. McGuire MK, Nunn ME. Prognosis versus actual outcome. III: The effectiveness of clinical parameters in accurately predicting tooth survival. J Periodontol 1996;67:666–674.

11. Ramseier CA, Lang NP. Die Parodontalbetreuung. Ein Lernprogramm zur Qualitätssicherung in der Parodontologie (CD-Rom). Berlin: Quintessence, 2007.

12. Vermylen K, De Quincey GN, Wolffe GN, van 't Hof MA, Renggli HH. Root proximity as a risk marker for periodontol disease: A case-control study. J Clin Periodontol 2005;32:260–265.

13. Svärdström G, Wennström JL. Periodontal treatment decisions for molars: An analysis of influencing factors and long-term outcome. J Periodontol 2000;71:579–585.

14. Basten CH, Ammons WF Jr, Persson R. Long-term evaluation of root-resected molars: A retrospective study. Int J Periodontics Restorative Dent 1996;16:206–219.

15. Carnevale G, Pontoriero R, di Febo G. Long-term effects of root-resective therapy in furcation-involved molars. A 10-year longitudinal study. J Clin Periodontol 1998;25:209–214.

16. Langer B, Stein SD, Wagenberg B. An evaluation of root resections. A ten-year study. J Periodontol 1981;52:719–722.

17. Bühler H. Evaluation of root-resected teeth. Results after 10 years. J Periodontol 1998;59:805–810.

18. Muzzi L, Nieri M, Cattabriga M, Rotundo R, Cairo F, Pini Prato GP. The potential prognostic value of some periodontal factors for tooth loss: A retrospective multilevel analysis on periodontal patients treated and maintained over 10 years. J Periodontol 2006;77:2084–2089.

19. Nieri N, Muzzi L, Cattabriga M, Rotundo R, Cairo F, Pini Prato GP. The prognostic value of several periodontal factors measured as radiographic bone level variation: A 10-year retrospective multilevel analysis of treated and maintained periodontal patients. J Periodontol 2002;73:1485–1493.

20. Stavropoulos A, Karring T. Long-term stability of periodontal conditions achieved following guided tissue regeneration with bioresorbable membranes: Case series results after 6-7 years. J Periodontol 2004;31:939–944.

21. Sculean A, Kiss A, Miliauskaite A, Schwarz F, Arweiler NB, Hannig M. Ten-year results following treatment of intra-bony defects with enamel matrix proteins and guided tissue regeneration. J Clin Periodontol 2008;35:817–824.

22. Araújo MG, Sukekava F, Wennström JL, Lindhe J. Ridge alterations following implant placement in fresh extraction sockets: An experimental study in the dog. J Clin Periodontol 2005;32:645–652.

23. Araújo MG, Lindhe J. Dimensional ridge alterations following tooth extraction. An experimental study in the dog. J Clin Periodontol 2005;32:212–218.

24. Nevins M, Camelo M, De Paoli S, et al. A study of the fate of the buccal wall of extraction sockets of teeth with prominent roots. Int J Periodontics Restorative Dent 2006;26:19–29.

25. Cortellini B, Tonetti MS. Long-term survival following regenerative treatment of intrabony defects. J Periodontol 2004;75:672–678.

26. Cortellini P, Stalpers G, Mollo A, Tonetti MS. Periodontal regeneration versus extraction and prosthetic replacement of teeth severely compromised by attachment loss to the apex: 5-year results of an ongoing randomized clinical trial. J Clin Periodontol 2011;38:915–924.

27. Cortellini P, Tonetti MS. A minimally invasive surgical technique with an enamel matrix derivative in the regenerative treatment of intra-bony defects: A novel approach to limit morbidity. J Clin Periodontol 2007;34:87–93.

28. Misch CE, Al-Shammari KF, Wang HL. Creation of interimplant papillae through a split-finger technique. Implant Dent 2004;13:20–27.

29. Schropp L, Wenzel A, Kostopoulos L, Karring T. Bone healing and soft tissue contour changes following single-tooth extraction. A clinical and radiographic 12-month prospective study. Int J Periodontics Restorative Dent 2003;23:313–323.

30. Tan WL, Wong TL, Wong MC, Lang NP. A systematic review of post-extractional alveolar hard and soft tissue dimensional changes in humans. Clin Oral Implants Res 2012;23(suppl 5):1–21.

31. Fiorellini JP, Nevins ML. Localized ridge augmentation/preservation. A systematic review. Ann Periodontol 2003;8:321–327.

32. Aghaloo TL, Moy PK. Which hard tissue augmentation techniques are the most successful in furnishing support for implant placement? J Oral Maxillofac Implants 2007:22(suppl):49–70.

33. Matuliene G, Studer R, Lang NP, et al. Significance of periodontal risk assessment in the recurrence of periodontitis and tooth loss. J Clin Periodontol 2010;37:191–199.

34. Schou S, Holmstrup P, Worthington HV, Esposito M. Outcome of implant therapy in patients with previous tooth loss due to periodontitis. Clin Oral Implants Res 2006;17(suppl 2):104–123.

35. Karoussis IK, Müller S, Salvi GE, Heitz-Mayfield LJA, Brägger U, Lang NP. Association between periodontal and peri-implant conditions: A 10-year prospective study. Clin Oral Implants Res 2004;15:1–7.

36. Lindquist LW, Carlsson GE, Jemt T. Association between marginal bone loss around osseointegrated mandibular implants and smoking habits: A 10-year follow-up study. J Dent Res 1997;76:1667–1674.

37. Karoussis IK, Kotsovilis S, Fourmousis I. A comprehensive and critical review of dental implant prognosis in periodontally compromised partially edentulous patients. Clin Oral Implants Res 2007;18:669–679.

38. Wen X, Liu R, Li G, et al. History of periodontitis as a risk factor for long-term survival of dental implants: A meta-analysis. Int J Oral Maxillofac Implants 2014;29:1271–1280.

39. Hardt CR, Gröndahl K, Lekholm U, et al. Outcome of implant therapy in relation to experienced loss of periodontal bone support: A retrospective 5-year study. Clin Oral Implants Res 2002;13:488–494.

40. Karoussis IK, Salvi GE, Heitz-Mayfield LJ, et al. Long-term implant prognosis in patients with and without a history of chronic periodontitis: A 10-year prospective cohort study of the ITI Dental Implant System. Clin Oral Implants Res 2003;14:329–339.

41. Evian CI, Emling R, Rosenberg ES, et al. Retrospective analysis of implant survival and the influence of periodontal disease and immediate placement on long-term results. Int J Oral Maxillofac Implants 2004;19:393–398.

42. Mengel R, Flores-de-Jacoby L. Implants in patients treated for generalized aggressive and chronic periodontitis: A 3-year prospective longitudinal study. J Periodontol 2005;76:534–543.

43. De Boever AL, Quirynen M, Coucke W, et al. Clinical and radiographic study of implant treatment outcome in periodontally susceptible and non-susceptible patients: A prospective long-term study. Clin Oral Implants Res 2009;20:1341–1350.

44. Roccuzzo M, De Angelis N, Bonino L, et al. Ten-year results of a three-arm prospective cohort study on implants in periodontally compromised patients. Part 1: Implant loss and radiographic bone loss. Clin Oral Implants Res 2010;21:490–496.

45. Anner R, Grossmann Y, Anner Y, et al. Smoking, diabetes mellitus, periodontitis, and supportive periodontal treatment as factors associated with dental implant survival: A long-term retrospective evaluation of patients followed for up to 10 years. Implant Dent 2010;19:57-64.

119

46. García-Bellosta S, Bravo M, Subirá C, Echeverría JJ. Retrospective study of the long-term survival of 980 implants placed in a periodontal practice. Int J Oral Maxillofac Implants 2010;25:613–619.

47. Matarasso S, Rasperini G, Iorio Siciliano V, et al. A 10-year retrospective analysis of radiographic bone-level changes of implants supporting single-unit crowns in periodontally compromised vs. periodontally healthy patients. Clin Oral Implants Res 2010;21:898–903.

48. Aglietta M, Siciliano VI, Rasperini G, et al. A 10-year retrospective analysis of marginal bone-level changes around implants in periodontally healthy and periodontally compromised tobacco smokers. Clin Oral Implants Res 2011;22:47–53.

49. Levin L, Ofec R, Grossmann Y, et al. Periodontal disease as a risk for dental implant failure over time: A long-term historical cohort study. J Clin Periodontol 2011;38:732–737.

50. Swierkot K, Lottholz P, Flores-de-Jacoby L, et al. Mucositis, periimplantitis, implant success, and survival of implants in patients with treated generalized aggressive periodontitis: 3- to 16-year results of a prospective long-term cohort study. J Periodontol 2012;83:1213–1225.

51. Jiang BQ, Lan J, Huang HY, et al. A clinical study on the effectiveness of implant supported dental restoration in patients with chronic periodontal diseases. Int J Oral Maxillofac Surg 2013;42:256–259.

52. Holm-Pedersen P, Lang NP, Müller F. What are the longevities of teeth and oral implants? Clin Oral Implants Res 2007;18(suppl 3):15–19.

53. Tonetti MS, Lang NP, Cortellini P, et al. Enamel matrix proteins in the regenerative therapy of deep intrabony defects. J Clin Periodontol 2002;29:317–325.

54. Lulic M, Brägger U, Lang NP, Zwahlen M, Salvi GE. Ante's (1962) law revisited: A systematic review on survival rates and complications of fixed dental prostheses (FDPs) on severely reduced periodontal tissue support. Clin Oral Implants Res 2007;18(suppl 3):63–72.

55. Jung BA, Wehrbein H, Hopfenmüller W, et al. Early loading of palatal implants (ortho-type II) a prospective multicenter randomized controlled clinical trial. Trials 2007;8:24.

56. Pjetursson BE, Tan K, Lang NP, Brägger U, Egger M, Zwahlen M. A systematic review of the survival and complication rates of fixed partial dentures (FPDs) after an observation period of at least 5 years. Clin Oral Implants Res 2004;15:667–676.

57. Lang NP, Pjetursson BE, Tan K, Brägger U, Egger M, Zwahlen M. A systematic review of the survival and complication rates of fixed partial dentures (FPDs) after an observation period of at least 5 years. II. Combined tooth-implant-supported FPDs. Clin Oral Implants Res 2004;15:643–653.

58. Ante IH. The fundamental principles of abutments. Mich State Dent Soc Bull 1926;8:14–23.

59. Pjetursson BE, Brägger U, Lang NP, Zwahlen M. Comparison of survival and complication rates of tooth-supported fixed dental prostheses (FDPs) and implant-supported FDPs and single crowns (SCs). Clin Oral Implants Res 2007;18(suppl 3):97–113.

60. Jung RE, Pjetursson BE, Glauser R, Zembic A, Zwahlen M, Lang NP. A systematic review of the 5-year survival and complication rates of implant-supported single crowns. Clin Oral Implants Res 2008;19:119–130.

61. Choquet V, Hermans M, Adriaenssens P, Daelemans P, Tarnow D, Malevez C. Clinical and radiographic evaluation of the papilla level adjacent to single-tooth dental implants. A retrospective study in the maxillary anterior region. J Periodontol 2001:72:1364–1371.

62. Tarnow D, Cho S, Wallace SS. The effect of inter-implant distance on the height of inter-implant bone crest. J Periodontol 2000;71:546–549.

63. Garber DA, Salama MA, Salama H. Immediate total tooth replacement. Compend Contin Educ Dent 2001;22:210–218.

64. Berglundh T, Lindhe J. Dimension of the periimplant mucosa. Biological width revisited. J Clin Periodontol 1996;23:971–973.

65. Esposito M, Grusovin MG, Maghaireh H, Coulthard P, Worthington HV. Interventions for replacing missing teeth: Management of soft tissues for dental implants. Cochrane Database Syst Rev 2007;18:CD006697.

66. Esposito M, Maghaireh H, Grusovin MG, Ziounas I, Worthington HV. Soft tissue management for dental implants: What are the most effective techniques? A Cochrane systematic review. Eur J Oral Implantol 2012;5:221–238.

67. Zadeh HH, Daftary F. Minimally invasive surgery: An alternative approach for periodontal and implant reconstruction. J Calif Dent Assoc 2004;32:1022–1030.

68. Bengazi F, Wennström JL, Lekholm U. Recession of the soft tissue margin at oral implants. A 2-year longitudinal prospective study. Clin Oral Implants Res 1996;7:303–310.

69. Warrer K, Buser D, Lang NP, Karring T. Plaque-induced periimplantitis in the presence or absence of keratinized mucosa. An experimental study in monkeys. Clin Oral Implants Res 1995;6:131–138.

70. Rompen E, Domken O, Degidi M, Pontes AE, Piattelli A. The effect of material characteristics, of surface topography and of implant components and connections on soft tissue integration: A literature review. Clin Oral Implants Res 2006;17(suppl 2):55–67.

71. Chung DM, Oh TJ, Shotwell JL, Misch CE, Wang HL. Significance of keratinized mucosa in maintenance of dental implants with different surfaces. J Periodontol 2006;77:1410–1420.

72. Zigdon H, Machtei EE. The dimensions of keratinized mucosa around implants affect clinical and immunological parameters. Clin Oral Implants Res 2008;19:387–392.

73. Bouri A Jr, Bissada N, Al-Zahrani MS, Faddoul F, Nouneh I. Width of keratinized gingiva and the health status of the supporting tissues around dental implants. Int J Maxillofac Implants 2008;23:323–326.

74. Kim BS, Kim YK, Yun PY, et al. Evaluation of peri-implant tissue response according to the presence of keratinized mucosa. Oral Surg Oral Med Oral Pathol Oral Radiol Endod 2009;107(3):e24–e28.

75. Adibrad M, Shahabuei M, Sahabi M. Significance of the width of keratinized mucosa on the health status of the supporting tissue around implants supporting overdentures. J Oral Implantol 2009;35:232–237.

76. Schrott AR, Jimenez M, Hwang JW, Fiorellini J, Weber HP. Five-year evaluation of the influence of keratinized mucosa on peri-implant soft-tissue health and stability around implants supporting full-arch mandibular fixed prostheses. Clin Oral Implants Res 2009;20:1170–1177.

77. Boynueğri D, Nemli SK, Kasko YA. Significance of keratinized mucosa around dental implants: A prospective comparative study. Clin Oral Implants Res 2013;24:928–933.

78. Burkhardt R, Joss A, Lang NP. Soft tissue dehiscence coverage around endosseous implants: A prospective cohort study. Clin Oral Implants Res 2008;19:451–457.

79. Wachtel H, Schlee M, Körner G. ZMK - Live Sonderedition – DGP Frühjahrstagung. Berlin: Quintessence, 2004.

120

"Learn the rules like a pro so you can break them like an artist."

PABLO PICASSO

7

Adjacent Implants

/ Tomohiro Ishikawa, Arndt Happe

One of the greatest challenges in dental implantology is the successful replacement of two adjacent missing teeth in the anterior dentition.[1] Owing to the specific biologic circumstances between adjacent implants, the interimplant papilla does not form correctly in most cases (see chapter 1). This is particularly problematic if the teeth are missing on one side while the contralateral natural papilla is fully developed. A study by Kokich et al[2] showed that patients are more likely to tolerate symmetric changes to the soft tissue height than asymmetric changes. Most patients will view a noticeably asymmetric soft tissue contour as a failure.[2]

However, the preservation and regeneration of hard and soft tissues is only a first step toward creating the conditions for papillae to be established that will both appear esthetic and remain stable in the long term. A natural-looking pink and white esthetic depends on several variables that need to be respected and monitored.

This chapter explores theoretical considerations and possible treatment options for rehabilitation after loss of two adjacent teeth in the esthetic zone. When facing this clinical situation, both biologic and clinical aspects must be taken into consideration.

Biologic Aspects

Size of papilla

When placing directly adjacent implants, the available interimplant space is going to be limited. The small amount of space for natural tissue leads to a reduced blood supply from the narrow bony base and an anatomical situation around implants that is completely different from that around natural teeth. For instance, supracrestal fibers inserting in the cementum are absent, and there is no periodontal space with a periodontal ligament and blood vessels to guarantee an adequate blood supply. Without a sufficient blood supply, the papilla will start to shrink.

Salama et al[3] published data clearly showing that the papilla to be expected between adjacent implants is markedly smaller than between natural teeth (see Table 1-1 in chapter 1). In light of this publication, Tarnow et al[4] conducted a study demonstrating that the average expected papilla height between adjacent implants is 3.4 mm.

Crestal bone resorption due to postrestorative bone remodeling

As soon as the implant is exposed and the restoration is functioning, the inflammatory cell infiltrate in the microgap between implant and abutment leads to resorption of the peri-implant bony ridge, a phenomenon known as *postrestorative bone remodeling*. It is more pronounced at horizontal non-platform-switched connections between implant and abutment than at connections with platform switching (eg, conical connections; see chapter 11).

Because this physiologic bone remodeling occurs on both sides of the interimplant bony ridge, it is vital to maintain an adequate distance between the two adjacent implants. If the distance is too small (ie, < 3 mm), resorptions on both sides will overlap and lead to loss of the original or regenerated interimplant crestal height. Resorption of the interimplant bony ridge therefore depends on the distance between the adjacent implants: The larger the distance, the less pronounced the resorption will be. In an animal study, Scarano et al[5] showed that, from the histology viewpoint, a larger interimplant distance (ie, up to 5 mm) can result in better preservation of the papillae (Table 7-1). All the implants healed with coverage, and the implant shoulders (microgaps) were placed at the height of the alveolar ridge. Admittedly, a distance of 5 mm between two implants is an esthetic impossibility under clinical conditions. The study by Tarnow et al[4] (analyzing

Table 7-1 Correlation between the interimplant distance and the condition of the papilla*

Interimplant distance (mm)	Vertical bone loss (mm)
2	1.98
3	1.78
4	1.01
5	0.23

*Data from Scarano et al.[5]

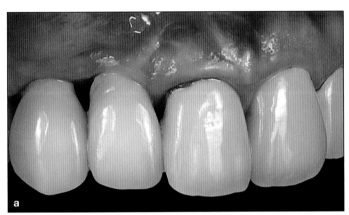 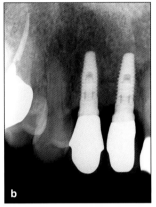

Fig 7-1 / *(a and b)* This case was an esthetic failure because the distance between the two implants was too small. Before implant placement, augmentation was performed with autogenous bone grafts. The patient reported that the soft tissue around the implants had gradually receded over a period of several years. The radiograph does show an interimplant distance of 3 mm, but the bony ridge lies 1 mm apical to the implant platforms. The case illustrates a common esthetic problem with adjacent implants: The interimplant papilla recedes, causing a nonesthetic result with a prominent black triangle. Both implants appear well osseointegrated on the radiograph, but remodeling of the bone is occurring in the ridge area around the implant-abutment connection. The result is typical of adjacent implants if steps are not taken to prevent tissue loss.[6]

123

radiographs) defined the guide value of 3 mm, which is accepted as the standard minimum interimplant distance.

The two observations made previously about soft tissue and bone lead to the conclusion that a flat papilla over a low bony ridge is found between two implants if the interimplant distance is too small, and this will impair the esthetic outcome (Fig 7-1).[6] If two implants are placed directly adjacent to each other, tissue loss is unavoidable. This is why therapeutic approaches to adjacent implants need to involve special techniques that support restoration of a natural-looking papilla.

Clinical Aspects

Clinically speaking, the top priority is to try and fulfill the patient's esthetic wishes and expectations but also to inform the patient of the real biologic limitations.

Bilateral tooth loss

As previously mentioned, patients tend to tolerate symmetric changes to the soft tissue height more than asymmetric changes. If there are no natural teeth on the contralateral side, an esthetic soft tissue contour can be created with better predictability even in the case of adjacent implants.

Clinical case

An elderly patient presented with an edentulous maxilla containing intraosseous and extraosseous defects (Fig 7-2a). The implants were placed with simultaneous guided bone regeneration (GBR). Single-tooth implants were used for tooth-by-tooth replacement, and papillae were established in all of the reconstructed interproximal areas (Fig 7-2b). The size of the papillae varies depending on the interimplant distance, the submucosal abutment contour, and the available volume of soft tissue. The regenerated

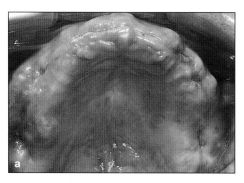
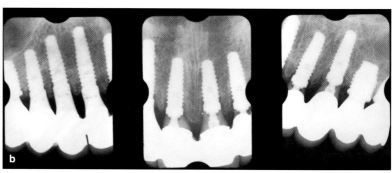
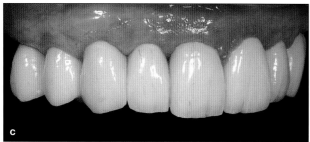
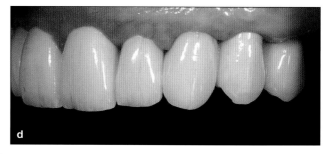
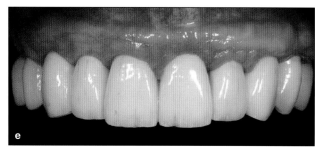

Fig 7-2 / *(a)* Edentulous maxilla in an elderly patient. *(b)* Radiographs after completion of treatment. *(c to e)* Intraoral views of the end result. (Laboratory work performed by Y. Nishimura.)

124

papillae were stable 4 years after treatment. Despite the less-than-ideal papilla heights, the patient was satisfied because the symmetric, harmonious relative heights of all the papillae created an overall appearance that was esthetically pleasing (Figs 7-2c to 7-2e). The radiographs show the heights of the interimplant bone. The interimplant bone crest is determined by the interimplant distance, and the degree of remodeling is mainly determined by the difference in this distance.

Unilateral tooth loss

When there is unilateral tooth loss, it is far more difficult to produce an attractive soft tissue esthetic than it is with bilateral missing teeth. It proves particularly challenging if there is a prominent contralateral papilla to compare with the compromised interimplant papilla.

Clinical case

A 20-year-old patient with unilateral trauma-related tooth loss presented after an accident (Fig 7-3a). The radiographs show that nearly all the interdental bone septa were intact (Figs 7-3b to 7-3d). The maxillary left central incisor was classified as worth preserving despite the unavoidable root canal treatment. Unfortunately, the right lateral incisor together with its vestibular bony wall had been lost, and the fracture line of the horizontal fracture of the right central incisor extended 2 mm subcrestally. It was therefore decided to replace both right incisors with implants. After completion of the treatment, the interimplant papilla between the implant crowns did not completely match the corresponding contralateral papilla, but the patient was very satisfied with the result despite the asymmetric papillae (Fig 7-3e). The radiograph reveals slight resorption of the interimplant bone (Fig 7-3f).

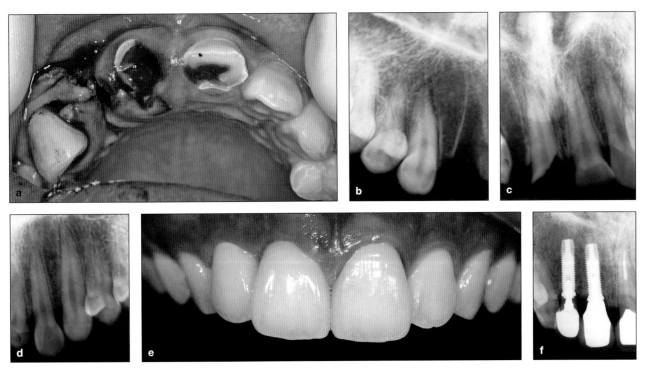

Fig 7-3 / *(a)* Occlusal view at initial visit. *(b to d)* The radiographs show that nearly all of the interdental bone septa were intact. *(e)* The papilla between the implant crowns does not fully match the corresponding contralateral papilla. *(f)* Radiograph shows slight resorption. (Laboratory work performed by K. Nakajima.)

Interimplant distance

The minimum distance required between two implants is 3 mm. It is always advisable to use the largest possible interimplant distance because this parameter has a direct impact on the potential height of the interimplant papilla.[7,8] The papillae between the central and lateral incisors as well as the lateral incisors and canines in both arches can be compared with their contralateral papillae. This means that there is a natural comparative size that must be achieved for a balanced esthetic result.

Limited mesiodistal space and a natural papilla on the contralateral side, which allows for comparison, create a difficult esthetic situation prior to treatment. If the interimplant distance is small, it is usually only possible to create small papillae. If there is sufficient space, however, the interimplant bony ridge can normally be preserved, and a natural-looking interimplant papilla can be established.

Clinical case with 3-mm interimplant distance

A 37-year-old patient presented after traumatic tooth loss (Fig 7-4a). Both central incisors with their vestibular bony

wall had been lost. Two implants were placed without the appropriate measures being taken to reduce postrestorative bone remodeling. As a result of bone remodeling processes in the area of the abutment-implant interface, the interimplant bone resorbed, and the interdental papilla in this area appeared distinctly reduced and visibly flatter than the papillae between implants and adjacent natural teeth. If the papilla is smaller between the central incisors, it is often still esthetically acceptable because the bilateral symmetry is not disturbed (Figs 7-4b and 7-4c).

Clinical case with 4-mm interimplant distance

A 55-year-old patient had lost both maxillary central incisors a few years before treatment. Although the ridge was already very narrow, there was no vertical deficit. The implants were placed in the ideal prosthetic position, and the alveolar ridge was augmented horizontally with GBR (Figs 7-5a and 7-5b). The horizontal bone augmentation laid the foundation for an esthetic papilla. After successful osseointegration, it was possible to develop an interimplant papilla to a height that was comparable with the interdental papillae of the adjacent natural teeth (Fig

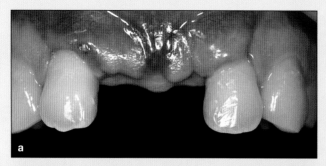

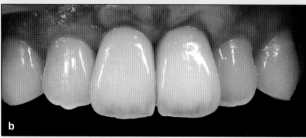

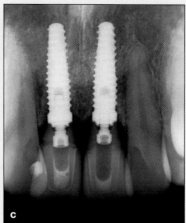

Fig 7-4 / *(a)* Preoperative view at first visit. *(b)* Bilateral symmetry can compensate for an undersized papilla. *(c)* Radiograph 6 years after treatment. The interimplant bony ridge has lost height because of the onset of postoperative bone remodeling. (Laboratory work performed by K. Nakajima.)

126

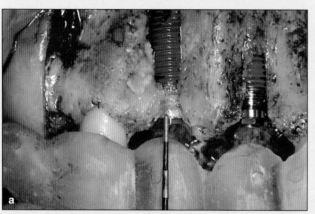

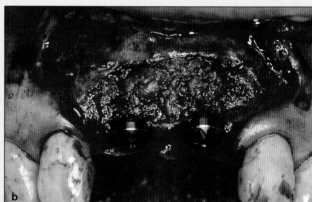

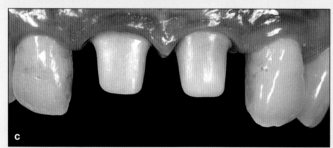

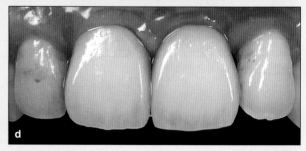

Fig 7-5 / *(a)* Two implants in situ in the region of the maxillary central incisors. Despite the narrowness of the ridge, its height remained preserved. *(b)* The implants were placed in the ideal prosthetic position. The missing vestibular tissue was regenerated by means of GBR. The horizontal bone augmentation laid the foundation for an esthetic papilla. *(c)* It was possible to develop the interimplant papilla up to a height that was comparable with the interdental papillae of the adjacent natural teeth. *(d and e)* The interimplant distance of 4 mm resulted in stability of the peri-implant soft tissue 10 years after the treatment. (Laboratory work performed by K. Nakajima.)

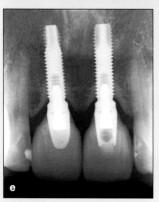

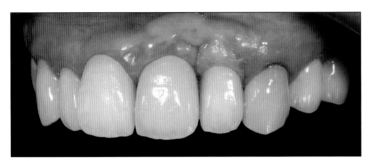

Fig 7-6 / Long-term papilla preservation: Although the space for the lateral incisor was narrower than normal, the papilla completely fills the interimplant space 5 years after treatment. (Laboratory work performed by K. Nakajima.)

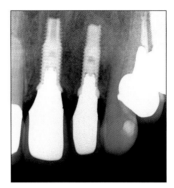

Fig 7-7 / Platform switching allowed closer placement of the implants. Although the interimplant distance was less than 3 mm (2.8 mm), the bony ridge between the implants was preserved over 5 years.

7-5c). The tissue is still stable 10 years after restoation. An interimplant distance of 4 mm or more results in a bone level that is stable in the long term (Figs 7-5d and 7-5e). Even without preservation techniques, the alveolar ridge tends to maintain its original or augmented height at this interimplant distance.

Solutions

Prevent crestal bone remodeling

There are several possible ways to prevent crestal bone loss. Even if these methods are not fully understood scientifically, they should be used because they produce good results and have no drawbacks for patients.

Modify the implant-abutment connection

Inflammatory infiltrate in the microgap after implant exposure is one of the main causes of peri-implant bone resorption. Because this appears to be more common with non-platform-switched connections, the following modifications have been proposed:

* Platform switching[9–12] (Figs 7-6 and 7-7)
* Sealing with a conical connection[13]
* Single-piece implants[14,15]

Loosen the implant-abutment connection as infrequently as possible

Whenever a fixed abutment is detached or disconnected, this leads to some tissue loss. Therefore, the treatment plan should be organized to minimize abutment disconnection and reconnection.[16–18] The problem of abutment disconnection and reconnection can be entirely avoided if the abutment is connected definitively just once (one abutment–one time concept).[19] However, in this case the future crown margin at the abutment must be anticipated, bearing in mind the scalloped soft tissue contour and soft tissue recession. Excessive soft tissue recession can expose the margin, while too little recession causes a deep submucosal margin, which makes it difficult to remove excess cement. One solution to this problem can be to use shoulderless abutments with gradual conditioning of the soft tissue[20–23] (Fig 7-8). However, there is some doubt about sufficient removal of excess cement with this method, and there is no general scientific consensus in favor of the method.

Free-end pontic

Instead of two adjacent implants, one logical solution is a cantilever partial denture with a free-end pontic on one implant. The narrower the tooth space, the safer it is to use a free-end pontic instead of forcing two implants into a narrow space.[8,24]

127

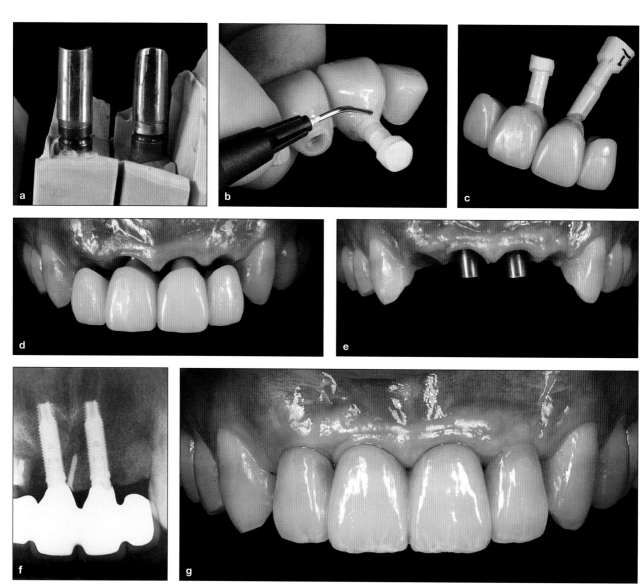

Fig 7-8 / (a) Shoulderless abutments have no defined border for the crown. (b and c) The subgingival contour is adapted with composite. If the abutment is not disconnected again, the clinician can adapt the prosthetic border and the subgingival contour to the analog of the borderless abutment. (d and e) The tissue was adapted week by week. If this type of abutment is used in cases with adjacent anterior implants, it is imperative to ensure an ideal implant position and parallelism between the two implants so that the abutments can be given enough length to stabilize the crown. (f) Radiograph of the situation. A root submergence technique was employed at the region of the right lateral incisor. (g) Result 2 years after placement. (Laboratory work performed by M. Hinoshita.)

Clinical case

A 20-year-old patient had lost both mandibular central incisors and the left canine together with the vestibular bone lamella 11 months before she first presented for treatment (Fig 7-9a). Typically, the distance between the mandibular lateral incisors is about 11 mm, but in this case the gap was much narrower than normal. From an esthetic viewpoint, the choice was between overlapping the central incisors over the lateral incisors or having very narrow central incisors. A GBR technique involving titanium mesh

and collagen membrane was chosen for reconstruction. In the region of the left central incisor, a narrow 3.25-mm implant was placed in the ideal three-dimensional (3D) position. In addition, hard and soft tissue augmentation was carried out. Because of the limited space, the teeth were reconstructed slightly unevenly (Fig 7-9b). Five years after the definitive restoration, the esthetic outcome is very good (Fig 7-9c). The radiograph 5 years after treatment clearly reveals the lack of space (Fig 7-9d). Bone remodeling led to ridge resorption despite platform switching. The lack of prosthetic space between the natural lateral incisors

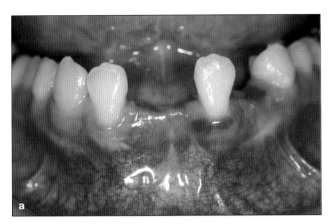
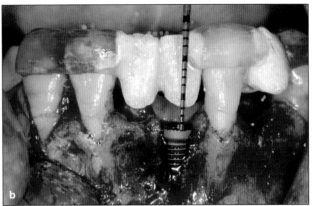
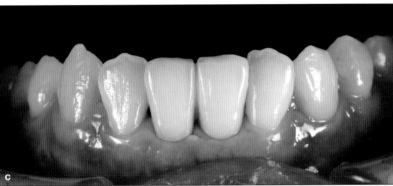
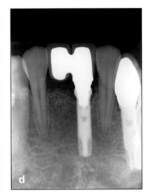

Fig 7-9 / *(a)* Very narrow gap and insufficient ridge width. *(b)* Ideal 3D position of the implant checked with a surgical template prior to bone augmentation. *(c and d)* Result 5 years after placement of the definitive restoration. (Laboratory work performed by K. Nakajima.)

would have prevented an esthetic papilla if two implants had been placed.[24,25]

Preservation of natural teeth

Intact roots or slightly destroyed roots with the periodontal ligament still present should be preserved as much as possible. To ensure long-term stability in these cases, enough ferrule length must be present or created (ie, 1.5 to 2.0 mm).[14,26] The required length can be created by surgical extrusion or by orthodontic extrusion and crown lengthening (see Fig 7-10).

To avoid damage to the periodontal ligament, the extraction for surgical extrusion should be performed very gently. When this method is used, the root should be placed back in its socket within 18 minutes to maintain the vitality of the periodontal ligament. Generally, a transplanted tooth is stabilized for 1 to 2 months, but the time required for stabilization also depends on the congruence of root and socket.[27–32]

In the long term and from the esthetic perspective, the use of natural abutment teeth should be preferred

to an implant solution, whenever possible, in view of the unavoidable craniofacial growth and esthetic limitations that will affect any reconstruction involving two adjacent implants.[33]

Clinical case

A 52-year-old patient presented with a vertical root fracture of the maxillary left lateral incisor and subgingival caries at the left canine (Figs 7-10a and 7-10b). The radiograph shows the minimal residual tooth substance (Fig 7-10c). Bone and soft tissue architecture were still almost intact. Preserving bone, soft tissues, and teeth should be a priority when the treatment is chosen. After extraction of the lateral incisor, the surfaces of the removed fragments were carefully assessed (Figs 7-10d and 7-10e), and the tooth fragment was discarded. The rest of the root was rotated 180 degrees and replanted in the socket of the lateral incisor (Fig 7-10f). This made it possible to establish a better clinical crown length, which allowed for a ferrule more than 2 mm wide, as required for a long-term crown restoration. Five months later, the root was fitted with a provisional restoration that served as anchorage for the

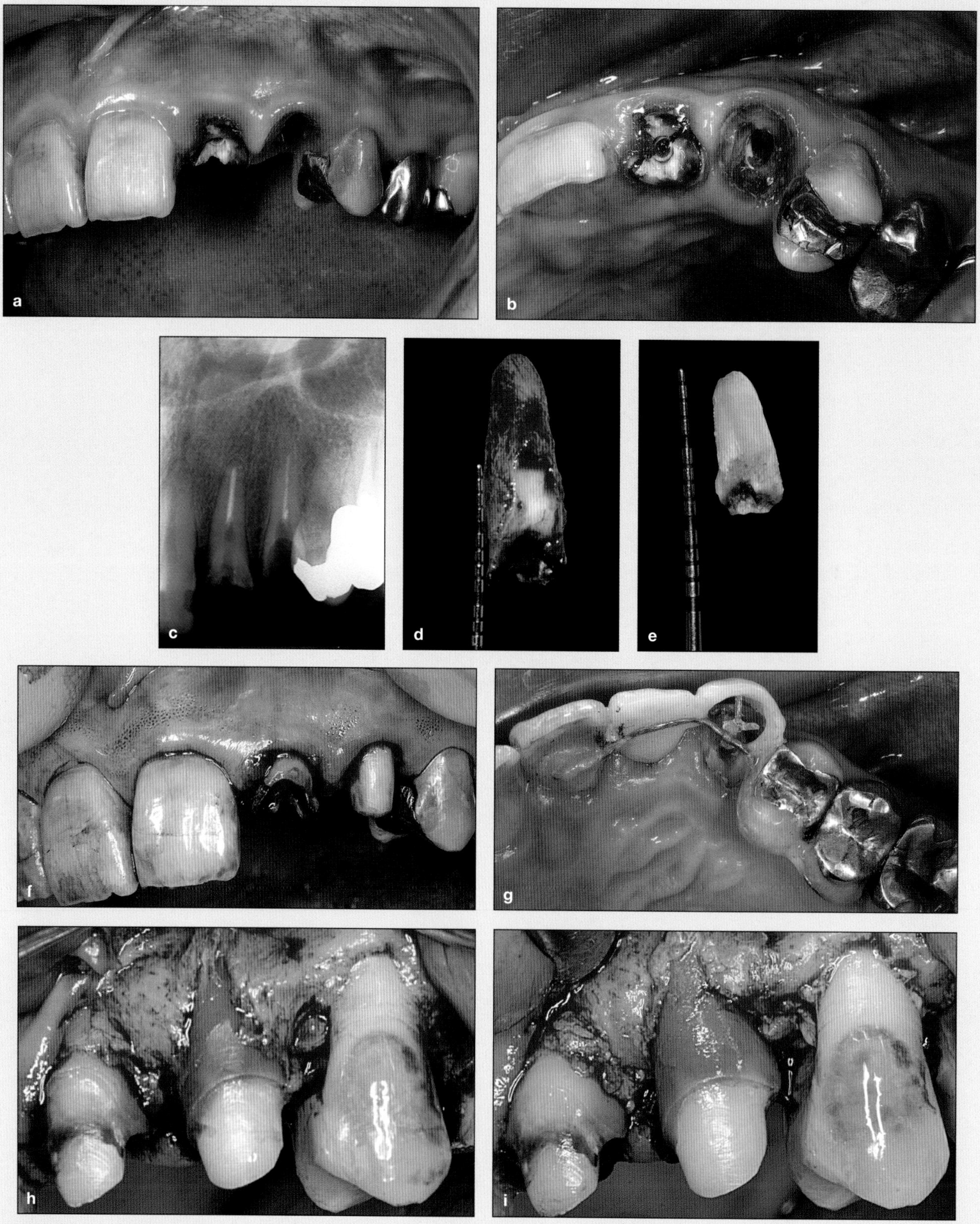

Fig 7-10 / *(a and b)* Intraoral situation at the first visit. *(c)* Radiograph of the preoperative situation. *(d and e)* After extraction of the left lateral incisor, the surfaces of the removed fragments were carefully assessed. *(f)* The replanted tooth roots of the lateral incisor and canine. *(g)* The root remnant of the canine was extruded using a simple appliance. *(h and i)* The situations before and after crown lengthening. ⟶

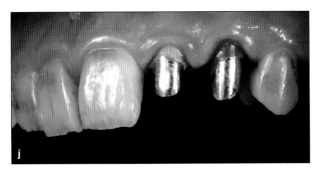

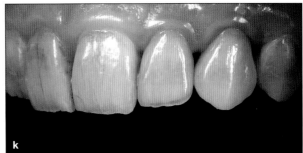

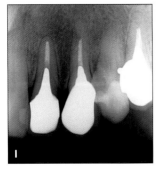

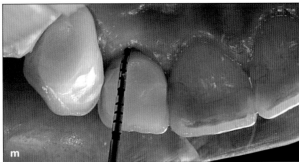

Fig 7-10 *cont.* / *(j)* Condition 1 year after crown lengthening. *(k)* Definitive restoration with zirconia crowns. *(l)* The radiograph after treatment shows the favorable root-crown relationship of the re-planted roots. *(m)* Over the old fracture surface, the sulcus depth was 4 mm with no bleeding on probing. (Laboratory work performed by M. Hinoshita.)

extrusion of the root of the canine with the aid of a simple appliance (Fig 7-10g). The canine was extruded by 3 mm over a period of 3 months. After the 3-month stabilization phase, surgical crown lengthening was performed (Figs 7-10h and 7-10i). One year after the crown lengthening, the condition of the abutment teeth was not ideal but much better than the pretreatment condition (Fig 7-10j). Zirconia crowns were cemented as the definitive restorations. A natural, healthy appearance was created with the definitive restorations (Figs 7-10k and 7-10l). This outcome is relatively easy to achieve with natural teeth, but it is very difficult with two adjacent implants.

The sulcus depth in the area of the fracture line was 4 mm at the lateral incisor. The deep sulcus formed because the replanted tooth had also lost the attachment apparatus in this area with the removed tooth fragment. Despite the palatal probing depth of 4 mm, no bleeding on probing was observed (Fig 7-10m).

Immediate implant placement with soft tissue augmentation

Immediate implant placement is more likely to result in a larger interimplant papilla than delayed implant placement.[34] Even if bone and soft tissues are intact, soft tissue augmentation is advisable to achieve an esthetic outcome

that is stable in the long term. It is probable that the soft tissue volume and the papilla size around implants are influenced by the quality and quantity of the grafted soft tissue itself[24,25,27–38] (see Fig 4-9 in chapter 4).

Clinical case

Figure 7-11 demonstrates such a typical clinical case. The maxillary central incisors could not be preserved because of endodontic problems. Because the buccal lamella was preserved, it was possible to perform immediate implant placement with a simultaneous connective tissue graft (CTG). To support the soft tissues, a bonded fixed partial denture served as a provisional restoration during the incorporation period. The situation 3 months after immediate implant placement shows favorable peri-implant soft tissue conditions with preserved interdental papilla (see Fig 7-11g). The patient was sent back to the referring dentist for prosthodontic treatment.

Socket shield technique (partial extraction therapy)

If a proximal aspect of a failing adjacent tooth is intact, the tooth fragment has tremendous potential for interproximal tissue preservation and can contribute to esthetic results,

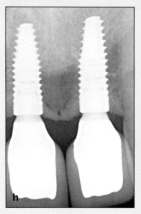

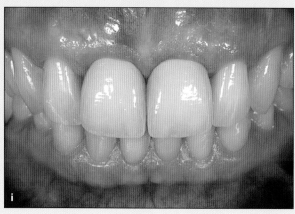

Fig 7-11 / *(a and b)* Condition before implant placement. *(c)* Immediate implant placement in the sites of the maxillary central incisors. *(d)* CTG from the palatal region of the left first premolar to first molar. *(e)* Condition after implant placement and insertion of CTG labial to the buccal lamella using the tunneling technique. *(f)* Healing after 1 week with provisional bonded fixed partial denture. *(g)* Condition 3 months after surgery before the prosthetic phase; the interdental papilla was preserved. *(h)* Radiograph 1 year after implant placement. *(i)* All-ceramic superstructure 1 year after implant placement. (Surgery performed by A. Happe; prosthodontics performed by B. van den Bosch; laboratory work performed by A. Nolte.)

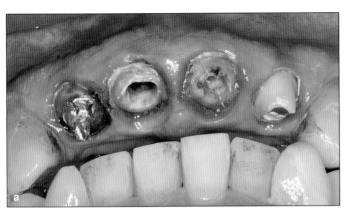
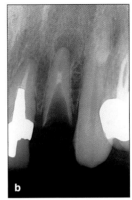
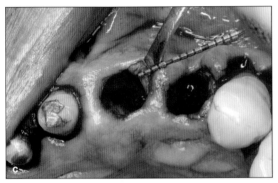
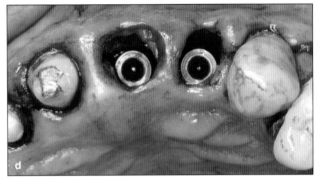

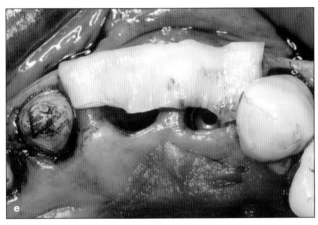
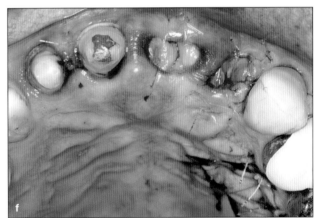

Fig 7-12 / *(a and b)* The maxillary left central incisor shows a buccopalatal fracture line, and the lateral incisor has limited tooth substance and a poor prognosis. If these teeth were extracted and the sites left to heal, advanced bone and soft tissue augmentation would be necessary. *(c)* The healthy proximal portion of the central incisor was severed at less than 1 mm above the bone crest. *(d)* A 4-mm-diameter implant was placed in the ideal position, not contacting the fragment. *(e and f)* Anorganic bovine bone material was grafted up to the bone height, and a CTG was placed to cover the buccal and occlusal aspects of the crest.

especially in adjacent implant sites. This concept was first introduced by Hürzeler et al[39] in 2010 and subsequently investigated histologically and clinically.[40] The position of the available periodontal attachment of the tooth fragment should be evaluated carefully to ensure an esthetic result before submergence. However, because there is not yet evidence of long-term success with this technique, the clinician should take extra care in choosing this procedure; meticulous maintenance will be essential.[41–46]

Clinical case

This 64-year-old patient requested a treatment as minimally invasive as possible and with a result as esthetic as possible. After the consultation and considering the high smile line, the proximal socket shield technique with a CTG was chosen (Fig 7-12).

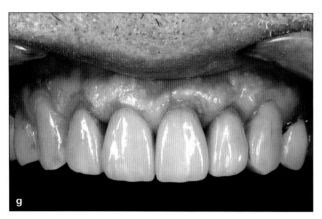
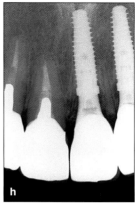

Fig 7-12 *cont.* / *(g and h)* One year after treatment, the interimplant papilla between the left incisors looks very natural compared with the contralateral side. The preserved tooth fragment seems to be maintaining the interproximal bone crest between the adjacent implants.

Hard and soft tissue augmentation

It is particularly challenging to achieve an esthetic result in cases with adjacent implants if there are hard and soft tissue defects.[1,4] In this situation, the treatment team in collaboration with the patient must determine what type of tooth replacement is desirable and explore whether the necessary conditions for an optimal esthetic outcome can be created with 3D augmentation of the bone and soft tissue.[47,48] To achieve a good esthetic result and satisfy the patient, the surgical and prosthetic working steps in the treatment plan must then be implemented meticulously.

Clinical case

The patient in Fig 7-13 had lost the maxillary right lateral incisor and canine in a traffic accident. After avulsion, both central incisors had been replanted in an incorrect position. Subsequently, these ankylosed with the alveolar bone 20 weeks after replantation. The high smile line increased the esthetic challenge (see Figs 7-13a and 7-13b). Overall, the esthetic problems in this trauma case arose from the malocclusion and the high lip position when smiling. The radiograph showed pronounced bone loss in the region of the right incisors (see Figs 7-13c and 7-13d). The alveolar bone around the existing teeth was intact. The radiograph of the central incisors shows progressive root resorption at the left central incisor.

The patient was also concerned about the mandibular prognathism visible in profile. Analysis of the lateral cephalogram revealed that the maxillary and mandibular position relative to the cranium was within the average range, but the mandible was advanced relative to the maxilla (see Figs 7-13e and 7-13f). The maxilla was too narrow to correct crowding with orthodontic flaring. Therefore, the treatment team planned an orthognathic surgical operation (see Figs 7-13g and 7-13h).

During the orthodontic treatment, the ankylosed central incisors served as anchors. The occlusion was surgically corrected by retral movement and counterclockwise rotation of the mandible. This movement reduced the required volume of vertical and horizontal augmentation. The occlusal relationship was markedly improved after the orthodontic treatment (see Fig 7-13i). The maxillary right first premolar had taken the position of the missing canine. The replacement resorption of the central incisor roots had advanced further, and larger parts of the roots were exposed (see Figs 7-13j and 7-13k). After extraction of the malpositioned central incisors, the site was left to heal for 6 months (see Fig 7-13l). Following careful planning with the aid of cone beam computed tomography (CBCT), extensive bone augmentation was performed with GBR. Preoperative analysis revealed that 5 mm vertical and 4 mm horizontal bone augmentation were preconditions for an attractive esthetic outcome (see Figs 7-13m to 7-13u). The autogenous bone graft was harvested from the base of the anterior nasal spine and the base of the zygoma, and the incisive canal was packed with a mix of autogenous bone and bovine bone substitute (see Figs 7-13v to 7-13y). Orthodontic correction of the tooth axis of the left lateral incisor was carried out during the bone maturation (see Figs 7-13z and 7-13aa).

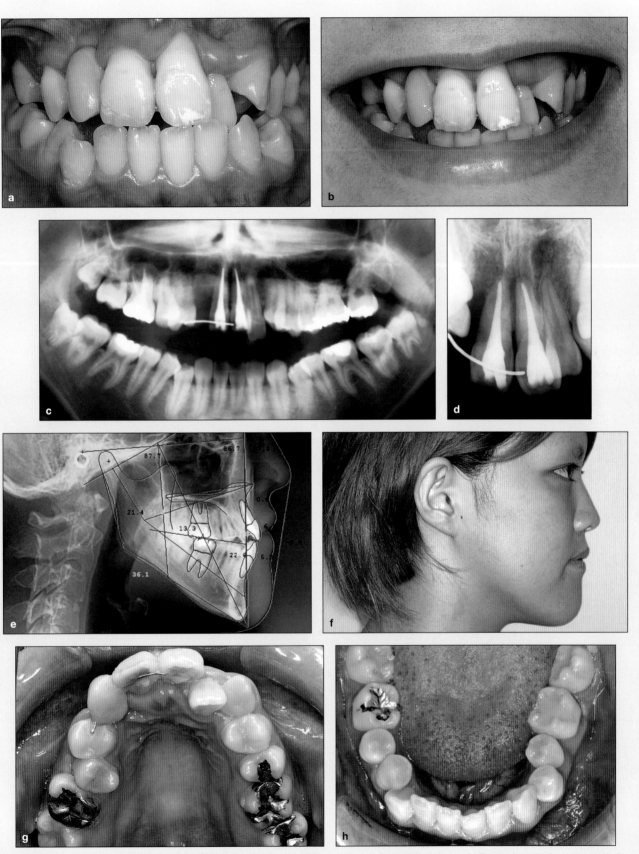

Fig 7-13 / *(a)* Preoperative view with incorrectly positioned maxillary central incisors after avulsion. *(b)* The high smile line increased the esthetic challenge. *(c)* Panoramic radiograph of the preoperative situation. *(d)* Periapical radiograph of the anterior dentition. *(e and f)* Lateral cephalogram and profile view. *(g and h)* Occlusal views of the preoperative situation in both arches.

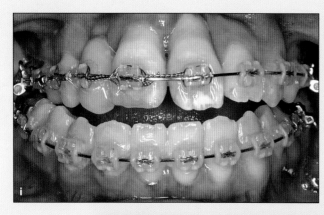

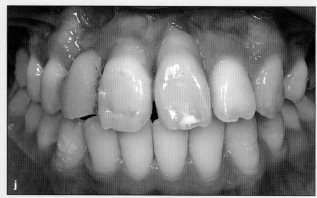

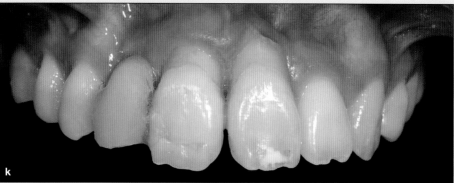

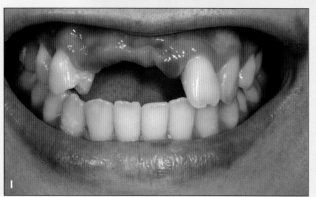

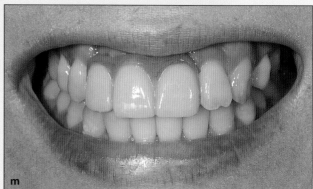

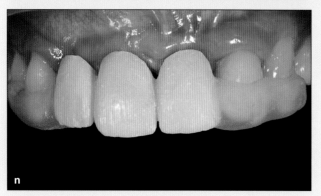

Fig 7-13 *cont.* / *(i)* Situation after completion of the orthodontic pretreatment. *(j)* The occlusal relationship after the orthodontic treatment. *(k)* Even after the orthodontic correction, it is still a complex task to create a pleasing esthetic. *(l)* Situation before bone augmentation. The high smile line, in particular, made the treatment challenging. *(m)* Bonded provisional restoration. The provisional with its pink gingival portion provided a preview of the intended end result. *(n)* A diagnostic template was fabricated to plan the tissue augmentation. This made it clear that a 3D ridge reconstruction was imperative for an esthetic outcome. →

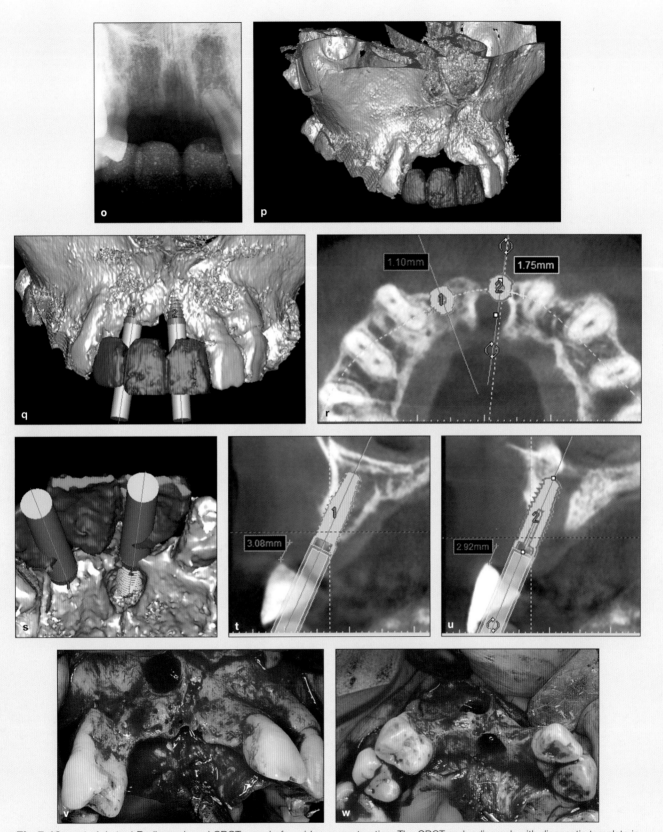

Fig 7-13 *cont.* / *(o to r)* Radiograph and CBCT scan before ridge reconstruction. The CBCT and radiograph with diagnostic template in place showed that the alveolar ridge had significant 3D hard and soft tissue defects. *(s to u)* The computer simulation prior to bone augmentation shows that the space for implant placement in the region of the right lateral incisor and left central incisor is inadequate. Furthermore, the angulation of the left lateral incisor and the prominent incisive canal prevent an ideal implant position. *(v and w)* The root eminences show the incorrect inclination of the teeth bordering the gap. The bone was cleaned of soft tissue, and the neurovascular bundle was removed from the incisive canal.

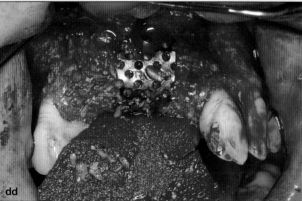

Fig 7-13 *cont.* / *(x and y)* To create the necessary bony foundation for implant placement, a mix of autogenous bone and bovine bone material in combination with a stiff, cross-linked collagen membrane was used for augmentation. *(z and aa)* Comparison of the situations before and after correction of the tooth axis of the left lateral incisor, which was completed orthodontically during the first healing phase after GBR. *(bb to dd)* Precise implant positioning and second esthetic GBR: A titanium mesh that was filled with particulate bone graft material was fixed with the aid of the gingiva former. →

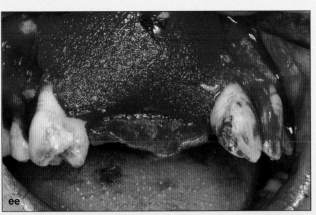

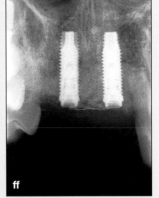

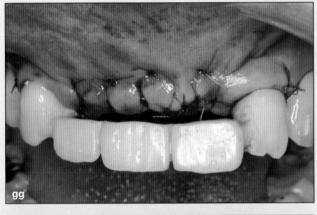

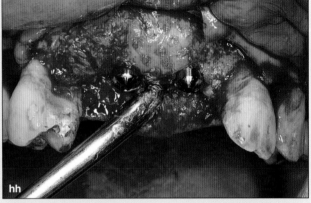

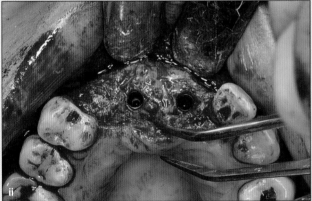

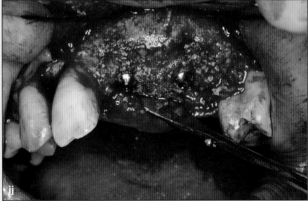

Fig 7-13 *cont.* / *(ee)* Esthetic GBR: The entire site was covered with a collagen membrane. *(ff)* Radiograph after implant placement. *(gg)* Immediately after the surgical procedure, the provisional restoration should be adapted to allow enough clearance for any postoperative edema. *(hh and ii)* The augmented ridge 7 months after implant placement. *(jj and kk)* Additional GBR for improved esthetics.

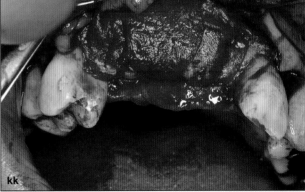

140

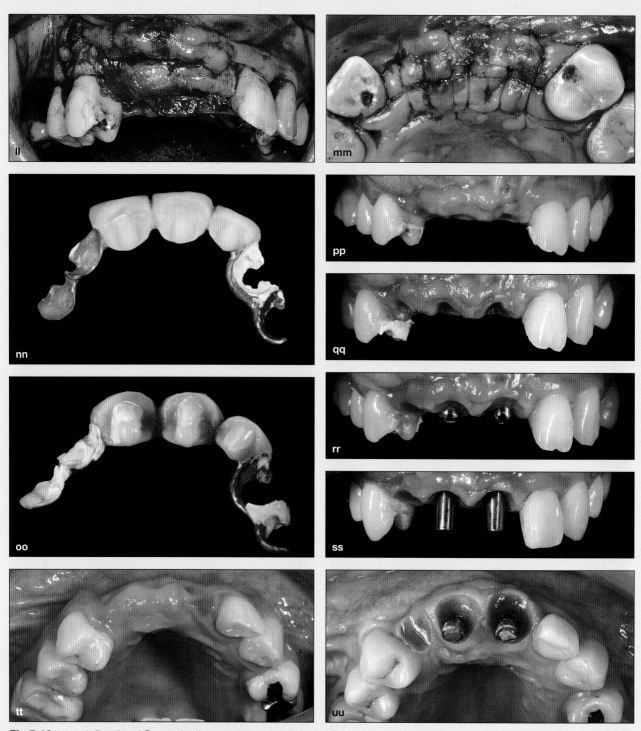

Fig 7-13 *cont.* / *(ll and mm)* Connective tissue augmentation. *(nn to ss)* The soft tissue was conditioned by gradual application of composite, initially to the bonded partial denture, then to the subgingival contour of the provisional prosthesis after placement of shoulderless abutments. *(tt and uu)* Comparison of the situations before and after the horizontal tissue augmentation. After three GBR procedures and one soft tissue augmentation, there was markedly more soft tissue and bone volume available. ⟶

141

Fig 7-13 *cont.* / *(vv and ww)* Definitive restoration. *(xx to aaa)* Comparison of lateral views before augmentation and after completion of treatment. *(bbb)* Radiograph of the final situation. The regenerated interimplant bony ridge appears stable after 2 years of functioning. *(ccc)* Follow-up radiograph after 3 years showing hard tissue maturation.

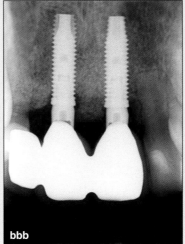

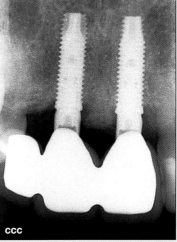

⟶ Solutions

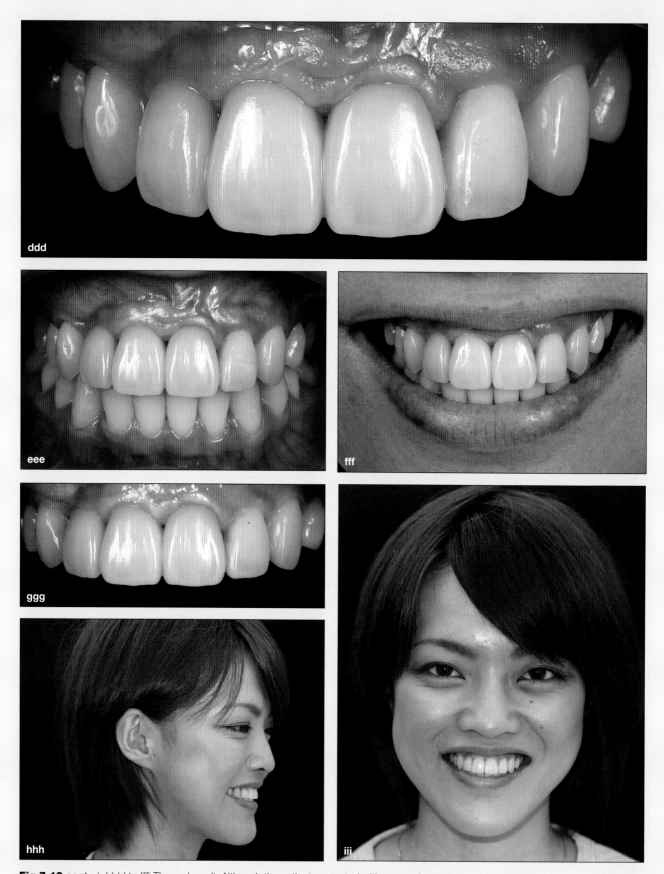

Fig 7-13 *cont.* / *(ddd to fff)* The end result. Although the patient presented with severe tissue damage, adequate tissue and papilla reconstruction was achieved, resulting in restored esthetics and function. *(ggg)* Photograph after 3 years of function showing soft tissue formation. *(hhh and iii)* Portrait after the treatment. Despite the high smile line, the patient is able to smile with confidence. (Orthodontics performed by K. Kida; laboratory work performed by M. Hinoshita.)

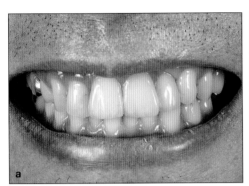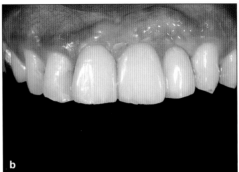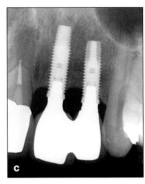

Fig 7-14 / *(a to c)* Natural-looking smile of a 40-year-old patient. Prosthetic papillae made of pink ceramic were created between each set of incisors. One year after treatment, the soft tissue conditions are stable, and the reconstruction provides a healthy, esthetic appearance. (Laboratory work performed by K. Nakajima.)

One year after the first augmentation, implants were placed in conjunction with a second augmentation (see Figs 7-13bb to 7-13gg). Seven months after implant placement and the second GBR, the bone fulfilled the requirements to form the basis for an esthetic reconstruction. The regenerated tissue was sufficient to support the future interimplant papilla on the labial aspect. To compensate for any resorption and increase the hard tissue volume horizontally and vertically, a third GBR procedure was performed with deproteinized bovine bone mineral (DBBM) and a collagen membrane (see Figs 7-13hh to 7-13kk). To augment the labial soft tissue volume, a subepithelial CTG was placed between the resorbable membrane and the labial flap and sutured to the labial ridge (see Figs 7-13ll and 7-13mm).

After more than 2 months' healing and complete vascularization of the grafted tissue, soft tissue conditioning was performed using Borg's technique.[49] To do this, the pontics of the bonded partial denture were first lengthened gradually and, after insertion of shoulderless abutments, composite was applied to the subgingival contour of the provisional restoration on a weekly basis to shape the soft tissue (see Figs 7-13nn to 7-13uu). The subgingival contour of the provisional restoration was transferred to a zirconia framework with the use of computer-aided design (CAD) software.

The interdisciplinary therapeutic approach encompassed correction of the malocclusion, reconstruction of the tissue lost from the trauma, and rehabilitation with two implants and a pontic. The tissue reconstruction and preservation that was carefully planned and implemented enabled an esthetically pleasing result to be achieved with healthy soft tissue and natural-looking papillae (see Figs 7-13vv to 7-13iii).

Gingival prosthesis

If it is likely that adequate reconstruction of the lost tissue will not be possible, the use of prosthetic gingiva should be suggested to the patient (Fig 7-14).

Conclusion

Patients who have lost adjacent teeth in the esthetic zone pose a special challenge for implant therapy. An understanding of the patient's esthetic and practical wishes forms the starting point for treatment. Bearing these expectations in mind, the biologic and clinical limitations of treatment can be assessed, and the therapy or combination of treatments suitable for esthetic and functional rehabilitation to the patient's satisfaction can be selected. Clear decision-making guidelines make it easier to adapt the type of prosthetic restoration if the chosen option is not esthetically workable. Furthermore, such guidelines help to make the treatment decisions plausible from the patient's point of view.

143

References

1. Buser D, Martin W, Belser UC. Optimizing esthetics for implant restorations in the anterior maxilla: Anatomic and surgical considerations. Int J Oral Maxillofac Implants 2004;19(suppl):43–61.
2. Kokich VO, Kokich VG, Kiyak HA. Perceptions of dental professionals and laypersons to altered dental esthetics: Asymmetric and symmetric situations. Am J Orthod Dentofacial Orthop 2006;130:141–151.
3. Salama MA, Salama H, Garber DA. Guidelines for aesthetic restorative options and implant site enhancement: The utilization of orthodontic extrusion. Pract Proced Aesthet Dent 2002;14:125–130.
4. Tarnow D, Elian N, Fletcher P, et al. Vertical distance from the crest of bone to the height of the interproximal papilla between adjacent implants. J Periodontol 2003;74:1785–1788.
5. Scarano A, Assenza B, Piattelli M, et al. Interimplant distance and crestal bone resorption: A histologic study in the canine mandible. Clin Implant Dent Relat Res 2004;6:150–156.
6. Tymstra N, Meijer HJ, Stellingsma K, Raghoebar GM, Vissink A. Treatment outcome and patient satisfaction with two adjacent implant-supported restorations in the esthetic zone. Int J Periodontics Restorative Dent 2010;30:307–316.
7. Tarnow DP, Cho SC, Wallace SS. The effect of inter-implant distance on the height of inter-implant bone crest. J Periodontol 2000;71:546–549.
8. Gastaldo JF, Cury PR, Sendyk WR. Effect of the vertical and horizontal distances between adjacent implants and between a tooth and an implant on the incidence of interproximal papilla. J Periodontol 2004;75:1242–1246.
9. Rodriguez-Ciurana X, Vela-Nebot X, Segalà-Torres M, et al. The effect of interimplant distance on the height of the interimplant bone crest when using platform-switched implants. Int J Periodontics Restorative Dent 2009;29:141–151.
10. Vela X, Méndez V, Rodríguez X, Segalá M, Tarnow DP. Crestal bone changes on platform-switched implants and adjacent teeth when the tooth-implant distance is less than 1.5 mm. Int J Periodontics Restorative Dent 2012;32:149–155.
11. Elian N, Bloom M, Dard M, Cho SC, Trushkowsky RD, Tarnow D. Radiological and micro-computed tomography analysis of the bone at dental implants inserted 2, 3 and 4 mm apart in a mini-pig model with platform switching incorporated. Clin Oral Implants Res 2014;25:e22–e29.
12. Atieh MA, Ibrahim HM, Atieh AH. Platform switching for marginal bone preservation around dental implants: A systematic review and meta-analysis. J Periodontol 2010;81:1350–1366.
13. Schmitt CM, Nogueira-Filho G, Tenenbaum HC, et al. Performance of conical abutment (Morse Taper) connection implants: A systematic review. J Biomed Mater Res A 2014;102:552–574.
14. Broggini N, McManus LM, Hermann JS, et al. Persistent acute inflammation at the implant-abutment interface. J Dent Res 2003;82:232–237.
15. Hermann JS, Buser D, Schenk RK, Schoolfield JD, Cochran DL. Biologic width around one- and two-piece titanium implants. Clin Oral Implants Res 2001;12:559–571.
16. Abrahamsson I, Berglundh T, Lindhe J. The mucosal barrier following abutment dis/reconnection. An experimental study in dogs. J Clin Periodontol 1997;24:568–572.
17. Rompen E. The impact of the type and configuration of abutments and their (repeated) removal on the attachment level and marginal bone. Eur J Oral Implantol 2012;5(suppl):S83–S90.
18. Rodríguez X, Vela X, Méndez V, Segalà M, Calvo-Guirado JL, Tarnow DP. The effect of abutment dis/reconnections on peri-implant bone resorption: A radiologic study of platform-switched and non-platform-switched implants placed in animals. Clin Oral Implants Res 2013;24:305–311.
19. Canullo L, Bignozzi I, Cocchetto R, Cristalli MP, Iannello G. Immediate positioning of a definitive abutment versus repeated abutment replacements in post-extractive implants: 3-year follow-up of a randomised multicentre clinical trial. Eur J Oral Implantol 2010;3:285–296.
20. Cocchetto RL, Loi I. Surgical-prosthetic interactions in the immediate loading of implants in the esthetic zone. In: Testori T, Galli F, del Fabbro M (eds). Immediate loading: A new era in oral implantology. London: Quintessence, 2011:361–375.
21. Loi I, Cocchetto R, Di Felice A. Abutment morphology and peri-implant soft tissues. In: Canullo L, Cocchetto R, Loi I (eds). Peri-Implant Tissue Remodeling: Scientific Background and Clinical Implications. Milan: Quintessence, 2012:107–126.
22. Cocchetto R, Canullo L. The "hybrid abutment": A new design for implant cemented restorations in the esthetic zones. Int J Esthet Dent 2015;10:186–208.
23. Canullo L, Cocchetto R, Marinotti F, Oltra DP, Diago MP, Loi I. Clinical evaluation of an improved cementation technique for implant-supported restorations: A randomized controlled trial. Clin Oral Implants Res 2016;27:1492–1499.
24. Tymstra N, Raghoebar GM, Vissink A, Meijer HJ. Dental implant treatment for two adjacent missing teeth in the maxillary aesthetic zone: A comparative pilot study and test of principle. Clin Oral Implants Res 2011;22:207–213.
25. Cordaro L, Torsello F, Mirisola Di Torresanto V, Rossini C. Retrospective evaluation of mandibular incisor replacement with narrow neck implants. Clin Oral Implants Res 2006;17:730–735.
26. Libman WJ, Nicholls JI. Load fatigue of teeth restored with cast posts and cores and complete crowns. Int J Prosthodont 1995;8:155–161.
27. Andreasen JO. Effect of extra-alveolar period and storage media upon periodontal and pulpal healing after replantation of mature permanent incisors in monkeys. Int J Oral Surg 1981;10:43–53.
28. Andreasen JO. Periodontal healing after replantation and autotransplantation of incisors in monkeys. Int J Oral Surg 1981;10:54–61.
29. Andreasen JO. A time-related study of periodontal healing and root resorption activity after replantation of mature permanent incisors in monkeys. Swed Dent J 1980;4:101–110.
30. Dryden JA, Arens DE. Intentional replantation. A viable alternative for selected cases. Dent Clin North Am 1994;38:325–353.
31. Tsukiboshi M. Autogenous tooth transplantation: A reevaluation. Int J Periodontics Restorative Dent 1993;13:120–149.
32. Rouhani A, Javidi B, Habibi M, Jafarzadeh H. Intentional replantation: A procedure as a last resort. J Contemp Dent Pract 2011;12:486–492.
33. Daftary F, Mahallati R, Bahat O, Sullivan RM. Lifelong craniofacial growth and the implications for osseointegrated implants. Int J Oral Maxillofac Implants 2013;28:163–169.
34. Kourkouta S, Dedi KD, Paquette DW, Mol A. Interproximal tissue dimensions in relation to adjacent implants in the anterior maxilla: Clinical observations and patient aesthetic evaluation. Clin Oral Implants Res 2009;20:1375–1385.
35. Grunder U. Crestal ridge width changes when placing implants at the time of tooth extraction with and without soft tissue augmentation after a healing period of 6 months: Report of 24 consecutive cases. Int J Periodontics Restorative Dent 2011;31:9–17.

144

36. Lee DW, Park KH, Moon IS. Dimension of keratinized mucosa and the interproximal papilla between adjacent implants. J Periodontol 2005;76:1856–1860.

37. Kan JY, Rungcharassaeng K, Umezu K, Kois JC. Dimensions of peri-implant mucosa: An evaluation of maxillary anterior single implants in humans. J Periodontol 2003;74:557–562.

38. Chen ST, Buser D. Esthetic outcomes following immediate and early implant placement in the anterior maxilla: A systematic review. Int J Oral Maxillofac Implants 2014;29(suppl):186–215.

39. Hürzeler MB, Zuhr O, Schupbach P, Rebele SF, Emmanouilidis N, Fickl S. The socket-shield technique: A proof-of-principle report. J Clin Periodontol 2010;37:855–862.

40. Bäumer D, Zuhr O, Rebele S, Schneider D, Schupbach P, Hürzeler M. The socket-shield technique: First histological, clinical, and volumetrical observations after separation of the buccal tooth segment—A pilot study. Clin Implant Dent Relat Res 2015;17:71–82.

41. Kan JY, Rungcharassaeng K. Proximal socket shield for interimplant papilla preservation in the esthetic zone. Int J Periodontics Restorative Dent 2013;33:e24–e31.

42. Siormpas KD, Mitsias ME, Kontsiotou-Siormpa E, Garber D, Kotsakis GA. Immediate implant placement in the esthetic zone utilizing the "root-membrane" technique: Clinical results up to 5 years postloading. Int J Oral Maxillofac Implants 2014;29:1397–1405.

43. Bäumer D, Zuhr O, Rebele S, Hürzeler M. Socket shield technique for immediate implant placement: Clinical, radiographic and volumetric data after 5 years. Clin Oral Implants Res 2017;28:1450–1458.

44. Gluckman H, Salama M, Du Toit J. Partial extraction therapies (PET) part 1: Maintaining alveolar ridge contour at pontic and immediate implant sites. Int J Periodontics Restorative Dent 2016;36:681–687.

45. Gluckman H, Salama M, Du Toit J. Partial extraction therapies (PET) part 2: Procedures and technical aspects. Int J Periodontics Restorative Dent 2017;37:377–385.

46. Gluckman H, Salama M, Du Toit J. A retrospective evaluation of 128 socket-shield cases in the esthetic zone and posterior sites: Partial extraction therapy with up to 4 years follow-up. Clin Implant Dent Relat Res 2018;20:122–129.

47. Grunder U, Gracis S, Capelli M. Influence of the 3-D bone-to-implant relationship on esthetics. Int J Periodontics Restorative Dent 2005;25:113–119.

48. Ishikawa T, Salama M, Funato A, et al. Three-dimensional bone and soft tissue requirements for optimizing esthetic results in compromised cases with multiple implants. Int J Periodontics Restorative Dent 2010;30:503–511.

49. Vela X, Méndez V, Rodríguez X, Segalà M, Gil JA. Soft tissue remodeling technique as a non-invasive alternative to second implant surgery. Eur J Esthet Dent 2012;7:36–47.

145

"If it's important to you, you will find a way.
If not, you will find an excuse."

UNKNOWN

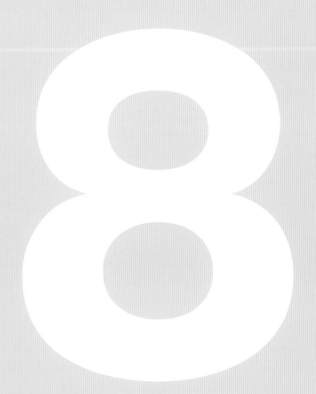

8
Soft Tissue
Augmentation

/ Arndt Happe, Gerd Körner

Soft tissue grafts are very often used in the esthetic zone to achieve an additional gain in volume but also to thicken the soft tissue itself. Subepithelial connective tissue grafts (CTGs) from the palate are commonly chosen. Palatal CTGs have been used in implantology for many years.[1,2] As opposed to free mucosal grafts (FMGs), these involve epithelium-free soft tissue grafts that ideally consist largely of connective tissue with only small portions of fatty and glandular tissue (Fig 8-1).

The palatal mucosa is thickest in the premolar area. Song et al[3] and Barriviera et al[4] each studied sizeable groups of patients and published the average thicknesses of palatal mucosa (Table 8-1). Müller and Eger[5] showed, conversely, that the mucosal thickness on the palate also correlates with the periodontal biotype (ie, phenotype). This means that patients who have a thin biotype (ie, those who most need thickening) also have thin palatal mucosa and therefore usually have little material available for autogenous augmentation.

Soft tissue grafts can be used as subepithelial CTGs, as described, or as full-thickness grafts with epithelium, hence as FMGs. FMGs can be obtained using scalpel or punch methods (see Figs 8-9c and 8-9d).

Technique

The graft material is usually harvested under local anesthesia. The entire donor site should be infiltrated with anesthetic solution with a 1:100,000 vasoconstrictor additive to ensure adequate hemostasis. The injections should infiltrate the area between the palatine artery and the donor site so that, in addition to the vasoconstrictor effect, short-term hemostasis can also be achieved by a slight increase in tissue pressure (Fig 8-2).

Before the graft is harvested, the dimensions of the planned graft should be simulated using a template (eg,

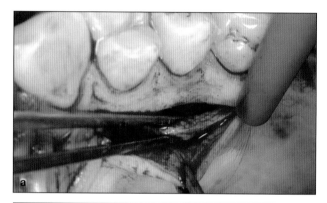

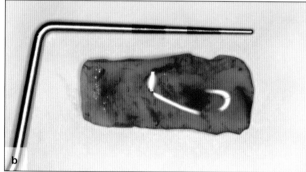

Fig 8-1 / *(a)* Harvesting a subepithelial CTG. *(b)* View of subepithelial CTG.

Table 8-1 Average mucosal thicknesses on the palate (mm) according to different studies

Region	Song et al[3]	Barriviera et al[4]
Canines	3.46	2.92
First premolars	3.66	3.11
Second premolars	3.81	3.28
First molars	3.13	2.89
Second molars	3.39	3.15

sterile paper from surgical tray or suture pack) and transferred to the donor site (Figs 8-3 and 8-4). The first incision is made with a size 15 blade vertically about 4 mm paramarginally and about 1.5 to 2 mm deep from distal to mesial. The blade ends in a slight curve resembling

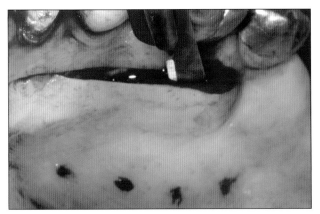

Fig 8-2 / Harvesting a CTG. Note the bleeding points medial to the donor site, which define the puncture sites for the local anesthesia.

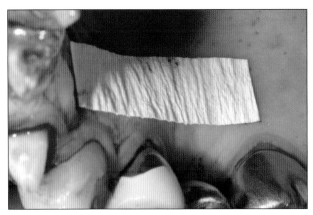

Fig 8-3 / Sterile paper serves as a template to transfer the dimensions of the graft to the donor site.

a hockey-stick shape, which makes it easier to remove the tissue. The scalpel is then rotated 90 degrees, and a mucosal flap 1.5- to 2-mm thick is dissected to gain access to the connective tissue (Fig 8-5a). The graft of the required size is then delineated with the scalpel; in the process, the second vertical incision is made about 1 mm medial to the access incision. This will form a fold for the mucosal flap to lie on after harvesting (Fig 8-5b). In addition, a circular incision of the graft is made mesially, distally, and in the medial direction (Figs 8-5c and 8-5d). The CTG together with periosteum is removed with the aid of a raspatory (Figs 8-5e to 8-5h).

Harvesting the graft will inevitably damage branches of the palatine artery and cause varying degrees of bleeding. Repeated infiltration medial to the donor site can help to staunch the blood. The space can (but must not necessarily) be filled with collagen sponge to achieve more adequate hemostasis (Figs 8-5i and 8-5j). Crossed polytetrafluoroethylene (PTFE) 5-0 mattress sutures can be used for closure of the donor site. In addition, 6-0 microsurgical interrupted sutures can be used to appose the wound margins (Fig 8-5k).

The technique for harvesting CTGs is described briefly here for the sake of completeness. Harvesting subepithelial CTGs requires surgical training beyond the scope of a book: Clinicians should learn the technique in appropriate postgraduate courses before applying it to patients. Complications such as arterial bleeding, flap necrosis, and sensation disorders in the donor site are serious problems that can influence the postoperative morbidity (Figs 8-6 and 8-7).

The technique stems from periodontology methods for plastic reconstruction of soft tissues for the purpose of recession coverage or for augmentation of pontic areas.[6–10]

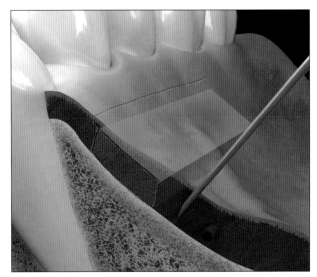

Fig 8-4 / Illustration of the donor region and anesthesia.

149

Langer and Calagna[11,12] were two of the first authors in the literature to describe subepithelial CTGs in connection with enhancing dentofacial esthetics. When dental implantology developed in the 1990s from the purely functional retention of tooth replacements into a valid technique for replacing missing teeth in the esthetic zone, periodontal surgery techniques for defect reconstruction were increasingly incorporated into implant dentistry.[13–15]

After the implementation of microsurgical techniques led to a paradigm shift in periodontal surgery, these techniques were soon adapted for use in implant surgery as well.[16–19] With the aid of fluorescence angiography, Burkhardt and Lang[20] showed in a comparative split-mouth clinical trial that vascularization immediately postopera-

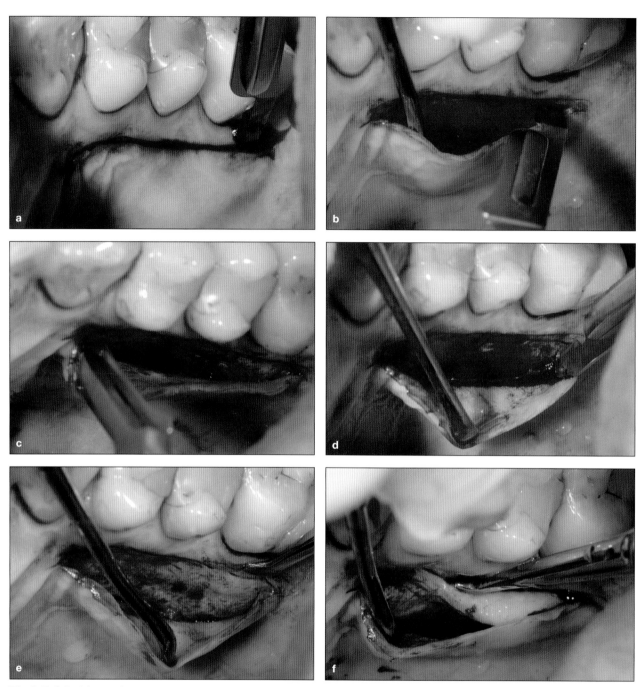

Fig 8-5 / Graft harvesting procedure: After the first incision, a mucosal flap is raised (a) and a parallel incision is made approximately 1 mm away to create a base (b). The graft is dissected mesially (c) and distally (d) before being detached with a micro raspatory (e and f).

tively and 1 week postoperatively was significantly better in the area that underwent microsurgery than in the macrosurgically treated area.

A fundamental study by Berglundh and Lindhe[21] showed that the thickness of the peri-implant soft tissue has an influence on crestal bone via development of the biologic width. Many authors recommend CTGs, especially in the esthetic zone[1,22–24]; these grafts help to reconstruct alve-

olar ridge defects and thicken the soft tissue. Soft tissue thickness has proven to be a prognostic factor for recessions occurring around implants and an important factor in whether restorative materials can be seen through the soft tissue, which can lead to soft tissue discoloration.[25–27]

In a split-mouth clinical trial, Wiesner et al[28] showed that thickening of soft tissue is possible: The authors report 1.3-mm average thickening 1 year postoperatively.

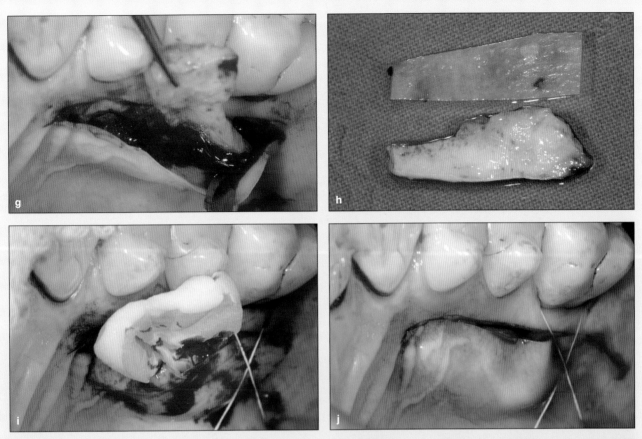

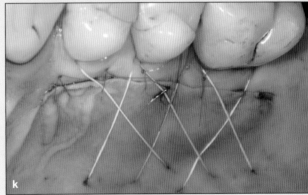

Fig 8-5 *cont.* / After removal of the graft *(g)*, a template made of sterile paper serves as a guide to the size and shape of the graft *(h)*. Collagen sponge is introduced into the donor site *(i and j)*, and the donor site is closed with sutures *(k)*.

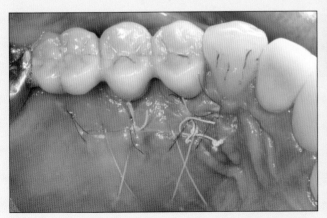

Fig 8-6 / Normal wound healing 1 week after harvesting the CTG.

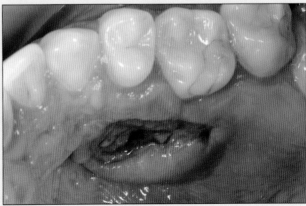

Fig 8-7 / Impaired wound healing after CTG harvesting with partial necrosis of the mucosal flap.

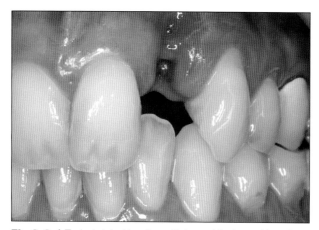

Fig 8-8 / Typical defect healing with loss of the buccal lamella.

Other authors report a thickness increase of 0.5 mm on average.[29] However, substitute materials are suitable for thickening soft tissues. In a 1-year clinical trial, Puišys and Linkevičius[30] demonstrated that mucosal thickness can be increased from 1.5 mm to 3.8 mm on average with an allogeneic dermis.[30] In the process, crestal bone resorption was significantly less in the group with increased soft tissue thickness than in the group with a nonaugmented thin mucosa. Admittedly, these results were collected in the posterior dentition. The results do show, however, that increasing soft tissue thickness is possible in principle.[30]

Despite all of this, the data pool of long-term results for augmentation with soft tissue grafts is rather small. A literature review by Thoma et al[31] concluded that only limited scientific studies are available. However, these few scientific studies clearly favor subepithelial CTGs. CTGs can be used as free or pedicle grafts at different stages of implantology treatment, as follows:

- At extraction (ie, prior to implant placement)
- At the time of implant placement
- As a separate procedure before implant exposure
- At the time of exposure
- As a corrective procedure following prosthetic restoration

It should be stressed at this point that soft tissue augmentation does have its limitations. This includes, for instance, soft tissue recession around implants. In the esthetic zone, soft tissue recession around implant superstructures is a complication that cannot be predictably corrected.[32]

Critical risk factors for the development of soft tissue recession around implants are described in the literature.

These include, for example, a thin periodontal biotype and the surgical approach for immediate implant placement (see chapter 4).[25,33] Correct three-dimensional (3D) positioning of the implant is another key factor.[34] If the implant is positioned too far buccally, surgery can no longer have a beneficial effect on soft tissue recession; therefore, careful planning of treatment and contouring of the emergence profile become particularly important.[13]

Soft Tissue Grafts at Extraction

Landsberg[35] coined the term *socket seal surgery* in connection with immediate implant placement as early as 1997. In 2004, Jung[36] picked up this term in relation to preimplantology management of extraction sockets and used FMGs in conjunction with a bone substitute material to create a favorable baseline situation for eventual implant placement and to avoid resorption asssociated with defect healing (Fig 8-8). Fickl et al[37] showed in an animal model that using soft tissue grafts in combination with substitute material can preserve tissue volume. Literature reviews also conclude that ridge preservation techniques can markedly reduce resorption postextraction.[38,39] The probability of requiring bone augmentation can be reduced by a factor of 10 (ie, 4% versus 42%) by using ridge preservation techniques in conjunction with bone substitute material.[38]

Clinical case 1

A patient in her early twenties presented with tooth trauma in the region of the maxillary central incisors (Fig 8-9). She had already sustained anterior tooth trauma to the left central incisor in the past, and the tooth had undergone endodontic treatment (see Fig 8-9a). When she presented for treatment, she had an extra-alveolar coronal fracture at the right central incisor and a longitudinal fracture of the root of the left central incisor. Immediate implant placement was not possible because of the patient's financial limitations. Because the buccal lamella at the left central incisor was intact, an inorganic bovine bone substitute was introduced into the socket (see Fig 8-9b), and the entrance to the socket was sealed with a mucosal punch graft from the palate at the region of the maxillary left premolars (socket seal) (see Figs 8-9c to 8-9e). After 3 months of uncomplicated healing (Fig 8-9f), the implant was placed in the fully healed bony alveolar process (see

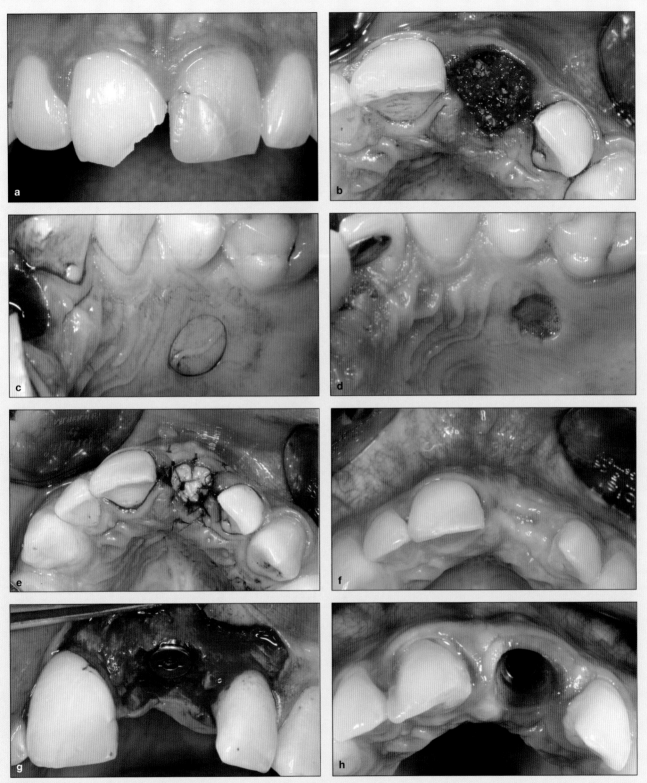

Fig 8-9 / *(a)* Preoperative view after two occasions of anterior dental trauma. *(b)* Given an intact buccal lamella, the bony socket of the maxillary left central incisor was filled with a bone substitute material. *(c)* Use of a punch to obtain the soft tissue graft. *(d)* Healing 1 week postoperative. *(e)* An FMG seals the entrance to the socket. *(f)* Fully healed site after 3 months. *(g)* Implant placement in the healed alveolar process. *(h)* Condition after minimally invasive exposure and tissue contouring.

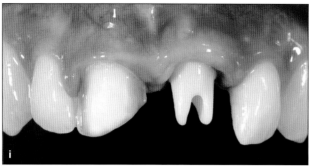

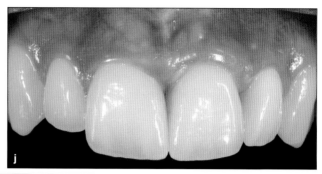

Fig 8-9 *cont.* / *(i and j)* The right central incisor was prepared for a veneer; a zirconia abutment can be seen in the site of the left central incisor. *(k to m)* Comparison of radiographs: preoperative situation *(k)*, after implant placement *(l)*, and after prosthetic restoration *(m)*.

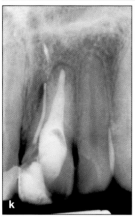

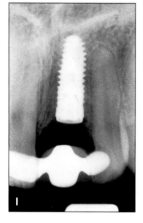

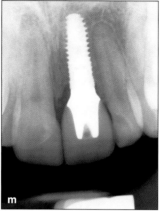

Fig 8-9g). The horizontal contour of the alveolar process was anatomically correct after minimally invasive implant exposure as a result of soft tissue displacement and maturation (see Fig 8-9h). The dentofacial esthetics were restored with a veneer on the right central incisor and a zirconia abutment with an all-ceramic crown on the left central incisor implant (see Figs 8-9i and 8-9j). However, the case also shows collapse of the papillae mesial and distal to the implant.

The use of soft tissue grafts can often improve the clinical situation, especially where there are hard or soft tissue defects of variable severity that are already evident prior to extraction (see Figs 8-9k to 8-9m). As a result, the baseline situation for the subsequent procedure is greatly improved because resorptive defect healing is prevented. There is also an enhanced baseline situation for further surgical interventions.

Clinical case 2

A young patient presented with a fistula and horizontal root fracture in the middle third of the maxillary right central incisor (Fig 8-10). Both facially and palatally, it was possible to palpate down to the apex with the periodontal probe. Buccal and palatal lamellae had been lost. To achieve a favorable preoperative situation for augmentation and prevent collapse of the tissue, the socket was filled with collagen, and the entrance to the socket was sealed with a free punch graft. The graft needed to be at least 3 mm thick, and the soft tissue alveolar margins had to be trimmed with a rotary diamond or scalpel. After about 6 weeks, the tissue had healed and matured enough to allow for unproblematic flap formation. In this case, augmentation ensued with autogenous bone grafts (bone chips) and a laser-perforated titanium membrane (Frios Bone Shield, Dentsply).

Clinical case with subepithelial CTG

After an anterior tooth trauma with complete luxation (avulsion) and reimplantation of the two central incisors in his youth, the patient presented several years later with massive external resorption at the maxillary left central incisor (Fig 8-11). The buccal bone lamella together with mucosa was absent, which resulted in a hard and soft tissue defect. The lack of fixed keratinized mucosa, in particular, makes adequate soft tissue management difficult in augmentation surgery and might cause functional problems in the peri-implant area in the long term. Im-

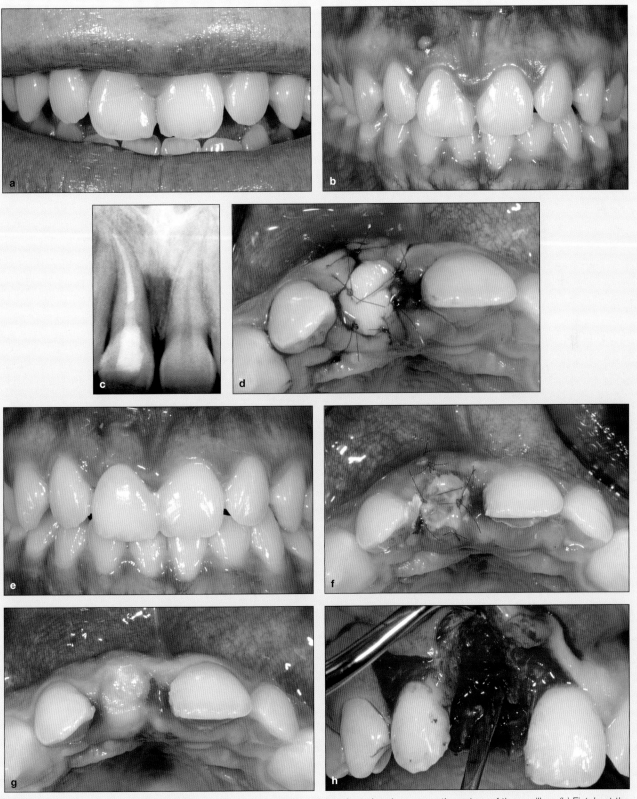

Fig 8-10 / *(a)* Lip appearance with relaxed top lip. In this position, the patient already exposes the apices of the papillae. *(b)* Fistula at the right central incisor with horizontal root fracture in the middle third. *(c)* Radiograph of preoperative situation. *(d)* Sealing the socket with an FMG (socket seal surgery). *(e)* Condition 1 week postoperatively with bonded partial denture. *(f)* After removal of the bonded partial denture. *(g)* Condition 6 weeks postoperatively prior to bone augmentation. *(h)* Defect at the right central incisor with complete loss of the buccal and palatal lamellae.

Fig 8-10 *cont.* / *(i)* Occlusal view of the defect. *(j)* Autogenous bone graft from the right retromolar region. *(k)* Augmented area with laser-perforated titanium membrane fixed with titanium pins. *(l)* Condition immediately after augmentation. Only one relieving incision was placed distal to the distal adjacent tooth. *(m)* After reopening and removal of the titanium membrane, regenerated alveolar ridge 3 months after augmentation can be observed. *(n)* Radiograph after augmentation. *(o)* Paralleling pin in place. *(p)* Placement of a 3.8-mm-diameter implant.

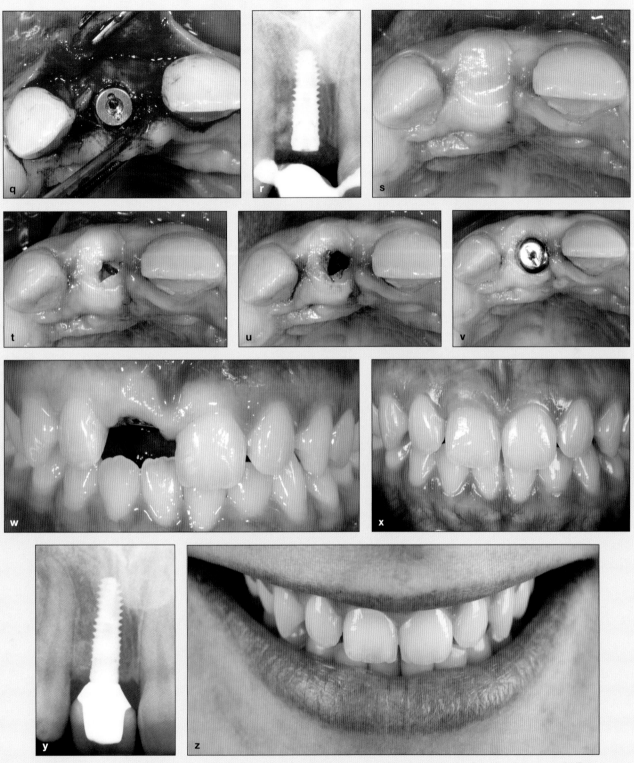

Fig 8-10 *cont.* / *(q)* Implant in place; there is sufficient bone available buccally. *(r)* Radiograph after implant placement. *(s)* Fully healed site 8 weeks after implant placement. *(t)* Exposure by excision of approximately 2 mm² mucosa. *(u)* After dilation of the opening, the cover screw can be removed (see "Keyhole access expansion technique" in chapter 10). *(v)* A prefabricated gingiva former was used. *(w)* Condition immediately after minimally invasive exposure. *(x)* Finished superstructure in situ. *(y)* Radiograph at restoration. *(z)* Smile after completion of the treatment. (Surgery and prosthodontics performed by A. Happe; laboratory work performed by A. Nolte.)

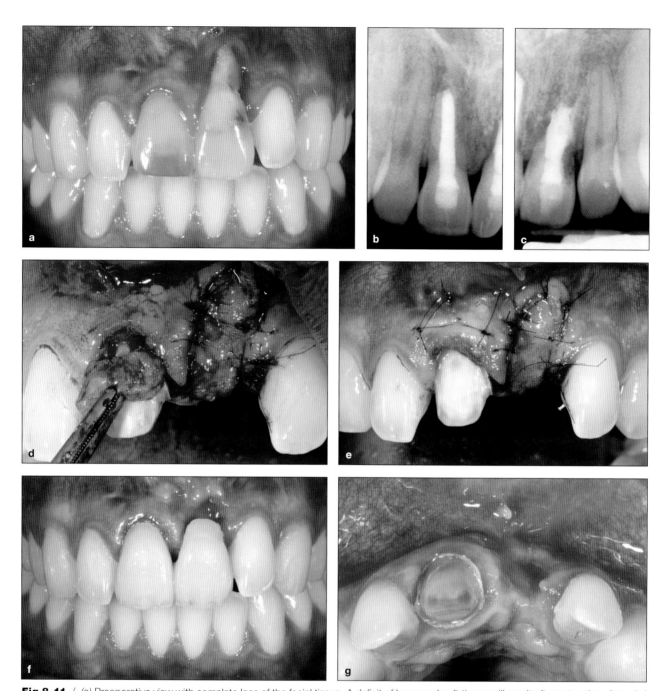

158

Fig 8-11 / *(a)* Preoperative view with complete loss of the facial tissue. A deficit of bone and soft tissue will result after extraction. *(b and c)* Radiographs of the maxillary central incisors. The left central incisor shows clear signs of external resorption. *(d)* The orifice of the extraction socket of the left incisor was sealed with a CTG, and the soft tissue defect was thereby reconstructed. *(e)* A vestibular pocket was created at the right central incisor to incorporate a graft with the aid of a vertical mattress suture. *(f)* Healed region of the left central incisor with fixed provisional restoration in place. *(g)* Healed left central incisor site with an alveolar ridge defect, which now constitutes a typical situation.

mediately after extraction, therefore, a subepithelial CTG was taken from the palate to reconstruct the soft tissue defect. A collagen matrix was introduced into the socket as the underlying base. (Hard materials would not be used today.) Bone regeneration is not expected in this situation; the material merely serves as a biocompatible underlay for the graft.

Using the envelope technique, another CTG was placed facial to the right central incisor for preprosthetic thickening of the soft tissue. These measures made it possible to change the tricky preoperative situation into a standard situation so that the bony defect could be regenerated with a combination of an autogenous bone graft from the retromolar region and layering with an inorganic bovine bone substitute and collagen membrane.

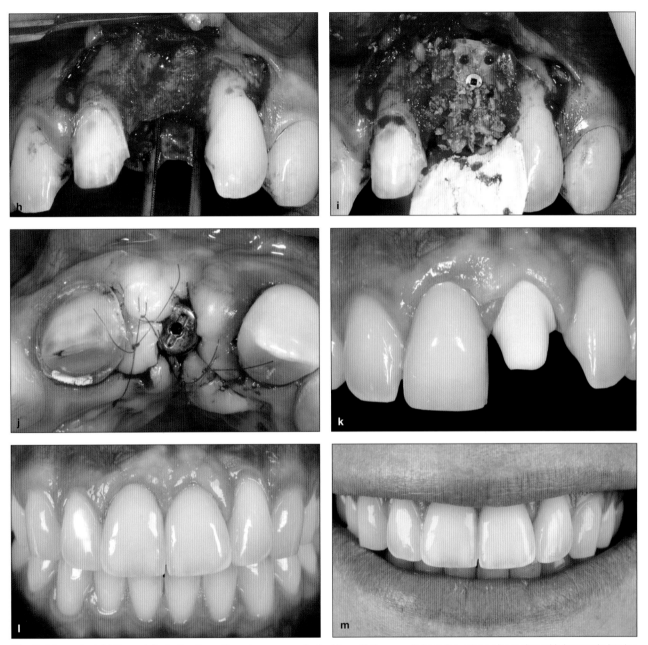

Fig 8-11 *cont.* / *(h)* Bony defect after formation of a mucoperiosteal flap. *(i)* Bone graft from the retromolar region with inorganic bovine bone substitute and collagen membrane. *(j)* Condition after microsurgical exposure. *(k)* Try-in of the customized zirconia abutment. After an implant-supported provisional restoration was worn for 1 year, the definitive restoration was placed. *(l and m)* Final appearance 1 year after the definitive restoration. (Surgery and prosthodontics performed by A. Happe; laboratory work performed by A. Nolte.)

CTGs Associated with Bone Augmentation

One of the most common complications associated with bone augmentation is dehiscence, resulting in exposure of the augmentation material and subsequent infection. Although this complication is primarily a soft tissue complication, it can lead to complete loss of the augmentation material.[40] Because the whole purpose of augmentation is to increase the bone volume, mobilization of enough soft tissue for coverage is one of the major challenges in these operations.

Several authors have described a palatal pedicle CTG, which allows two-layer coverage of the augmented site and should therefore reduce the risk of dehiscence[2,41] (Fig 8-12). For this purpose, in the same way as harvesting a CTG, an incision is made that opens into the deficient area (here the augmentation site). A CTG is then harvested,

159

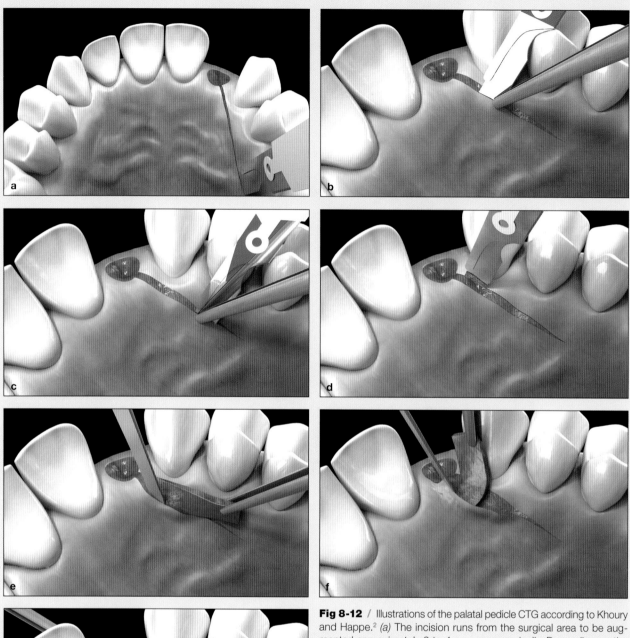

Fig 8-12 / Illustrations of the palatal pedicle CTG according to Khoury and Happe.[2] *(a)* The incision runs from the surgical area to be augmented approximately 3 to 4 mm paramarginally. Depending on the tissue requirement, it extends about two tooth widths from the anterior dentition distally and to a depth of about 1.5 mm. *(b)* The scalpel is rotated to dissect a mucosal flap roughly 1.5 mm thick. *(c)* The whole area must be carefully dissected. *(d)* The graft is incised 1 mm medial from the access incision. *(e)* A scalpel is used to make a complete incision around the graft, which is then loosened with a raspatory. *(f)* The graft is detached from distal to mesial. *(g)* The graft can now be rotated clockwise into the defect. ⟶

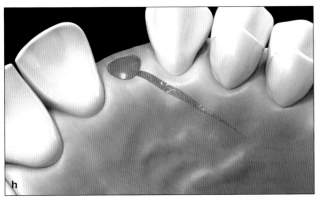
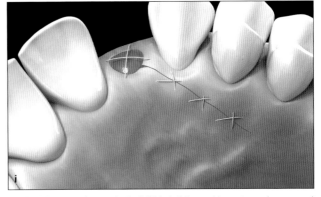

Fig 8-12 *cont.* / *(h)* Finally, the graft is exposed only in the deficient area (in this case, the socket). *(i)* This is followed by suture closure and fixing the graft in the defect.

Fig 8-13 / *(a)* Palatal pedicle CTG in the region of the maxillary right canine to second premolar. The donor site communicates with the defect area at the right lateral incisor. *(b)* The graft is rotated into the defect area.

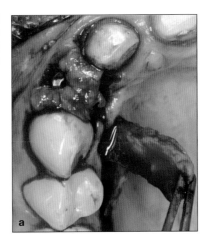
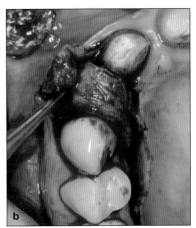

161

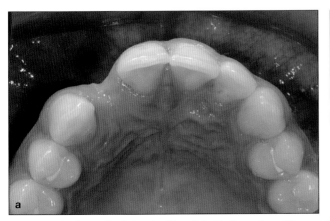
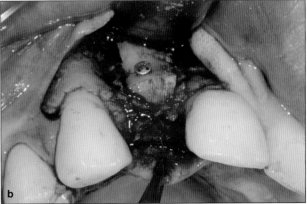

Fig 8-14 / *(a)* Localized alveolar ridge defect in the region of the maxillary right lateral incisor. *(b)* Augmentation with autogenous bone graft.

and it remains pedicled close to the defect and can be rotated and sunk into the deficient area. At the end of the operation, the donor site is completely covered again (Figs 8-13 and 8-14).

In a few cases, connective tissue healing of alveolar ridge defects is observed such that reflection of the mucoperiosteal flap results in an excess of tissue on the wound flap; this would make it difficult to appose the flap after augmentation, and it would have to be removed. In this case, this tissue can also be used to raise a buccally pedicled, tongue-like flap. This pedicle CTG can then be pulled into a pocket created palatally with the aid of a vertical mattress suture. Therefore, adequate soft tissue sealing can also be achieved (Fig 8-15).

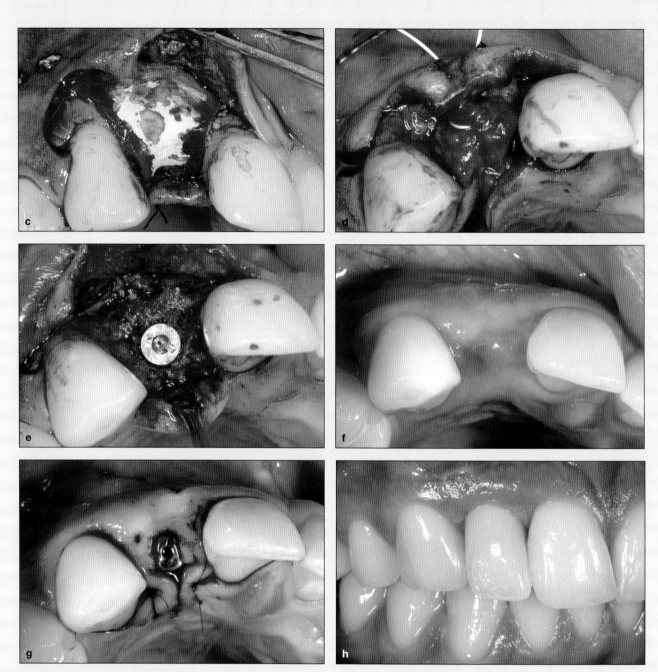

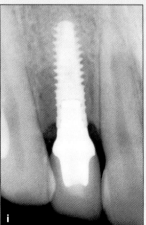

Fig 8-14 *cont.* / *(c)* The graft is covered with biomaterial and a collagen membrane. *(d)* Soft tissue augmentation with palatal pedicle CTG from the region of the right canine and premolars. *(e)* Implant placement 3 months after augmentation. *(f)* Healed site before exposure. *(g)* Microsurgical exposure by the split-finger technique. *(h and i)* Clinical view and radiograph 6 months after implant placement. (Surgery and prosthodontics performed by A. Happe; laboratory work performed by A. Nolte.)

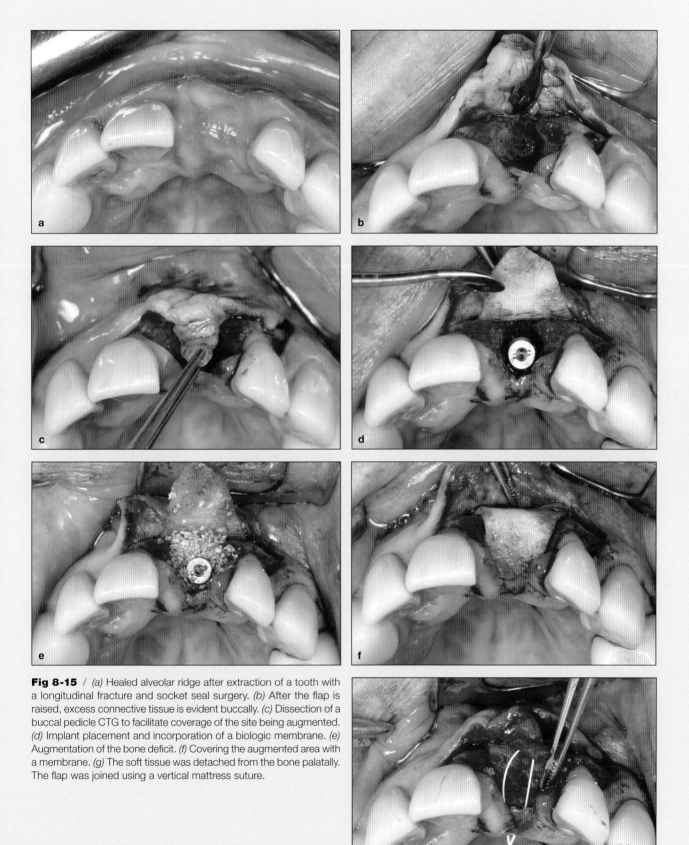

Fig 8-15 / *(a)* Healed alveolar ridge after extraction of a tooth with a longitudinal fracture and socket seal surgery. *(b)* After the flap is raised, excess connective tissue is evident buccally. *(c)* Dissection of a buccal pedicle CTG to facilitate coverage of the site being augmented. *(d)* Implant placement and incorporation of a biologic membrane. *(e)* Augmentation of the bone deficit. *(f)* Covering the augmented area with a membrane. *(g)* The soft tissue was detached from the bone palatally. The flap was joined using a vertical mattress suture.

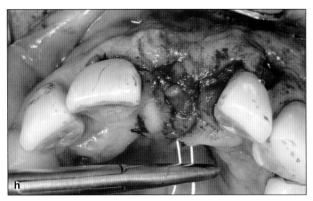
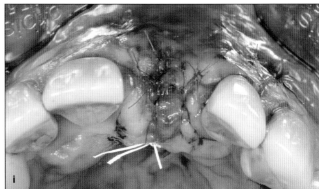

Fig 8-15 *cont.* / *(h)* The buccal pedicle flap is pulled into the palatal pocket with the vertical mattress suture, and the augmented area is sealed. *(i)* Lengthening the mucoperiosteal flap creates a tension-free, adequate soft tissue seal. *(j)* Fully healed site 2 weeks postoperatively.

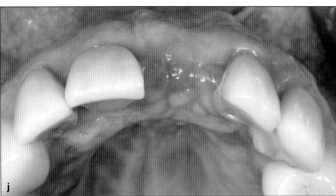

CTGs at Implant Placement

If bone has to be augmented before implantology treatment, connective tissue augmentation is likely to be performed together with implant placement in many cases.

Clinical case

The patient wanted an esthetic improvement in the maxillary right canine to left central incisor area, which had been restored with an old porcelain-fused-to-metal (PFM) partial denture (Figs 8-16a to 8-16c). A new partial denture was ruled out because the patient wanted single-tooth restorations. Bone augmentation was first carried out with a block graft from a retromolar location (Figs 8-16d and 8-16e). After uncomplicated healing, implants were placed in the region of the right incisors 3 months later (Figs 8-16f to 8-16k). Both implants were placed, and a combined CTG with mucosal portion (inlay graft) was placed (Figs 8-16l to 8-16o). The implants were exposed 2 months later after uncomplicated healing by the minimally invasive keyhole access expansion technique (see chapter 10). Because there was still not enough keratinized mucosa available in the region of the right central incisor, a mucosal graft with keratinized tissue was harvested from the first quadrant buccally and introduced into the region of the right incisors (Figs 8-16p to 8-16s). After incorporation, raised areas that had formed due to scarred healing were leveled and contoured with a rotary diamond (Figs 8-16t and 8-16u). The peri-implant tissue was first shaped with provisional restorations, and then definitive all-ceramic restoration took place after 6 months' maturation (Fig 8-16v).

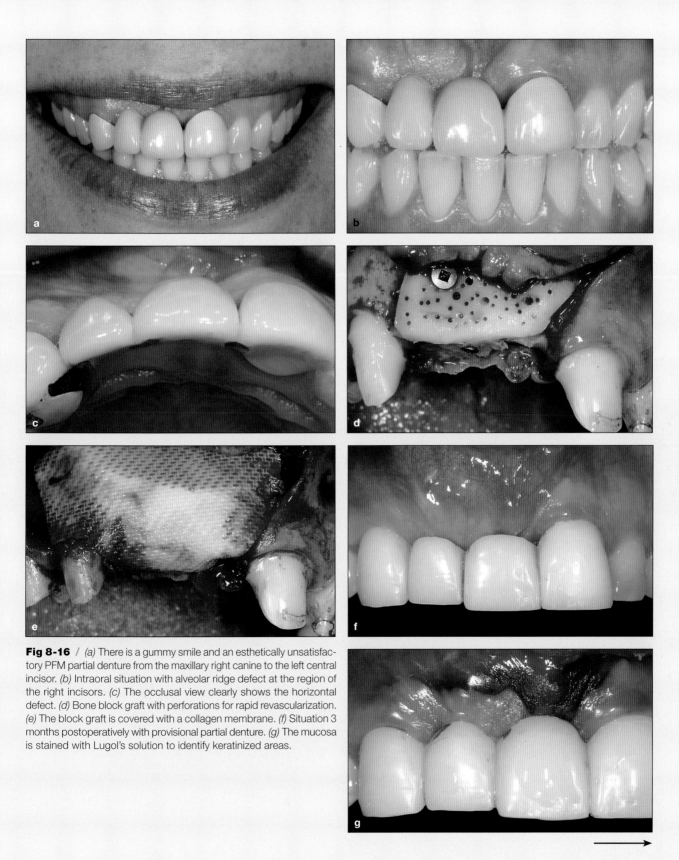

Fig 8-16 / *(a)* There is a gummy smile and an esthetically unsatisfactory PFM partial denture from the maxillary right canine to the left central incisor. *(b)* Intraoral situation with alveolar ridge defect at the region of the right incisors. *(c)* The occlusal view clearly shows the horizontal defect. *(d)* Bone block graft with perforations for rapid revascularization. *(e)* The block graft is covered with a collagen membrane. *(f)* Situation 3 months postoperatively with provisional partial denture. *(g)* The mucosa is stained with Lugol's solution to identify keratinized areas.

166

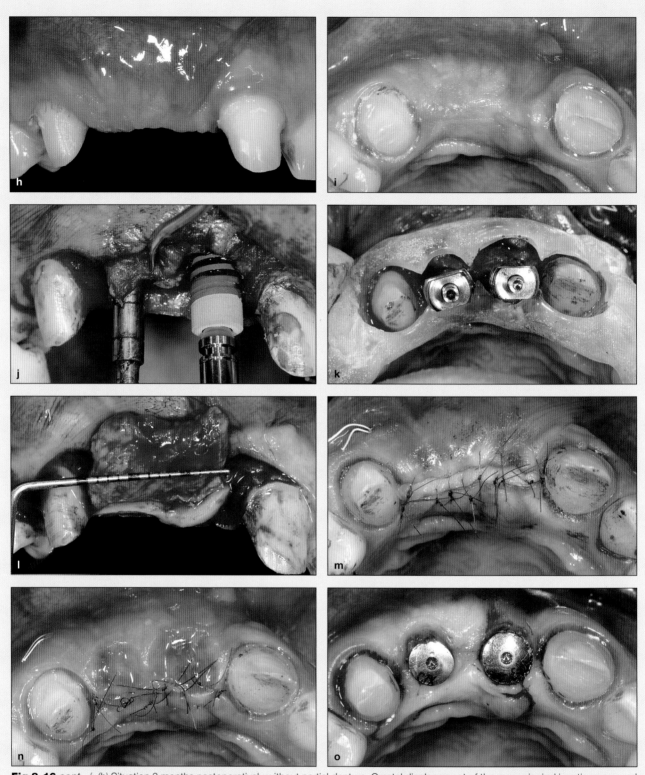

Fig 8-16 *cont.* / *(h)* Situation 3 months postoperatively without partial denture. Crestal displacement of the mucogingival junction occurred as a result of the augmentation surgery. *(i)* Occlusal view of the augmented alveolar ridge. *(j)* Implant placement at the sites of the right incisors. *(k)* The implants in situ with a surgical template. The position of the implants is displaced slightly palatally. *(l)* The soft tissue graft is fitted into the defect. The mucosal part is visible. *(m)* Condition after implant placement and soft tissue augmentation. *(n)* Situation 1 week postoperatively; the wound is free of irritation. *(o)* Exposed implants with gingiva formers.

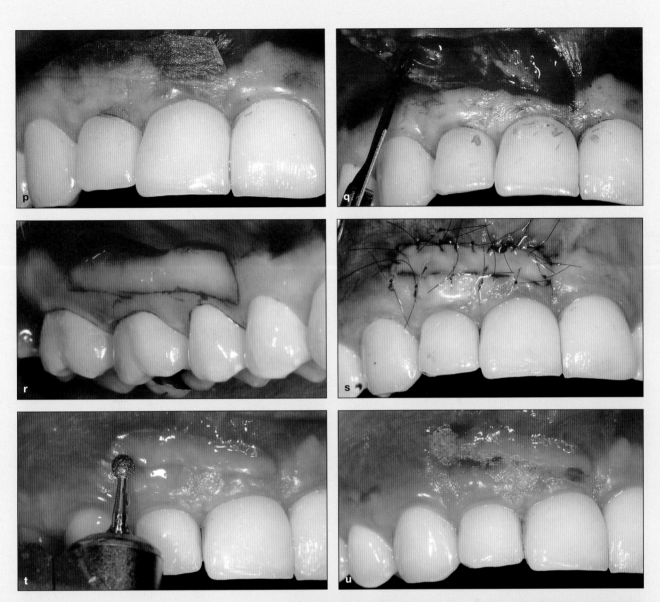

Fig 8-16 *cont.* / *(p)* A piece of sterile paper serves as a template for transferring the dimensions of the mucosal graft to the donor site. The mucosa is stained to identify keratinized areas. *(q)* The graft bed is prepared. *(r)* Harvesting the FMG buccally in the first quadrant. *(s)* The FMG is microsurgically fixed. *(t)* A few weeks after uncomplicated incorporation of the FMG, ablative tissue contouring is completed using a rotary diamond. *(u)* Condition after tissue abrasion. *(v)* Smile after treatment with definitive all-ceramic restoration of the anterior dentition with implants at the right incisors. (Surgery and prosthodontics performed by G. Körner; laboratory work performed by K. Müterthies.)

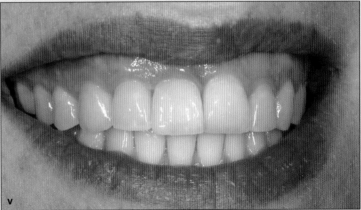

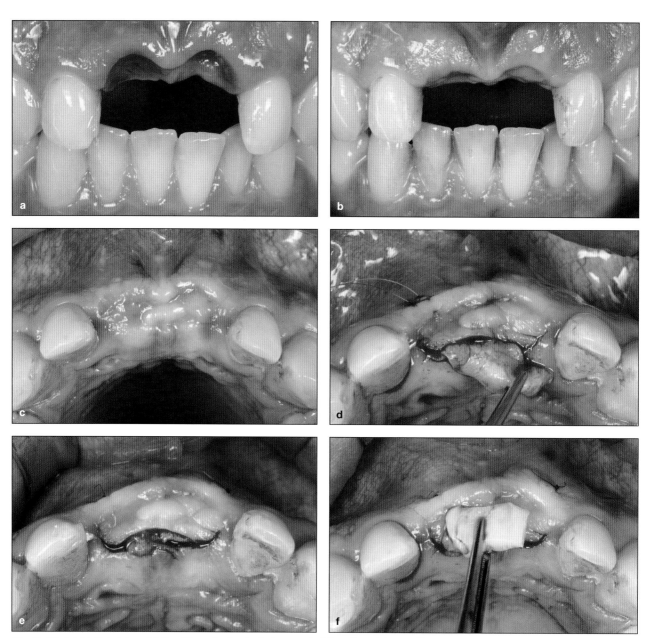

Fig 8-17 / *(a)* Initial status. *(b)* Condition after implant placement at the sites of the maxillary central incisors and bone augmentation by guided bone regeneration. *(c)* Condition before connective tissue augmentation. *(d)* The first graft is pulled into the pocket with the vertical mattress suture. *(e)* Two vertical mattress sutures are used to fix the first graft in the pocket buccal to the ridge. *(f)* The second graft from the tuberosity region.

⟶

CTG as a Separate Procedure

Clinical case

In a few cases, it may be best to carry out augmentation of connective tissue in a separate procedure and not combine it with other interventions. A man in his early twenties presented with an edentulous gap in the region of the maxillary right incisors and a 3D alveolar ridge defect (Fig 8-17a). After implant placement and augmentation, there

was still a lack of ridge volume (Figs 8-17b and 8-17c). Therefore, augmentation of connective tissue was performed about 8 weeks before the exposure procedure. A graft was harvested from the palate in the premolar region, and a second graft was taken from the tuberosity. Grafts from the tuberosity area are usually richer in connective tissue than grafts from the premolar region and also contain smaller fatty and glandular proportions. Therefore, grafts from the tuberosity region are generally more stable in terms of volume.

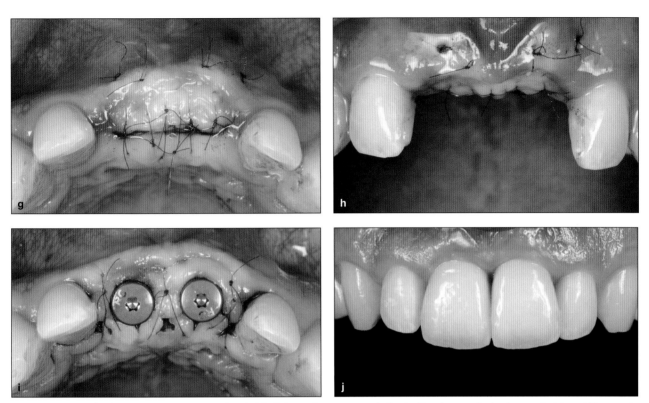

Fig 8-17 *cont.* / *(g)* The procedure is completed. All of the grafts are securely fixed with microsurgical suture material, and the area is sealed. *(h)* Frontal view. *(i)* Around 8 weeks after the soft tissue augmentation, the implants were microsurgically uncovered by the split-finger technique. *(j)* Final appearance after prosthetic restoration of the implants. (Surgery performed by A. Happe; prosthodontics performed by B. van den Bosch; laboratory work performed by P. Holthaus.)

Augmentation was performed through crestal access, through which the crestal and vestibular soft tissue at the central incisors was detached from bone. The first graft (from the premolar region) was placed facially (Figs 8-17d and 8-17e), and the second (from the tuberosity) was located crestally (Figs 8-17f to 8-17h) to facilitate the interdental papilla between the implants. After uncomplicated incorporation, implant exposure was performed by the split-finger technique (Fig 8-17i) (see also chapter 10). By this technique, additional tissue is brought from the palatal to the vestibular position. An acceptable result was achieved by the combination of hard and soft tissue augmentation (Fig 8-17j).

CTG at Exposure

The importance of the implant exposure operation is often underestimated. However, at this stage it is actually still possible to exert a decisive influence on the treatment outcome. Augmentation with connective tissue can still take place at the time of exposure.

The case illustrated in Fig 8-18 shows the placement of a CTG in combination with a split-finger technique according to Misch[42] (for complete case see chapter 9, Fig 9-20). The flap is preferably raised as a split flap, and the graft is placed between the periosteum, which remains on the bone, and the mucosa. If osteosynthesis material has to be removed and a full-thickness mucoperiosteal flap needs to be prepared, the graft can also be placed directly on the bone. A clinical trial by Puišys and Linkevičius showed that it is also possible to achieve mucosal thickening with the aid of substitute materials for connective tissue.[30] The case illustrated in Fig 8-19 shows the use of a porcine dermis for increasing soft tissue thickness on exposure by the split-finger technique.

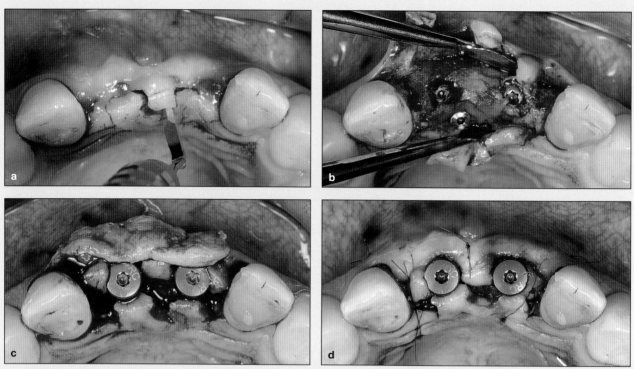

Fig 8-18 / *(a)* Microsurgical exposure of two implants in the region of the maxillary right incisors by the split-finger technique. *(b)* Access to the implants and removal of osteosynthesis material. *(c)* Subepithelial CTG is used to thicken the facial soft tissue. *(d)* Condition at the end of the exposure operation. Microsurgical suturing and complete coverage of the graft. (See Fig 9-20 for complete case.)

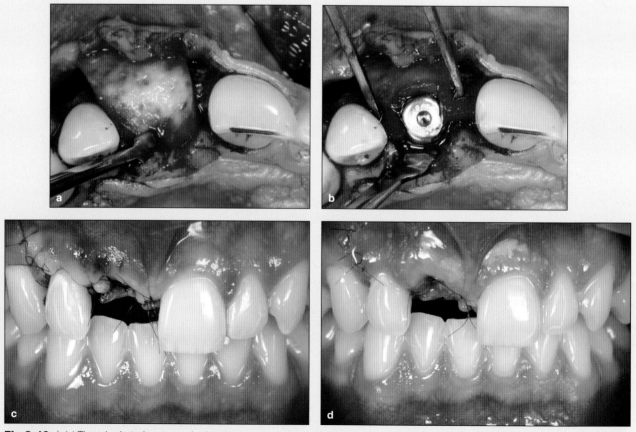

Fig 8-19 / *(a)* The rehydrated xenogeneic dermis was properly trimmed to the dimensions of the defect. *(b)* After exposure of the implant, the substitute material is introduced by means of mucosal flap formation according to the split-finger technique. *(c)* The mucosa is apposed with 6-0 monofilament sutures. *(d)* Frontal view of wound conditions on suture removal 1 week postoperatively.

References

1. Khoury F, Happe A. Soft tissue management in oral implantology: A review of surgical techniques for shaping an esthetic and functional peri-implant soft tissue structure. Quintessence Int 2000;31:483–499.

2. Khoury F, Happe A. The palatal subepithelial connective tissue flap method for soft tissue management to cover maxillary defects: A clinical report. Int J Oral Maxillofac Implants 2000;15:415–418.

3. Song JE, Um YJ, Kim CS, et al. Thickness of posterior palatal masticatory mucosa: The use of computerized tomography. J Periodontol 2008;79:406–412.

4. Barriviera M, Duarte WR, Januário AL, Faber J, Bezerra AC. A new method to assess and measure palatal masticatory mucosa by cone-beam computerized tomography. J Clin Periodontol 2009;36:564–568.

5. Müller HP, Eger T. Masticatory mucosa and periodontal phenotype: A review. Int J Periodontics Restorative Dent 2002;22:172–183.

6. Langer B, Langer L. Subepithelial connective tissue graft technique for root coverage. J Periodontol 1985;56:715–720.

7. Miller PD Jr. Root coverage using the free soft tissue autograft following citric acid application. III. A successful and predictable procedure in areas of deep-wide recession. Int J Periodontics Restorative Dent 1985;5:14–37.

8. Abrams L. Augmentation of the deformed residual edentulous ridge for fixed prosthesis. Compend Contin Educ Gen Dent 1980;1:205–213.

9. Allen EP, Gainza CS, Farthing GG, Newbold DA. Improved technique for localized ridge augmentation. A report of 21 cases. J Periodontol 1985;56:195–199.

10. Studer SP, Allen EP, Rees TC, Kouba A. The thickness of masticatory mucosa in the human hard palate and tuberosity as potential donor sites for ridge augmentation procedures. J Periodontol 1997;68:145–151.

11. Langer B, Calagna L. The subepithelial connective tissue graft. J Prosthet Dent 1980;44:363–367.

12. Langer B, Calagna LJ. The subepithelial connective tissue graft. A new approach to the enhancement of anterior cosmetics. Int J Periodontics Restorative Dent 1982;2:22–33.

13. Garber DA. The esthetic dental implant: Letting restoration be the guide. J Oral Implantol 1996;22:45–50.

14. Scharf DR, Tarnow DP. Modified roll technique for localized alveolar ridge augmentation. Int J Periodontics Restorative Dent 1992;12:415–425.

15. Israelson H, Plemons JM. Dental implants, regenerative techniques, and periodontal plastic surgery to restore maxillary anterior esthetics. Int J Oral Maxillofac Implants 1993;8:555–561.

16. Cortellini P, Tonetti MS. Microsurgical approach to periodontal regeneration. Initial evaluation in a case cohort. J Periodontol 2001;72:559–569.

17. Wachtel H, Schenk G, Böhm S, Weng D, Zuhr O, Hürzeler MB. Microsurgical access flap and enamel matrix derivative for the treatment of periodontal intrabony defects: A controlled clinical study. J Clin Periodontol 2003;30:496–504.

18. Zadeh HH, Daftary F. Minimally invasive surgery: An alternative approach for periodontal and implant reconstruction. J Calif Dent Assoc 2004;32:1022–1030.

19. Shanelec DA. Anterior esthetic implants: Microsurgical placement in extraction sockets with immediate plovisionals. J Calif Dent Assoc 2005;33:233–240.

20. Burkhardt R, Lang NP. Coverage of localized gingival recessions: Comparison of micro- and macrosurgical techniques. J Clin Periodontol 2005;32:287–293.

21. Berglundh T, Lindhe J. Dimension of the periimplant mucosa. Biological width revisited. J Clin Periodontol 1996;23:971–973.

22. Mankoo T. Single-tooth implant restorations in the esthetic zone—Contemporary concepts for optimization and maintenance of soft tissue esthetics in the replacement of failing teeth in compromised sites. Eur J Esthet Dent 2007;2:274–295.

23. Funato A, Salama MA, Ishikawa T, Garber DA, Salama H. Timing, positioning, and sequential staging in esthetic implant therapy: A four-dimensional perspective. Int J Periodontics Restorative Dent 2007;27:313–323.

24. Jung RE, Holderegger C, Sailer I, Khraisat A, Suter A, Hämmerle CH. The effect of all-ceramic and porcelain-fused-to-metal restorations on marginal peri-implant soft tissue color: A randomized controlled clinical trial. Int J Periodontics Restorative Dent 2008;28:357–365.

25. Lee A, Fu JH, Wang HL. Soft tissue biotype affects implant success. Implant Dent 2011;20:e38–e47.

26. Jung RE, Sailer I, Hämmerle CH, Attin T, Schmidlin P. In vitro color changes of soft tissues caused by restorative materials. Int J Periodontics Restorative Dent 2007;27:251–257.

27. Park SE, Da Silva JD, Weber HP, Ishikawa-Nagai S. Optical phenomenon of peri-implant soft tissue. Part I. Spectrophotometric assessment of natural tooth gingiva and peri-implant mucosa. Clin Oral Implants Res 2007;18:569–574.

28. Wiesner G, Esposito M, Worthington H, Schlee M. Connective tissue grafts for thickening peri-implant tissues at implant placement. One-year results from an explanatory split-mouth randomised controlled clinical trial. Eur J Oral Implantol 2010;3:27–35.

29. Schneider D, Grunder U, Ender A, Hämmerle CH, Jung RE. Volume gain and stability of peri-implant tissue following bone and soft-tissue augmentation: 1-year results from a prospective cohort study. Clin Oral Implants Res 2011;22:28–37.

30. Puišys A, Linkevičius T. The influence of mucosal tissue thickening on crestal bone stability around bone-level implants. A prospective controlled clinical trial. Clin Oral Implants Res 2015;26:123–129.

31. Thoma DS, Benić GI, Zwahlen M, Hämmerle CH, Jung RE. A systematic review assessing soft tissue augmentation techniques. Clin Oral Implants Res 2009;20(suppl 4):146–165.

32. Burkhardt R, Joss A, Lang NP. Soft tissue dehiscence coverage around endosseous implants: A prospective cohort study. Clin Oral Implants Res 2008;19:451–457.

33. Chen ST, Wilson TG Jr, Hämmerle CH. Immediate or early placement of implants following tooth extraction: Review of biologic basis, clinical procedures, and outcomes. Int J Oral Maxillofac Implants 2004;19(suppl):12–25.

34. Chen ST, Darby IB, Reynolds EC. A prospective clinical study of non-submerged immediate implants: Clinical outcomes and esthetic results. Clin Oral Implants Res 2007;18:552–562.

35. Landsberg CJ. Socket seal surgery combined with immediate implant placement: A novel approach for single-tooth replacement. Int J Periodontics Restorative Dent 1997;17:140–149.

36. Jung RE, Siegenthaler DW, Hämmerle CH. Postextraction tissue management: A soft tissue punch technique. Int J Periodontics Restorative Dent 2004;24:545–553.

37. Fickl S, Zuhr O, Wachtel H, Bolz W, Huerzeler MB. Hard tissue alterations after socket preservation: An experimental study in the beagle dog. Clin Oral Implants Res 2008;19:1111–1118.

38. Horváth A, Mardas N, Mezzomo LA, Needleman IG, Donos N. Alveolar ridge preservation. A systematic review. Clin Oral Investig 2013;17:341–363.

171

39. Weng D, Stock V, Schliephake H. Are socket and ridge preservation techniques at the day of tooth extraction efficient in maintaining the tissues of the alveolar ridge? Systematic review, consensus statements and recommendations of the 1st DGI Consensus conference in September 2010, Aerzen, Germany. Eur J Oral Implantol 2011;4(suppl):S59–S66.
40. Happe A, Khoury F. Complications and risk factors in bone grafting procedures. In: Khoury F, Antoun H, Missika P (eds). Bone Augmentation in Oral Implantology. Chicago: Quintessence, 2007:405–429.
41. Nemcovsky CE, Artzi Z, Moses O. Rotated palatal flap in immediate implant procedures. Clinical evaluation of 26 consecutive cases. Clin Oral Implants Res 2000;11:83–90.
42. Misch CE, Al-Shammari KF, Wang HL. Creation of interimplant papillae through a split-finger technique. Implant Dent 2004;13:20–27.

"Things don't just happen.
They are made to happen."

JOHN F. KENNEDY

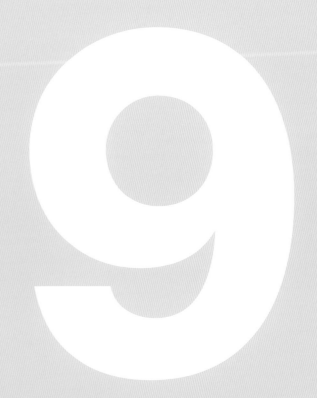

Bone Augmentation

/ Arndt Happe, Daniel Rothamel, Gerd Körner

I f there are alveolar ridge defects in the esthetic zone, tissue must be regenerated to restore bone to a stable volume with adequate anatomical architecture. This is the only way to achieve an esthetic, natural-looking result. The predictability of augmentation measures depends not only on the technique selected, but also on the nature of the defect and the quality of the tissue involved.

Apart from the technique and the patient's general state of health, the following factors also influence the outcome of augmentation procedures:

- Defect dimensions
- Configuration of the defect (eg, horizontal, vertical, three-dimensional, single-wall, two-wall, three-wall)
- Location of the defect (eg, maxilla, mandible, anterior region, posterior region)
- Bone quality
- Surgical skills (known as the *center effect*)

There is no universal approach to the treatment of ridge defects. Every defect is unique and has specific requirements in terms of hard and soft tissue reconstruction.[1]

Based on the scientific literature on bone augmentation, there is more evidence in favor of a two-stage procedure than for simultaneous augmentation with implant placement.[2] Autogenous bone grafts are the gold standard, but bone substitute materials function very well if they are used with suitable techniques for their specific indications.[3] For instance, there is little evidence for the use of substitute materials in vertical defects. They should be used solely for horizontal defects and preferably for defects within the jaw contour (ie, intrabony defect) rather than outside the contour (ie, contour-forming defect).[4] Benic and Hämmerle[5] developed a clear classification that links the specific preoperative clinical situations to a particular therapeutic approach (Table 9-1 and Figs 9-1 to 9-4).

Table 9-1 Description of defects and treatment*

Class	Morphology of defect	Treatment option
0	Optimal ridge contour, sufficient bone volume	GBR
1	Intra-alveolar defect between implant and bone	GBR
2	Peri-implant 5-wall defect, volume stability	GBR
3	Peri-implant 4-wall defect, no volume stability	GBR
4	Horizontal ridge defect	Additional stabilization
5	Vertical ridge defect	Additional stabilization

GBR, guided bone regeneration.
*Adapted from Benic and Hämmerle.[5]

174

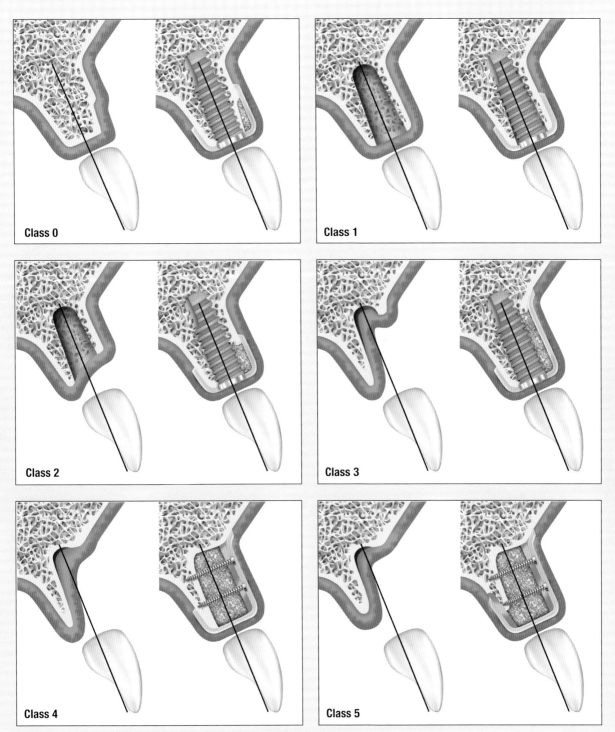

Fig 9-1 / Defect morphology and treatment option for alveolar ridge defects (adapted from Benic and Hämmerle[5]).

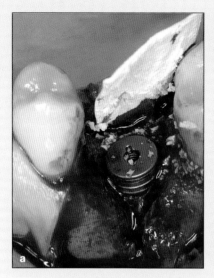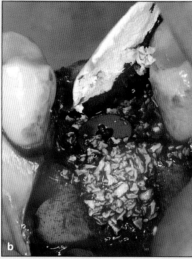

Fig 9-2 / *(a)* Example of a defect inside the alveolar ridge contour. *(b)* This can be treated with a xenogeneic substitute material and a collagen membrane.

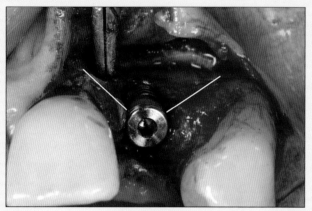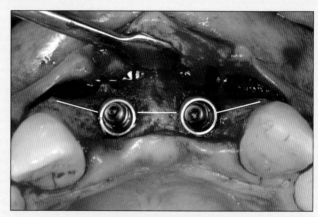

Fig 9-3 / Moderate lateral defect. The implant lies within the ridge contour.

Fig 9-4 / Challenging lateral defect with implants that lie partly outside the ridge contour.

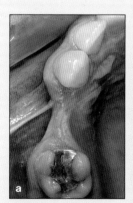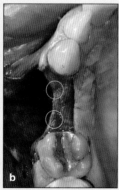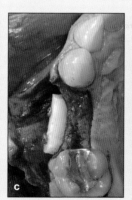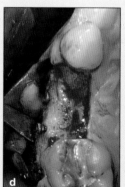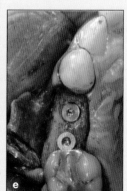

Fig 9-5 / *(a)* Horizontal ridge defect in the region of the maxillary right premolars. *(b)* The bone defect after preparation of a mucoperiosteal flap. *White circles* indicate the planned implant positions. *(c)* Monocortical autogenous bone graft from the mandibular ramus, fixed with osteosynthesis screws (1.2 mm in diameter). *(d)* Integration of the graft after 4 months. *(e)* The implants were placed without any problems.

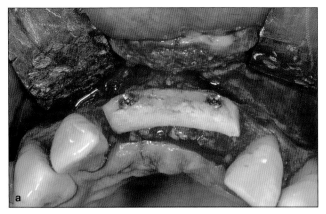

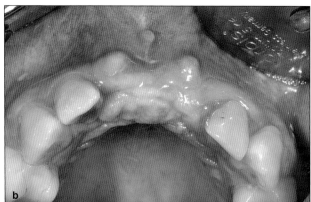

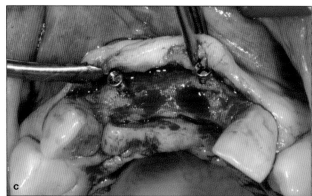

Fig 9-6 / *(a)* Monocortical graft in the region of the maxillary central incisors. *(b and c)* Clinical photographs 3 months after augmentation. More than 50% of the graft has been resorbed.

Reconstruction of Bony Ridge Defects

In recent decades, a large number of treatment options for ridge defects have been described and clinically tested, including guided bone regeneration (GBR), autogenous bone grafts, bone spreading, and distraction osteogenesis.[3,6] Other methods, such as tissue engineering and the use of bone morphogenetic proteins (BMPs) and growth factors, are still at the experimental stage and are not yet widely accepted in terms of clinical use, let alone routine use.

Autogenous bone grafts

The use of autogenous bone grafts for the treatment of intraoral bone defects continues to be seen as the gold standard for horizontal bone regeneration.[7] These grafts are usually harvested as bone blocks from the retromolar region or the mandibular symphysis, and they can be screwed onto the local bone as lateral or onlay grafts.[8–11]

Bone block grafts have demonstrated good bony integration (Fig 9-5), but depending on the technique chosen, they can have a tendency to resorb to various degrees.[3,6,12,13] An average resorption rate of up to 20% is reported in the literature[6] (Fig 9-6).

To reduce the loss of volume of augmented bone, a proposal was made to cover the autogenous, monocortical block graft with a xenogeneic material and a collagen membrane.[14] The authors reported an average 7% reduction in the mean total volume change with this technique. However, monocortical bone blocks do entail a risk of slow remodeling, so bone might still be inadequate at the time of implant placement (Figs 9-7 and 9-8). By contrast, particulate bone has a faster remodeling and revascularization rate.[15,16]

Khoury and Khoury[16] introduced a technique in which a thin autogenous cortical bone plate is used as a shield to reconstruct the cortical layer of the deficient bone. This plate creates a space between itself and the local bone, which is filled with bone chips (Fig 9-9). The technique serves the purpose of three-dimensional (3D)

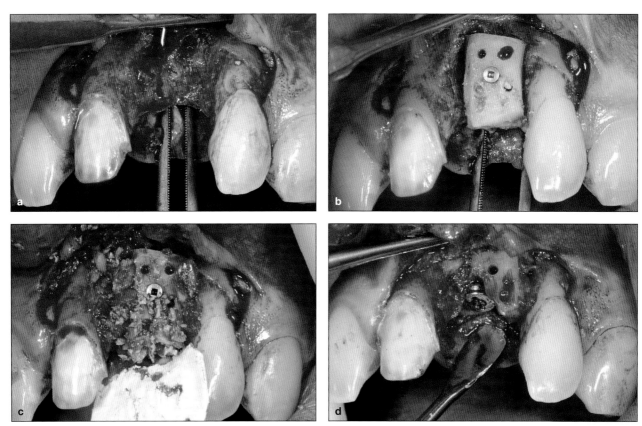

Fig 9-7 / *(a)* Challenging defect in the region of the maxillary left central incisor with loss of attachment mesial to the left lateral incisor. *(b)* Monocortical block fixed over the defect with perforations to facilitate revascularization. *(c)* Covering the graft with xenogeneic substitute material and a collagen membrane (technique according to von Arx and Buser[14]). *(d)* Clinical integration of the graft, given inadequate remodeling.

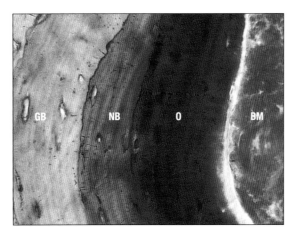

Fig 9-8 / Typical histologic picture of a bone block graft from the retromolar region: Devitalized parts with empty lacunae can clearly be seen. GB, grafted bone; NB, newly formed bone; O, osteoid; BM, bone marrow. (Courtesy of A. Ponte and A. Piatelli.)

reconstruction of substantial bone defects with the aid of autogenous bone, which is rapidly revascularized and remodeled.[16] The technique essentially mimics biology by combining a cortical plate for mechanical stability with a quasi-cancellous internal component, which facilitates good ingrowth of blood vessels. For augmentation in the case of 3D bone defects, one or more bone blocks are harvested—preferably from the ramus and less commonly from the body of the mandible. The cortical bone is separated from the block so that only a relatively thin plate (ie, 1 to 1.5 mm) is harvested. Depending on the size of the plate, one or more bone plates are cut from it

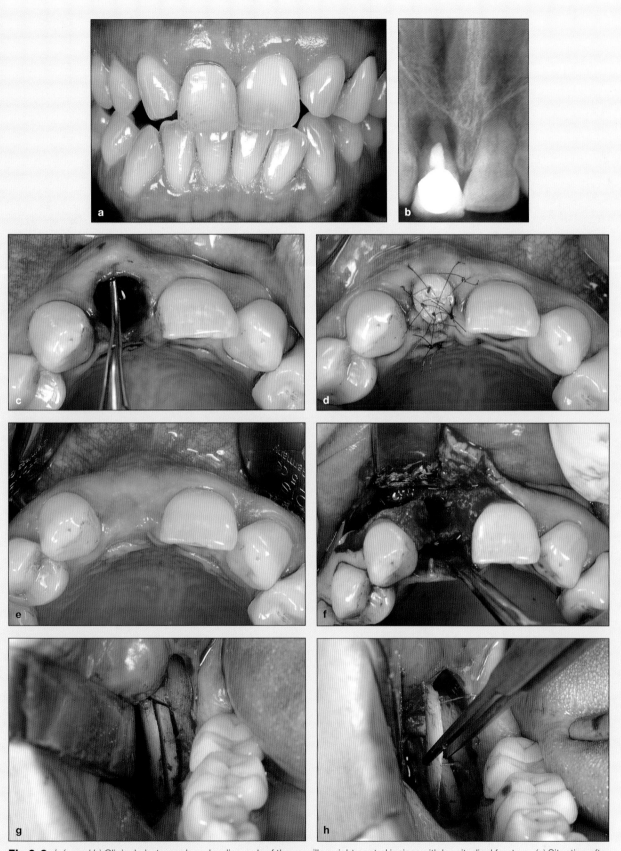

Fig 9-9 / *(a and b)* Clinical photograph and radiograph of the maxillary right central incisor with longitudinal fracture. *(c)* Situation after extraction with loss of buccal and palatal bone wall. *(d)* Free mucosal graft for ridge preservation. The space was filled with collagen sponge. *(e)* Situation after incorporation 6 weeks following extraction and ridge preservation. *(f)* Bone defect with total loss of the labial and palatal cortical lamella. *(g)* Exposure of the mandibular ramus. Two bone disks were cut using piezoelectric surgery. *(h)* With this technique, thin cortical bone disks can easily be harvested from the ramus.

180

Fig 9-9 *cont.* / *(i)* Reconstruction of the labial and palatal cortical bone. *(j)* Vertical height of the grafted labial bone plate. *(k)* The space between the two bone plates is filled with bone chips. *(l)* Flap closure with microsurgical sutures. *(m)* Radiograph after augmentation. *(n)* Situation after 3 mugnths of graft incorporation. *(o)* The implant in place. *(p)* Recontouring the crestal bone.

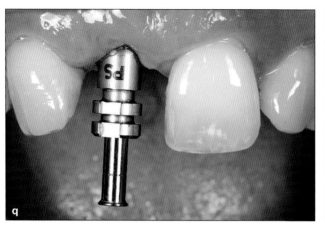
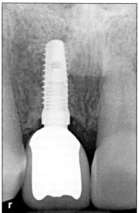

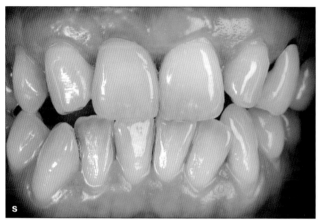
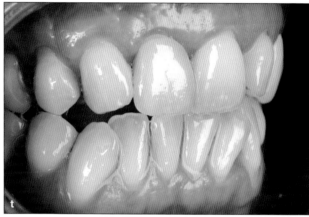

Fig 9-9 *cont.* / *(q)* Impression procedures are performed after the site has healed. *(r)* Radiograph of the definitive restoration. *(s and t)* Frontal and lateral views of the definitive restoration. (Surgery and prosthodontics performed by A. Happe; laboratory work performed by P. Holthaus.)

and shaped to fit onto the defect and replace the missing cortical bone. The space is filled with the crushed remnants of the block (see the textbook by Khoury et al[17] for a detailed description of this technique).

Because it is difficult to cut plates out of bone blocks and there is a certain risk of injury to the surgeon, some authors recommend using a bone mill to produce thin bone apertures.[18] These furthermore have the advantage of already being curved so that they fit to the curvature of the alveolar ridge.[18] However, the plates can also be cut directly from the mandibular ramus with piezoelectric surgical techniques (see Figs 9-9g and 9-9h). Admittedly, harvesting bone grafts from intraoral donor sites tends

to be associated with increased rates of complications and patient morbidity.[19,20] One alternative is to replace the autogenous cortical shell with a xenogeneic cortical plate or a partially demineralized porcine bone plate (Fig 9-10). This modified Khoury technique was the starting point for development of the bone lamina technique described later in this chapter.

The partially demineralized xenogeneic cortical lamella can be shaped after rehydration and adapted to the morphology of the defect. It serves as a space-forming resorbable biologic membrane. It can therefore be used in preimplantology augmentation (see Fig 9-10) or for augmentation in conjunction with implant placement (Fig 9-11).

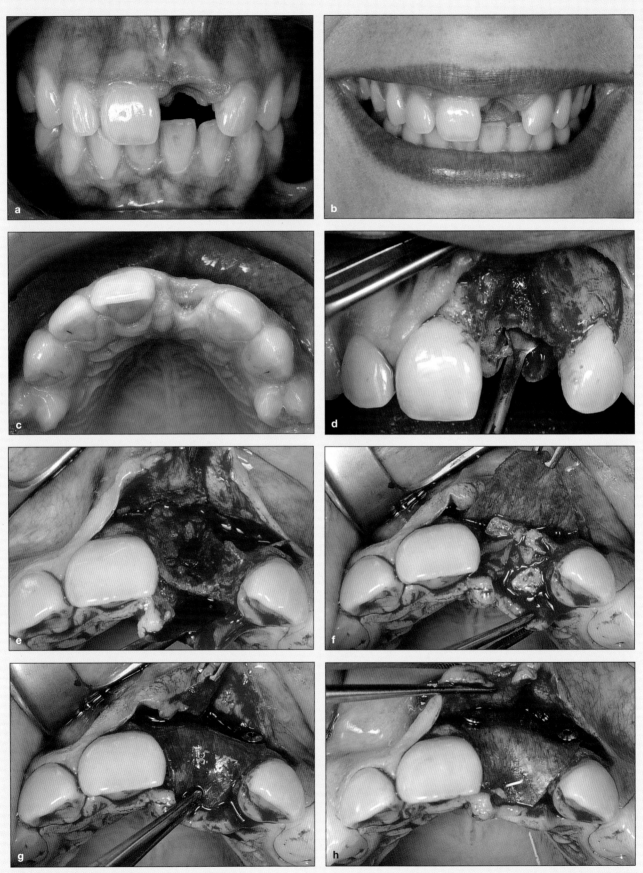

Fig 9-10 / *(a)* Edentulous gap at the region of the maxillary left central incisor. *(b)* The patient has a high smile line. *(c)* Clearly visible ridge defect. *(d and e)* Frontal and occlusal views of the bone defect. *(f)* Augmentation with autogenous bone grafts. *(g)* Covering the defect with a bone lamina. *(h)* The lamina is fixed with titanium pins on the vestibular side and stabilized palatally with a suture.

182

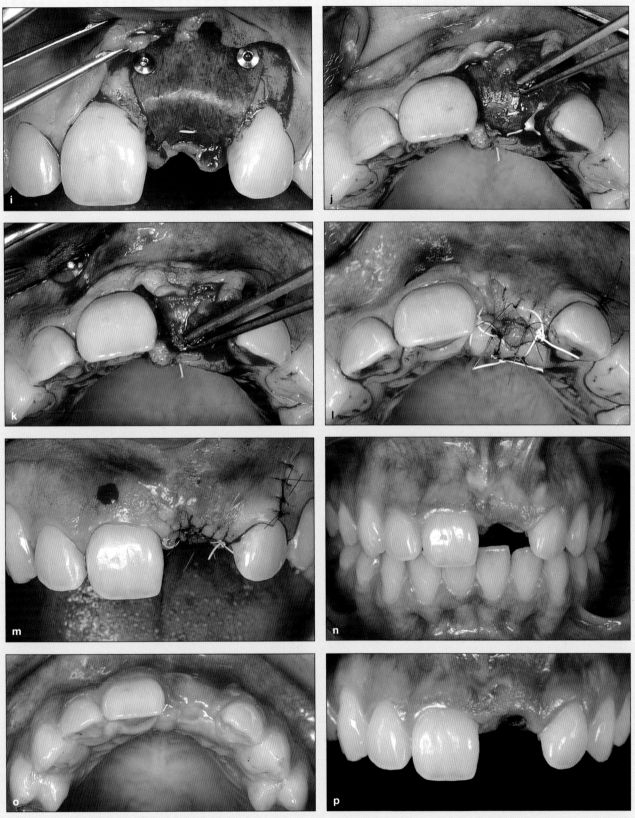

183

Fig 9-10 *cont.* / *(i)* Situation immediately after augmentation. *(j)* When the flap was prepared, connective tissue was mobilized from the flap. *(k)* The mobilized connective tissue allows double-layer soft tissue wound closure. *(l and m)* Microsurgical suture closure. *(n and o)* The healed situation in frontal and occlusal views. *(p)* Condition after complete healing 2 weeks after exposure operation.

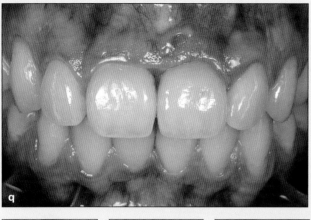

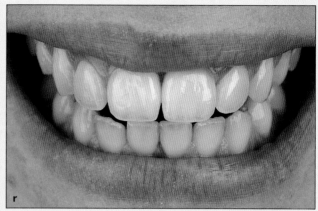

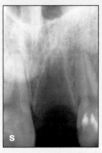
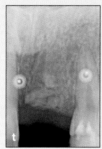
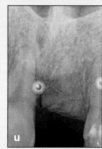
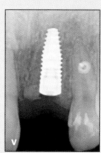
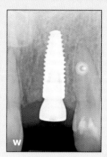
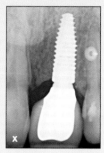

184

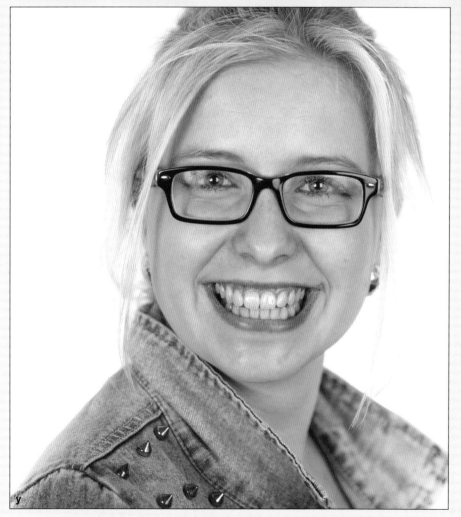

Fig 9-10 *cont.* / *(q and r)* Definitive restoration and smile after completion of treatment. *(s)* Pretreatment radiograph. *(t)* Radiograph of graft in place. *(u to x)* Radiographs after augmentation and at different stages of implant treatment. *(y)* Final portrait. (Surgery and prosthodontics performed by A. Happe; laboratory work performed by P. Holthaus.)

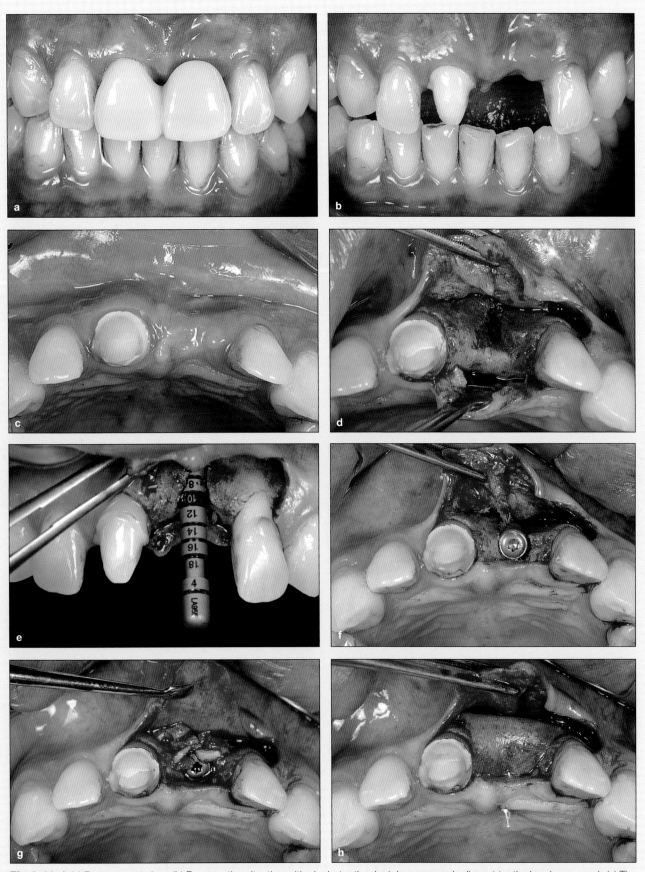

Fig 9-11 / *(a)* Pretreatment view. *(b)* Preoperative situation with single-tooth edentulous gap and adjacent tooth already prepared. *(c)* The occlusal view shows the localized horizontal alveolar ridge defect. *(d)* Condition after flap formation with distal releasing incision. *(e)* Checking the depth after preparation of the implant site. *(f)* An implant 4.1 mm in diameter was placed, taking the prosthetic aspects into account. *(g)* Augmentation with autogenous bone chips; the soft bone lamina was fixed with two pins. *(h)* The bone lamina was pulled under the flap in the palatal direction and fixed with a suture.

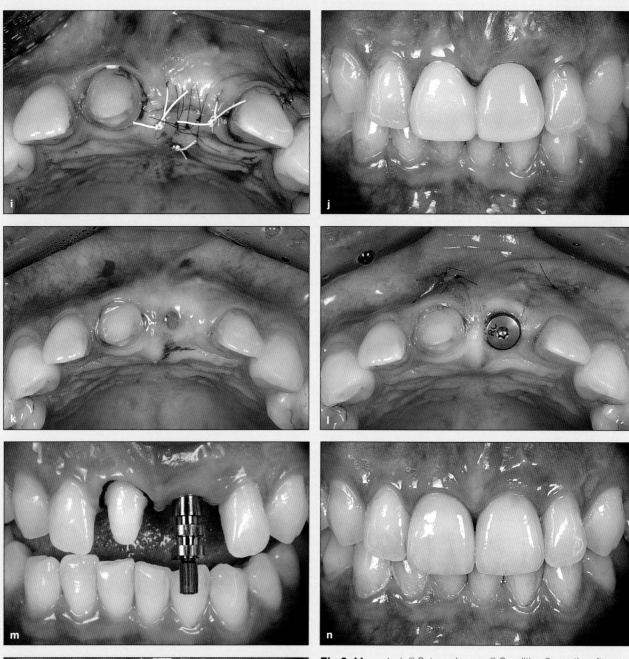

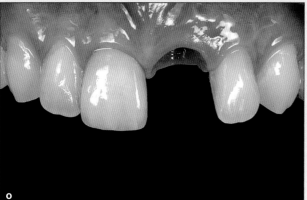

Fig 9-11 *cont.* / *(i)* Suture closure. *(j)* Condition 3 months after operation. Adequate volume was successfully regenerated. *(k)* Condition 3 months after implant placement and augmentation. *(l)* Minimally invasive exposure by the keyhole access expansion technique and removal of the pins. *(m)* At the time of impression for provisional restoration on tooth and implant. *(n)* The provisional restoration is used to contour the emergence profile and consolidate the augmented site. *(o)* Contoured emergence profile 3 months after placement of the provisional restoration.

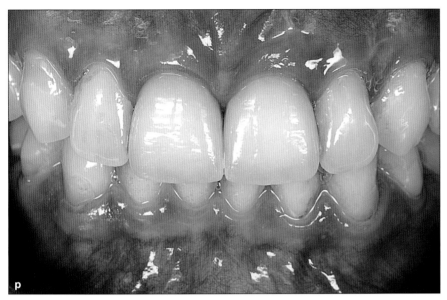

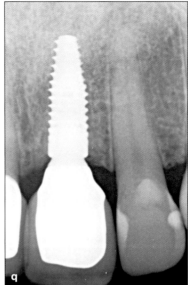

Fig 9-11 *cont.* / *(p and q)* Definitive restoration 6 months postoperatively.

Intraoral donor sites for bone grafts

The most commonly chosen region for intraoral bone graft harvesting is the retromolar region of the mandible (Fig 9-12). Harvesting is done with fissure drills, diamond disks, or ultrasonic instruments[10,21,22] (Fig 9-13). One of the advantages of this donor region is that relatively long grafts can be harvested, whereas grafts from the mandibular symphysis are usually thicker. Grafts 40 mm long and 10 to 15 mm wide can routinely be obtained from the retromolar region.[21] The thickness of these blocks is clearly defined by the dimensions of the anatomical structures of the mandible and the distance to the mandibular nerve. The distance to the nerve is usually 4 mm, and the thickness of the cortical plate is about 3.5 mm.[23,24] The volume of the graft harvested from the retromolar region ranges from 0.9 to 1.7 cm^3, according to several different sources.[10,21,22]

Grafts from the symphysis, on the other hand, are thicker but are shorter in length because of the limiting anatomical structures (ie, the apices of the anterior teeth and the mental foramen).[21] The vertical dimension is also markedly smaller in the symphysis region than in the retromolar region because it is imperative to maintain a minimum safety margin of 5 mm from the tooth roots and the lower edge of the mandible as well as the neurovascular bundles. As a result, the maximum graft size is about 25 × 15 mm.[25] Despite the anatomical limitations, larger graft volumes can be harvested in the symphysis area: in the region of 2.6 cm^3 on average[10] (Fig 9-14).

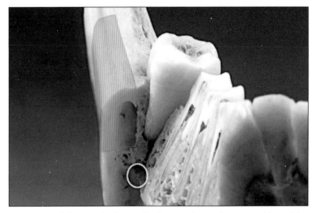

Fig 9-12 / Anatomical mandibular specimen shows marking of the retromolar region from where grafts are routinely harvested.

Apart from the typical surgical complications associated with implant surgery procedures and grafting techniques in the oral cavity (eg, bleeding, infection), the individual donor sites have a specific potential for complications depending on their anatomy.[26] Patients have to be told about these potential risks, which can include temporary or permanent neurosensory disturbances affecting the lips, teeth, or chin.[27,28] Harvesting from the chin causes the mandibular incisors to lose sensitivity in 12% of cases.[24] Retromolar harvesting can lead to painful restriction of mouth opening in the short term, but this does not seem to have any clinical relevance in the long term.[24] The most significant complication of harvesting bone blocks from the retromolar region is injury to the mandibular nerve

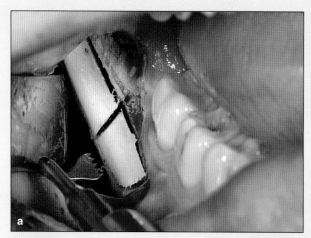

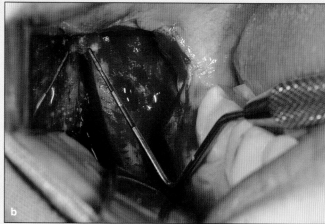

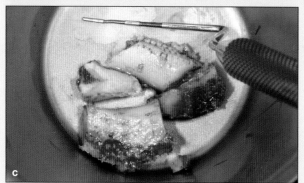

Fig 9-13 / *(a)* Osteotomy lines are created with a piezoelectric surgical instrument to harvest a graft from a retromolar region. *(b)* Situation after graft harvesting. *(c)* The bone blocks or bone grafts harvested on one side of the jaw.

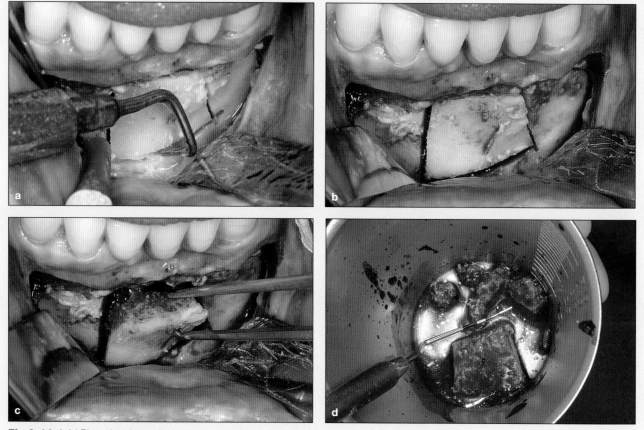

Fig 9-14 / *(a)* Piezoelectric surgical osteotomy in the chin region. *(b)* An incision is made around the perimeter of the graft. *(c)* After luxation with bone chisels, the graft can be harvested. *(d)* The bone grafts harvested from the chin.

with transient or permanent neurosensory disturbances. Some authors report an incidence of 4% for this serious complication. By contrast, the majority of authors do not list any disorders of this kind when reporting late complications.[16,21–24]

Harvesting grafts from the symphysis is frequently associated with neurosensory disturbances of the mandibular anterior teeth, the lower lip, and the chin. A few authors report a complication rate of 52% after 18 months in relation to sensory disturbances.[29] However, rates of 7% to 29% after 3 months are more commonly reported for this complication.[10,16,28]

If substantial bone grafts are required, clinicians have to resort to extraoral donor sites. The iliac crest is frequently used for harvesting sizeable quantities of autogenous bone.[30] Harvesting in this site cannot usually be performed on an outpatient basis and is associated with high postoperative morbidity and symptoms for the patient. The requirement of an additional surgical site for voluminous augmentations increases postoperative morbidity and carries an additional risk of severe complications. To avoid these complications, alternative surgical techniques have been explored that are not dependent on autogenous bone grafts. Biomaterials, such as xenografts and allografts, have proved their excellent clinical value in scientific studies and frequently make harvesting of autogenous grafts redundant.[31,32]

Collagen membranes

Various GBR techniques for reconstruction of ridge defects were developed in the past, including the use of particulate bone substitute materials that make it easy to reconstruct the ridge contours. However, a membrane was needed that would stabilize the substitute material locally and prevent the ingrowth of unwanted soft tissue cells.[33] For this purpose, various solutions have been introduced in recent years, including titanium films, expanded polytetrafluoroethylene (ePTFE) membranes with and without titanium reinforcement, as well as resorbable collagen and polylactide membranes.

The use of particulate substitutes with nonreinforced membranes is technically complex. Graft stability is more difficult to achieve than with bone block technqiues, and this stability is a prerequisite for rapid incorporation. Furthermore, nonresorbable membranes have to be removed prior to implant placement and carry the risk of exposure with subsequent wound infection.[34,35] However, collagen

membranes can provide a solution in cases of dehiscence and exposure of the graft to the oral cavity. After the operating site is covered with the membrane, the collagen matrix supports secondary closure of the soft tissue.[35] In cases of lateral augmentation with an inorganic bovine substitute, the use of collagen membranes led to stable long-term results over an observation period of 12 to 14 years, which did not differ significantly from the results with implants in local bone.[36]

Adequate durability could not be achieved with resorbable membranes, especially in vertical augmentations. New techniques were therefore developed to improve the durability of the collagen matrix or lengthen its resorption time.[37] Chemical cross-linking led to longer resorption times, but also to more severe inflammatory reactions of the surrounding tissue as well as higher complication rates.[38,39] The same applies to enzymatic modification with incorporated ribose molecules.[40] The current widespread techniques for improving the barrier function are using double-layer native collagen membranes or native membranes from porcine pericardia.[36,41,42] The best results in terms of vertical and horizontal defect filling and the lowest complication rates are achieved with collagen membranes rather than ePTFE membranes, polylactide membranes, or titanium membranes.[43]

Bone Lamina Technique

Depending on the defect, it may be possible with this technique to reduce the quantity of autogenous bone required or entirely avoid the use of autogenous bone. The objective is the regeneration of deficient ridge areas by bone substitute materials with or without autogenous bone in combination with a barrier that secures the space over a long enough period of time. The fundamental idea is to imitate nature by reconstructing the cortical bony plate with a xenogeneic lamella of cortical bone that is partially demineralized and therefore constitutes a special type of native collagen membrane. This membrane is rigid enough to secure the space for regeneration but is also flexible enough to be adapted to the defect. This so-called lamina is used like a GBR barrier membrane to inhibit the ingrowth of epithelial or connective tissue cells into the defect. At the same time, its mechanical properties allow it to secure the space and stabilize the augmentation material. As a biologic product, the lamina can be resorbed, although it maintains its barrier function for 5 to 6 months. There are

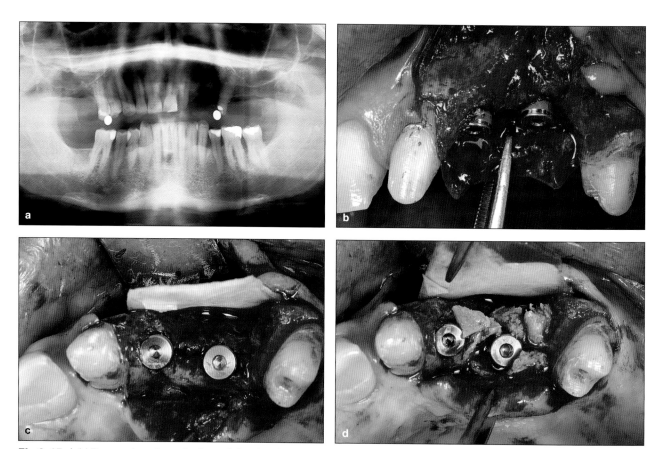

Fig 9-15 / *(a)* Panoramic radiograph of a partially edentulous patient with a vertical ridge defect in the region of the maxillary left canine and first premolar. *(b)* Situation after implant placement. The vertical defect can clearly be seen. *(c)* The bone lamina in position for reconstruction of the vestibular plate. *(d)* Augmentation with autogenous bone chips.

two types of lamina (OsteoBiol, Tecnoss). The soft type is 0.5 mm thick and is available for non-volume-stable defects. The hard type is approximately 1 to 1.5 mm thick; it is more rigid and can be screwed in place. However, it can still be bent to adapt to the defect.

Description of the technique

Once the defect has been filled with bone graft, it is covered with the cortical lamina (OsteoBiol): a stiff, dried lamina consisting of 100% cortical bone that becomes bendable after it is rehydrated. Defects with a vertical component always require an autogenous graft (Fig 9-15), whereas most horizontal defects can be reconstructed with xenografts or allografts (Fig 9-16).

A xenogeneic corticocancellous substitute material (eg, OsteoBiol mp3) is used as the augmentation material to fill the defect. This is used either on its own or in conjunction with autogenous bone, depending on the regeneration po-

tential of the defect.[44,45] This biomaterial, which consists of 90% collagenated corticocancellous porcine bone (CCPB) particles measuring 0.6 to 1 mm in diameter and 10% collagen gel, is intended for horizontal augmentation. Its production involves a unique biotechnology process that prevents ceramization of natural bone and maintains tissue collagen. Collagen is considered one of the key factors in bone regeneration because it can effectively activate platelets and cause aggregation to occur. Platelets play a necessary role during the initial phase of the healing process, which is characterized by increased activation of chemical signaling chains that are mediated via cytokines and growth factors. These include platelet-derived growth factor (PDGF), insluin-like growth factor 1 (IGF-1), IGF-2, and vascular endothelial growth factor (VEGF), whose activating effect on osteoblasts and osteoclasts is well known.[46]

Furthermore, collagen attracts stem cells located in the bone marrow for the second healing phase and plays a part in their differentiation.[47] Collagen is an insoluble substrate that is suitable as a carrier of osteoinductive messengers

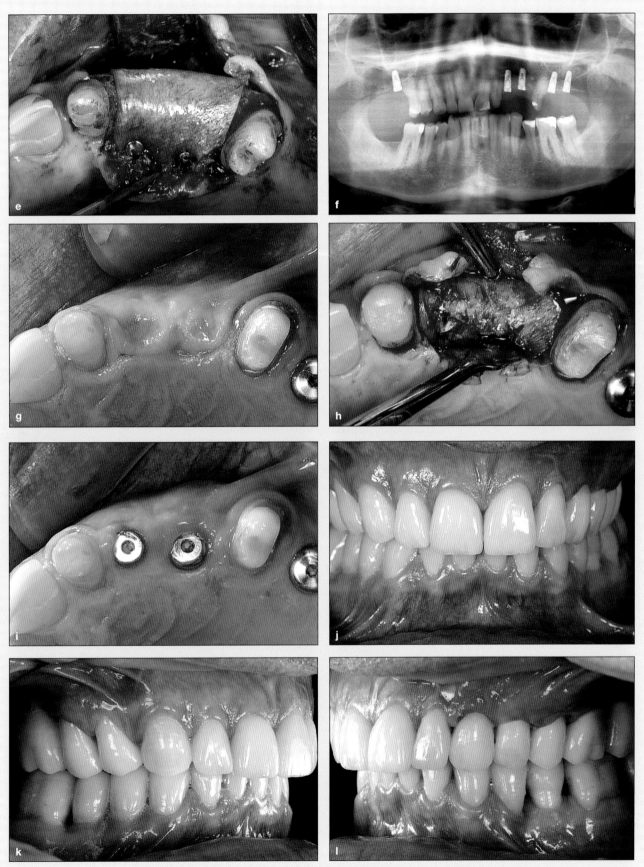

191

Fig 9-15 *cont.* / *(e)* The bone lamina is adapted to the augmentation material and fixed with titanium pins. *(f)* Postoperative panoramic radiograph. *(g)* The healed region of the defect. *(h)* Adequate bone regeneration at the time of implant exposure 3 months later. *(i)* Situation after surgical uncovering and soft tissue healing. *(j)* Frontal view after implant prosthetic restoration work. *(k and l)* Lateral views after completion of treatment.

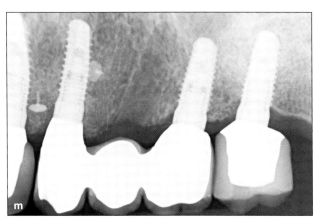

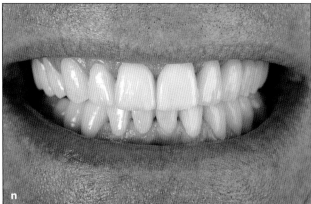

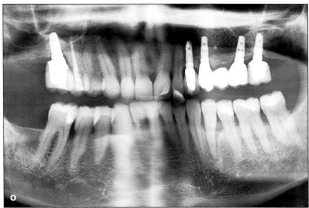

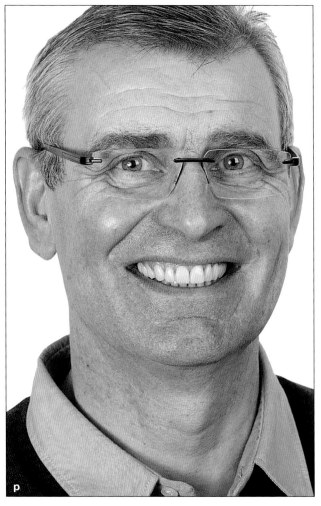

Fig 9-15 *cont.* / *(m and n)* Apical radiograph and smile 1 year after completion of treatment. *(o)* Panoramic radiograph 3 years after completion of treatment. *(p)* Final portrait. (Surgery and prosthodontics performed by A. Happe; laboratory work performed by D. Meyer.)

and can facilitate and guide the formation of new bone. It increases the proliferation rate of osteoblasts by two-thirds and stimulates the activation of platelets, osteoblasts, and osteoclasts in the process of tissue healing.[46]

The biocompatibility of porcine bone substitute materials was studied as early as 2007 by Trubiani et al[48] in an in vitro experiment using mesenchymal stem cells from the periodontal ligament. These stem cells showed great affinity for the 3D biomaterials, and they were capable of differentiating into osteoblasts in vitro. After 30 days' induction, the cells were separated from the substrate and were able to organize themselves. The corticocancellous composition facilitates progressive, osteoclast-type resorption with a similar rate of parallel formation of new bone.[45]

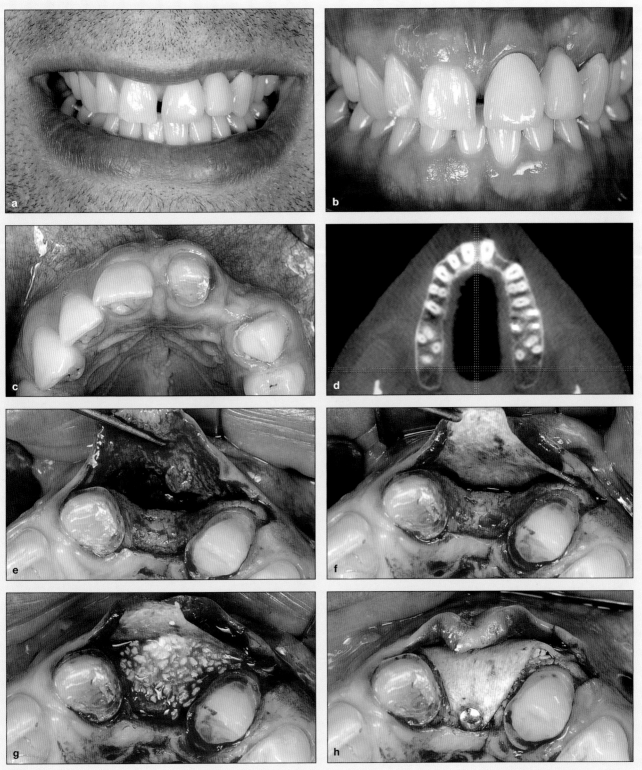

Fig 9-16 / *(a)* Appearance with a partial denture from the maxillary left central incisor to canine. *(b)* The treatment plan stipulates regeneration of the defect in the region of the left lateral incisor and implant placement in this site. *(c)* Occlusal view of the ridge defect. *(d)* Cone beam computed tomography (CBCT) shows the width of the residual bone to be 5.66 mm. *(e)* View of the bone defect after a full-thickness flap has been raised. *(f)* The bone lamina is cut to size and adapted to the defect. Two titanium pins are used for vestibular fixation. *(g)* The space between the lamina and the local bone is filled with OsteoBiol mp3. *(h)* The lamina is folded over the augmentation material to cover the mp3 particles occlusally.

194

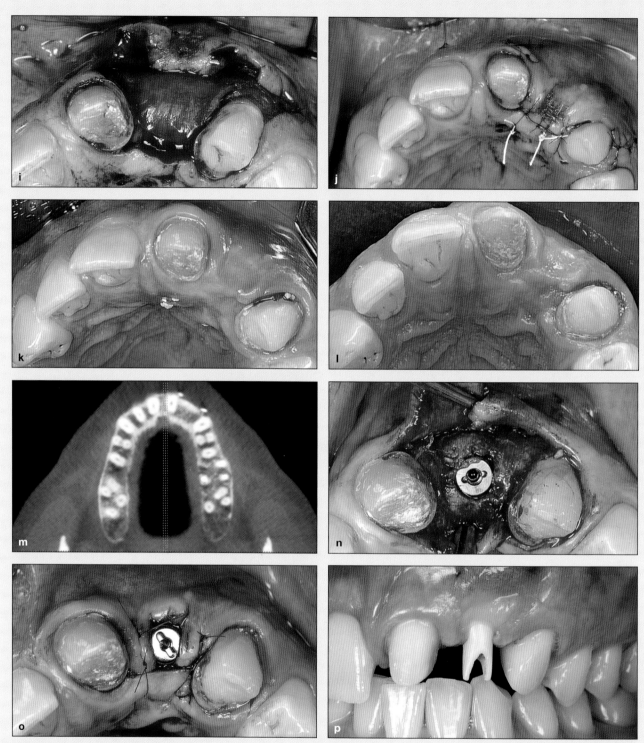

Fig 9-16 *cont.* / *(i)* The lamina is then covered with a collagen membrane (OsteoBiol Evolution), guaranteeing rapid soft tissue integration. *(j)* The soft tissue is carefully sutured for tension-free closure. *(k)* Soft tissue healing 4 weeks postoperatively. *(l)* Clinical view of the healed ridge after 6 months. *(m)* The CBCT taken 6 months postoperatively shows a new crestal width of 10.34 mm. The natural bone morphology with vestibular cortical plate and internal cancellous compartment can clearly be seen. *(n)* The appropriately dimensioned implant can be placed in the planned position. *(o)* The soft tissue is sutured around the gingiva former to allow transmucosal healing. *(p)* After a 3-month healing phase, the implant restoration is begun. First, a zirconia abutment is attached.

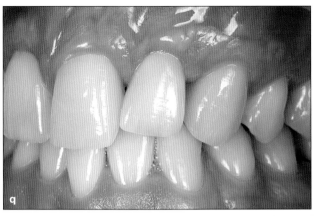 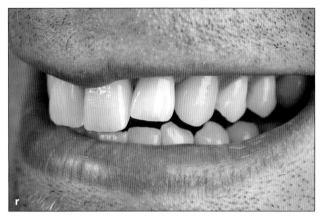

Fig 9-16 *cont.* / *(q)* This is followed by an all-ceramic lithium disilicate crown. *(r)* Smile with the definitive restoration. (Surgery and prosthodontics performed by A. Happe; laboratory work performed by D. Meyer.)

Clinical application

After 5 to 10 minutes' rehydration in sterile isotonic saline, the lamina should be formed into the correct size and shape. It has now achieved the desired plasticity and can be adapted to the bone defect. The shape of the lamina must leave a space between the local bone and the new vestibular plate that it represents (see Fig 9-16f). The lamina should be fixed with titanium pins.

The CCPB can be filled directly into the bone defect or the space enclosed by the lamina (see Fig 9-16g). CCPB contains collagen gel, which helps to stabilize the graft, and it is also hydrophilic, which allows rapid blood absorption and hence the required graft vascularization. The augmentation material must be covered with the lamina to prevent ingrowth of soft tissue (see Fig 9-16h). For a thin mucosa, it is advisable to cover the augmentation material and the lamina with a collagen membrane (eg, OsteoBiol Evolution) (see Fig 9-16i); this allows for rapid soft tissue integration. At the end of the procedure, careful, tension-free suture closure of the soft tissue is completed using microsurgical techniques[49] (see Fig 9-16j). The microsurgical approach is superior to macrosurgical techniques in terms of blood supply and revascularization of the soft tissue flap, which are crucial to the nutrition and healing of tissues.[50]

For antibiotic prophylaxis, clindamycin 600 mg (twice daily) or amoxicillin 500 mg (three times daily) is given orally perioperatively and for 1 week after treatment. In addition, a nonsteroidal anti-inflammatory drug (ibuprofen 600 mg) and a mouthwash (chlorhexidine 0.2%) are also prescribed.

After about 5 months, the CCPB particles become well integrated and form a single entity with the newly formed bone tissue parts.[45] Crespi et al[44] confirmed the high osteoconductivity of CCPB in a split-mouth study on alveolar ridge regeneration.

Figure 9-17 shows the typical histologic image of a large amount of newly formed bone and well-integrated particles of the xenograft with signs of resorption. By using this technique, moderate lateral defects can be fully regenerated without autogenous bone grafts (Fig 9-18).

A hard lamina 1 to 1.5 mm thick is available for defects that are not stable in volume. This primarily includes Benic and Hämmerle[5] class 4 to 5 defects, but it may include class 3 defects. These challenging defects require autogenous bone, an autogenous bone mixture, or allografts. The lamina is rigid so that it can be screwed, but it is still flexible enough to be adapted to the defect. The case depicted in Fig 9-19 demonstrates this clinical situation. After loss of the maxillary central incisors with a 3D defect, augmentation had to be performed before implant placement. The two implants (3.3 mm and 2.9 mm in diameter; Straumann BLT) were placed 3 months later.

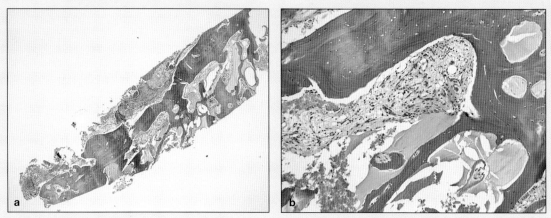

Fig 9-17 / *(a)* Histology of the newly formed bone with interposed particles of substitute material. *(b)* Greater magnification of the histologic image.

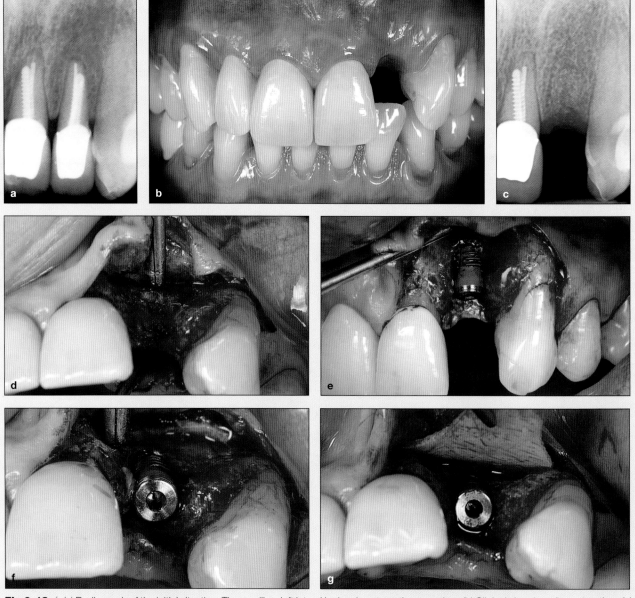

Fig 9-18 / *(a)* Radiograph of the initial situation. The maxillary left lateral incisor is not worth preserving. *(b)* Clinical situation after extraction. *(c)* Radiograph of the edentulous gap. *(d)* Clinical image of the bone defect after flap formation. *(e)* Implant in situ in the deficient bone with exposed titanium surface. *(f)* Buccal view of implant in place before augmentation. *(g)* Reconstruction of the buccal bone lamella with the bone lamina.

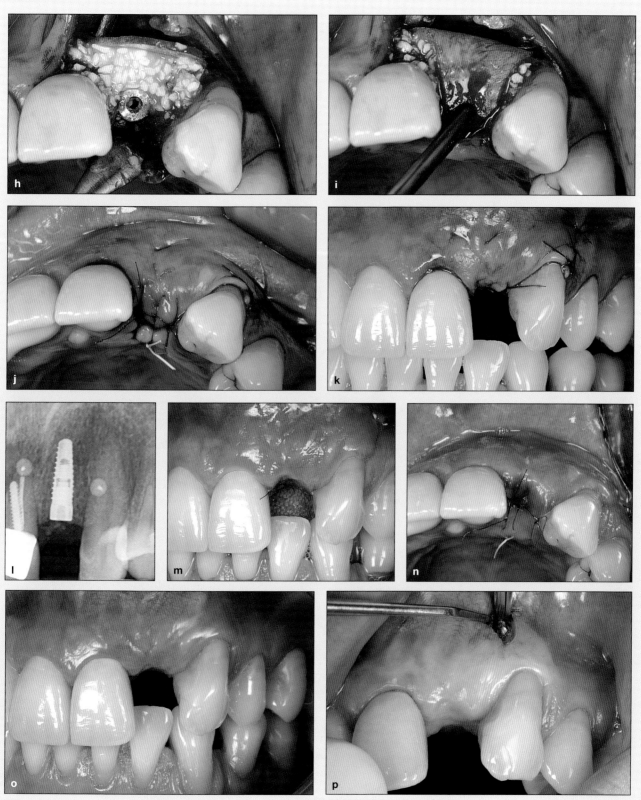

Fig 9-18 *cont.* / *(h)* The space between the lamina and the bone was filled with substitute material. *(i)* The lamina was folded over the material to cover the site completely. *(j)* Microsurgery was used to close the wound. *(k)* Buccal view postoperatively. *(l)* Radiograph of implant in place and titanium pins fixing the bone lamina. *(m and n)* Healing after 1 week. *(o)* Healed site 4 months after implant placement and augmentation; the clinical situation did not require further soft tissue augmentation. *(p)* Micro-invasive removal of the titanium pins. The pin is visible through the micro-incision.

→

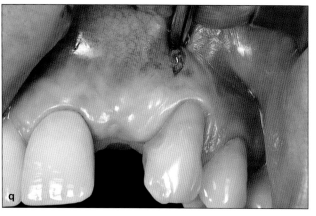
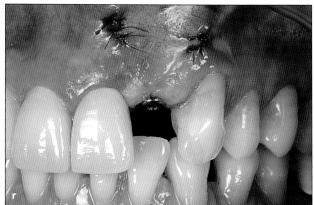
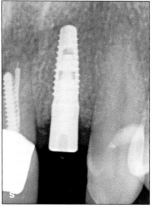
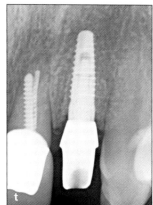
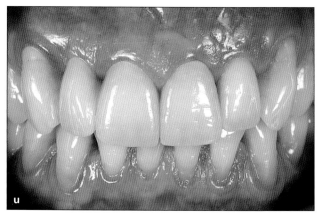

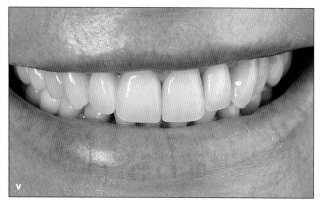

Fig 9-18 *cont.* / *(q)* Micro-invasive removal of the titanium pins. The pin is visible through the micro-incision. *(r)* After removal of the pins and micro-invasive implant exposure, the site was sutured, and the gingiva former was screwed in. *(s)* Radiograph of implant after the exposure operation. *(t)* Radiograph during the prosthetic treatment phase. *(u)* Clinical situation after completion of the treatment. *(v)* Smile after treatment. (Surgery and prosthodontics performed by A. Happe; laboratory work performed by A. Nolte.)

Allogeneic Bone Grafts

Allogeneic bone grafts are available in particulate form or as bone blocks. Particulate allografts require stabilization by a GBR membrane or bone lamina (Fig 9-20). Unlike particulate materials, the advantage of block grafts is that they can be easily fixed with osteosynthesis screws to provide stability.[51] With lag screws, corticocancellous grafts can be further immobilized by press fit.

Allogeneic bone block grafts have gained popularity in recent years. Various allogeneic graft materials have been developed as an alternative to autogenous grafts. Partially deproteinized allogeneic bone blocks, unlike demineralized freeze-dried bone allograft and deproteinized xenogeneic bone blocks, exhibit better graft stability and can be fixed better with osteosynthesis screws.[51]

In a small case series of five ridge defects in three patients, a freeze-dried allogeneic cancellous onlay graft was used with satisfactory results.[49,52] A case series involving 82 blocks showed predictable bone regeneration of alveolar ridge defects in 73 patients for corticocancellous, solvent-dried block allografts.[51] However, slight resorption in the area of contact surfaces between the bone block and the recipient site was observed with blocks that did

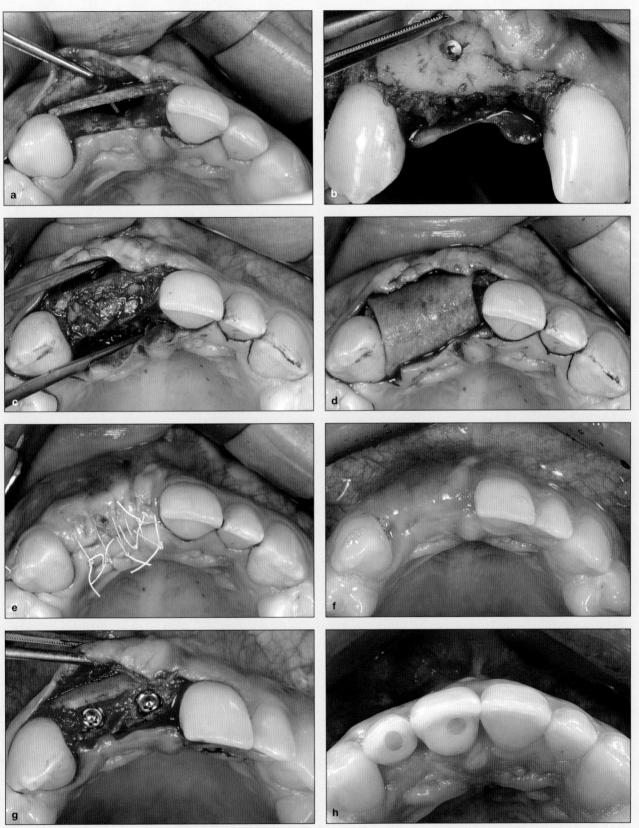

Fig 9-19 / (a) A 1-mm-thick rigid cortical lamina was screwed in, leaving a gap. (b) The lamina was fixed at the level of the crestal bone apices of the adjacent teeth, and the edges were rounded. (c) The gap was filled with autogenous bone chips. (d) The area was covered with a soft cortical lamina. (e) The area was closed with PTFE sutures immediately postoperatively. (f) Condition after 3 months' incorporation. (g) Two implants were placed into the healed augmented bone. (h) Final image with two screw-retained single crowns.

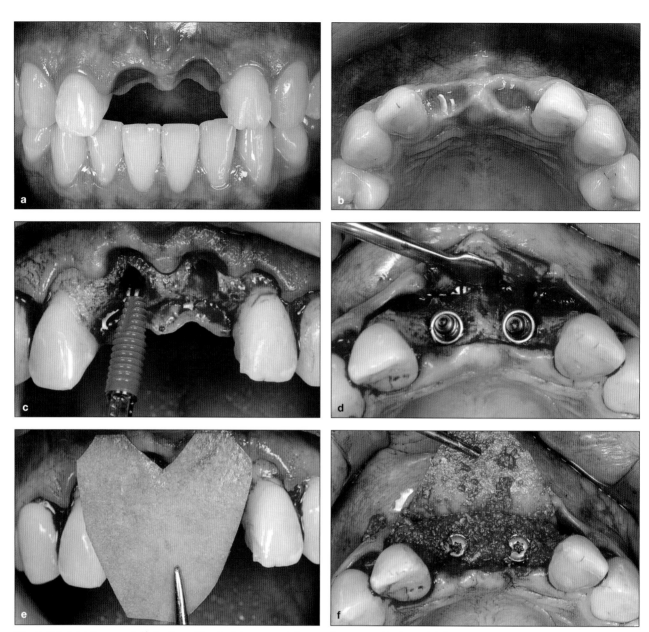

200

Fig 9-20 / *(a)* Preoperative situation with edentulous gap at the maxillary central incisors. *(b)* Occlusal view of the horizontal ridge defect. *(c)* The flap is designed without vertical releasing incisions, and the first implant is placed. *(d)* Both implants were placed with consideration given to the prosthodontic aspects. *(e)* Customized lamina with notch for the nasal spine. *(f)* The lamina in situ. The defect is augmented with allogeneic bone particles.

not fit perfectly to the defect contour. Although a donor site with possible complications was not necessary (as for autogenous bone blocks), the operating time was not significantly shortened because the blocks had to be fitted precisely to the defects.

To reduce the treatment time and the burden on the patient, the block allografts can be preshaped using stereolithographic (STL) models of the arch prior to the surgical procedure.[53] However, it must be kept in mind STL models are considered aseptic but not sterile, and there is no

validated method for storing preshaped blocks until the procedure is performed. Because the size of these blocks is also limited, several blocks are necessary for larger augmentations, which further complicates their preparation.[53] In the era of 3D implant therapy, computer-aided design/ computer-assisted manufacturing planning processing of block allografts is becoming more and more popular as a method of improving graft adaptation to the recipient site as well as shortening the operating time[54] (Fig 9-21).

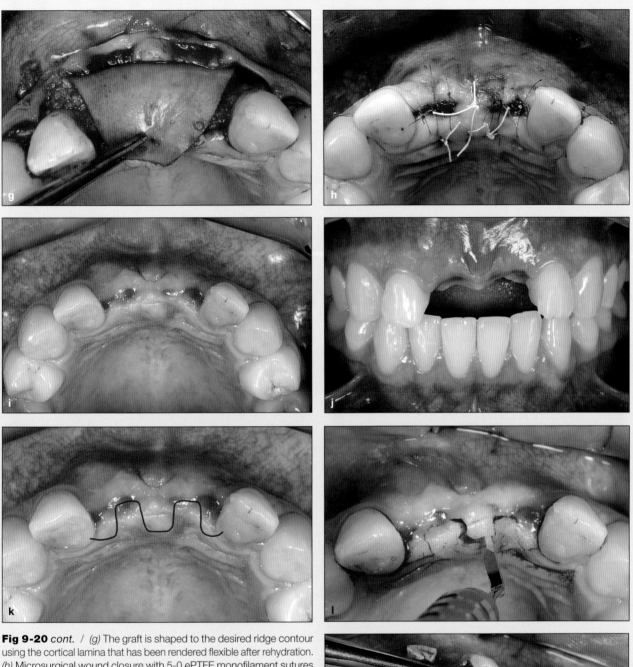

Fig 9-20 *cont.* / *(g)* The graft is shaped to the desired ridge contour using the cortical lamina that has been rendered flexible after rehydration. *(h)* Microsurgical wound closure with 5-0 ePTFE monofilament sutures and 6-0 polyvinylidene fluoride monofilament sutures (Seralene, Serag Wiessner). *(i and j)* Situation after 3 months of healing. *(k)* Planned incision for the implant exposure operation (split-finger technique). *(l)* Microsurgical flap preparation with an angled micro scalpel. *(m)* Supraperiosteal flap (split flap). The titanium pins are visible, and the ridge has been adequately regenerated.

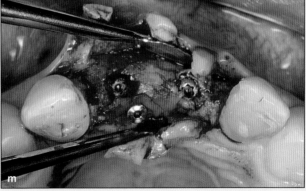

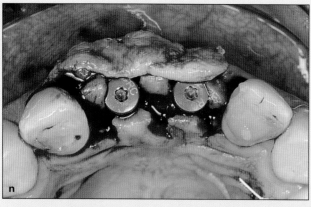

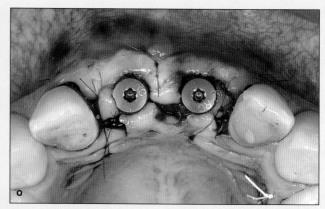

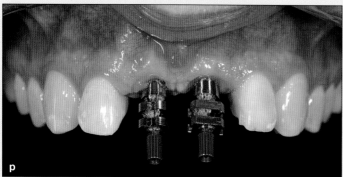

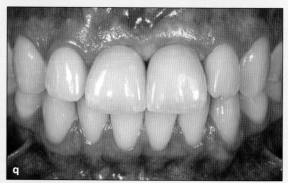

202

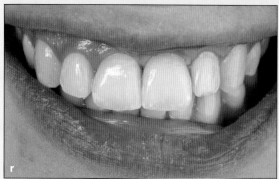

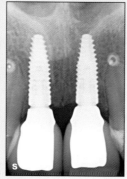

Fig 9-20 *cont.* / *(n)* A connective tissue graft harvested from the palate (region of the left premolar to first molar) is placed for vestibular soft tissue augmentation. *(o)* Microsurgical adaptation of the soft tissue around the gingiva former. *(p)* The impression posts in place. *(q and r)* Intraoral and smile views with the definitive restorations in place. *(s)* Radiograph with the completed restorations. *(t)* Patient's portrait after completion of treatment. (Surgery performed by A. Happe; prosthodontics performed by B. van den Bosch; laboratory work performed by P. Holthaus.)

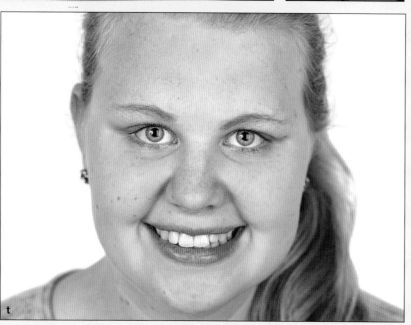

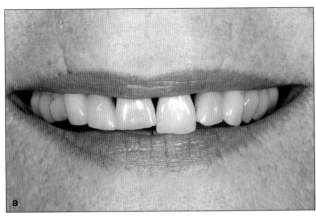
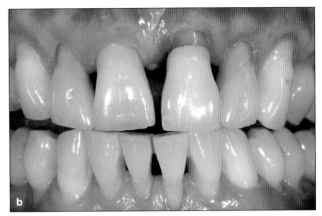
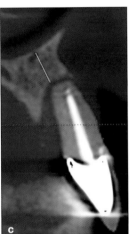
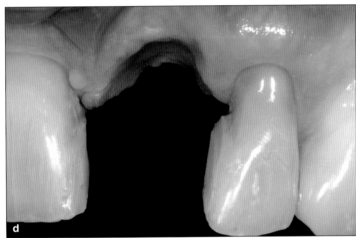
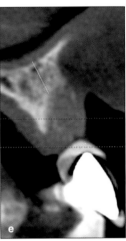

Fig 9-21 / (a) Smile before treatment. (b) Situation after completed periodontal treatment. The maxillary left central incisor is not worth preserving. (c) CBCT sagittal section of the left central incisor demonstrates extreme loss of attachment. (d) Site after extraction. (e) CBCT sagittal section of the deficient ridge at the extraction site.

Distraction Osteogenesis

Distraction osteogenesis, also known as *callus distraction*, was developed by Gavriil Ilizarov[55] to lengthen lower limbs by using external fixation. The technique has also been used for several years in oral and maxillofacial surgery.[56–58] To perform distraction osteogenesis, a bone segment is separated from the local bone and joined using an external distraction device. After 1 week of healing (soft tissue healing and callus formation), the segment is moved in the desired direction by turning the distraction screw. Depending on the distraction device, one turn of the screw may result in a 0.3-mm movement of the segment. The distraction protocol stipulates a total of 0.9 mm movement per day. As soon as the segment has reached the desired position, a 2-week retention phase begins in which no further movement takes place and the callus is allowed to mature. To enhance patient comfort, the distraction screw can be separated from the distractor after these 2 weeks. This is followed by another 12 weeks of healing before

implants can be placed. This technique is particularly suitable for augmentation in cases of vertical defects. After installation of the distractor, the soft tissue can be closed without being stretched. This is an advantage because this stretching normally causes complications such as dehiscence or necrosis. Instead, the soft tissue is stretched simultaneously with the callus. Furthermore, a vital bone segment is moved in an intact soft tissue envelope. Therefore, the complication rate is lower, and the survival rate of implants is higher, when compared with conventional augmentation techniques such as GBR or block grafts.[56,59] However, the ridge width cannot be increased simultaneously during vertical distraction. For this reason, horizontal bone augmentation is frequently required after distraction osteogenesis.

As with all other augmentation techniques, mechanical irritation due to the distractor or bone segment can cause unsatisfactory bone healing and must be avoided (Figs 9-22 and 9-23).

204

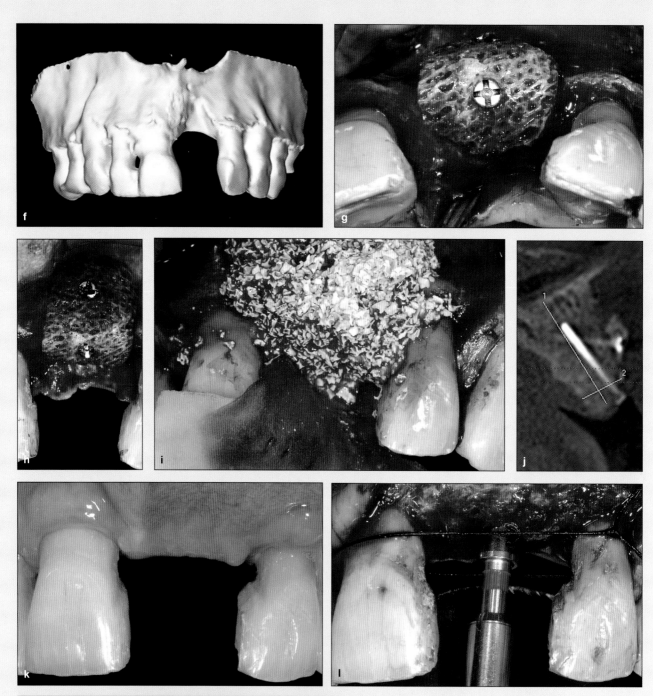

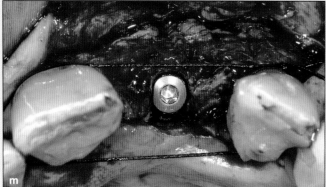

Fig 9-21 *cont.* / *(f)* The CBCT scan allowed for a block allograft (Maxgraft Bonebuilder, Botiss) to be individually milled. *(g and h)* The customized allogeneic bone block in situ. *(i)* The block is covered with xenograft and a collagen membrane. *(j)* CBCT sagittal section after 4 months' graft incorporation. *(k)* Clinical view of the healed site. *(l)* The implant is placed. *(m)* Implant in situ. ⟶

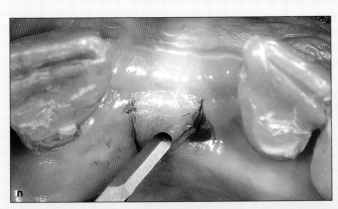

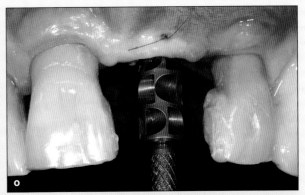

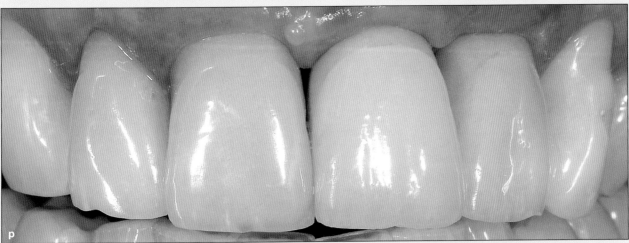

Fig 9-21 *cont.* / *(n)* Minimally invasive exposure with the roll flap technique. *(o)* The impression post is fitted during the prosthetic phase. *(p)* Intraoral view after the prosthodontic treatment with implant crown for the left central incisor and ceramic veneers on the adjacent teeth. *(q)* Portrait of the patient after treatment. (Surgery and prosthodontics performed by G. Körner; laboratory work performed by K. Müterthies.)

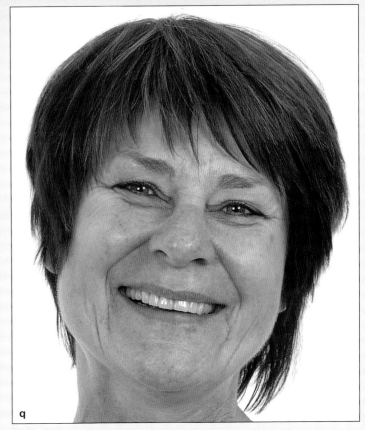

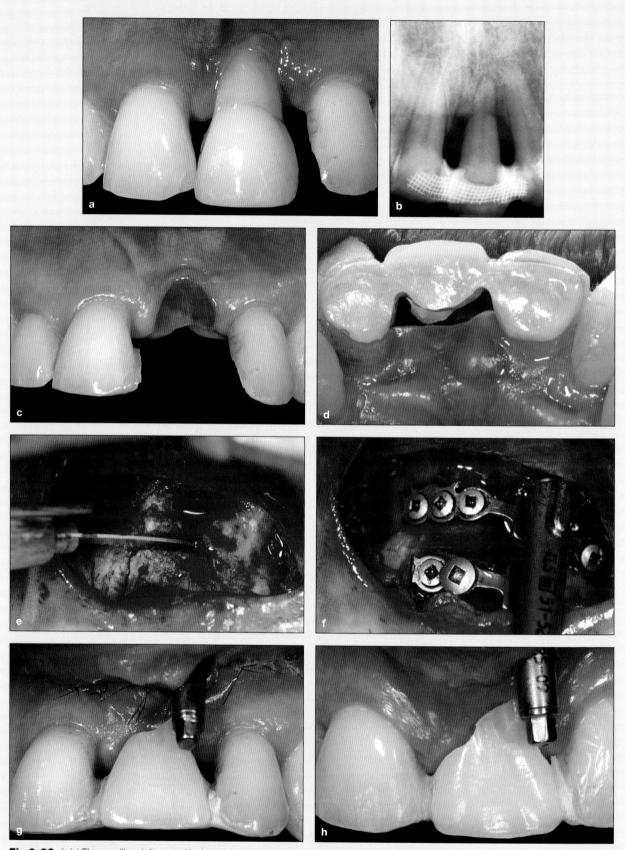

206

Fig 9-22 / *(a)* The maxillary left central incisor demonstrates extreme loss of attachment and is not worth preserving. *(b)* The radiograph shows the vertical tissue loss. *(c)* The healed ridge after extraction of the left central incisor. *(d)* Provisional bonded zirconia partial denture in situ. *(e)* Access to the alveolar bone was created via a paramarginal incision 4 mm apical to the soft tissue margin. An oscillating bone saw was used to incise around the segment. *(f)* The distractor fixed in situ with screws. *(g)* Situation after the procedure. The soft tissue is closed with sutures around the distraction element. *(h)* Situation after completion of the distraction phase with the provisional partial denture in place.

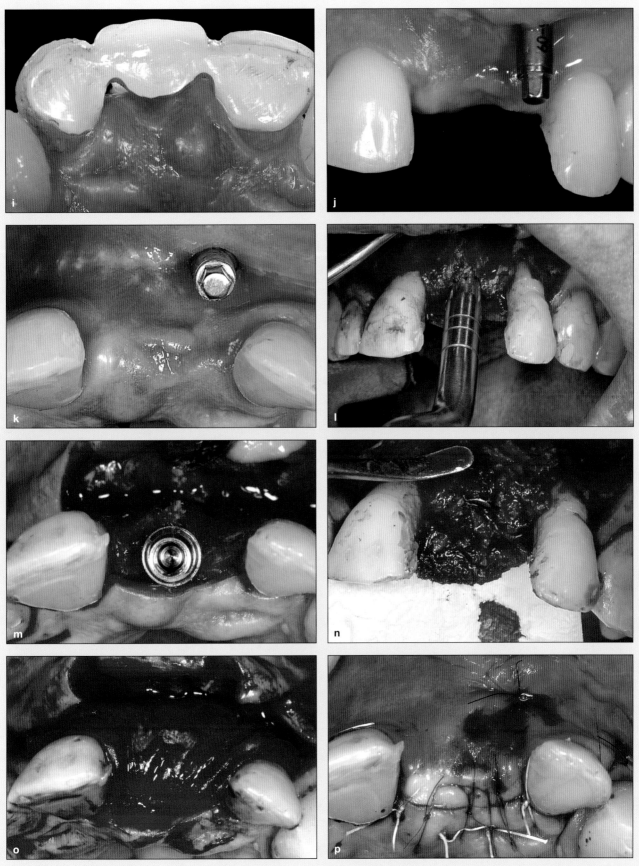

Fig 9-22 *cont.* / *(i)* Palatal view. *(j and k)* Frontal and occlusal views without partial denture. The vertical defect is overcompensated. *(l)* Horizontal ridge augmentation is completed with bone spreading. *(m)* Implant in situ. *(n)* Augmentation with bone chips obtained with drilling and a xenograft. *(o)* As with a GBR technique, a collagen membrane is used to cover the graft material. *(p)* Soft tissue closure after bone grafting.

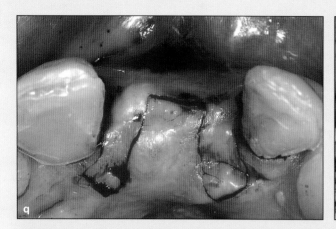

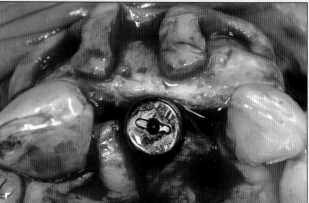

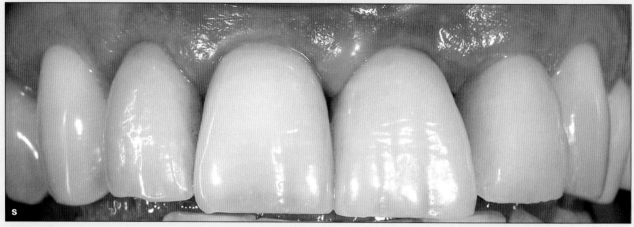

Fig 9-22 *cont.* / *(q)* After 3 months, the exposure operation is performed with a split-finger incision. *(r)* Occlusal view of the exposure with the CTG. *(s)* Definitive restorations: implant crown on the left central incisor and veneers on the left lateral incisor and both right incisors. (Surgery and prosthodontics performed by G. Körner; laboratory work performed by K. Müterthies.)

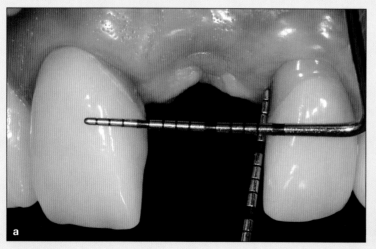

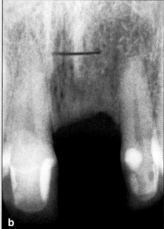

Fig 9-23 / *(a)* Edentulous gap at the maxillary left central incisor with loss of attachment mesial to the lateral incisor. *(b)* Radiograph of the situation. →

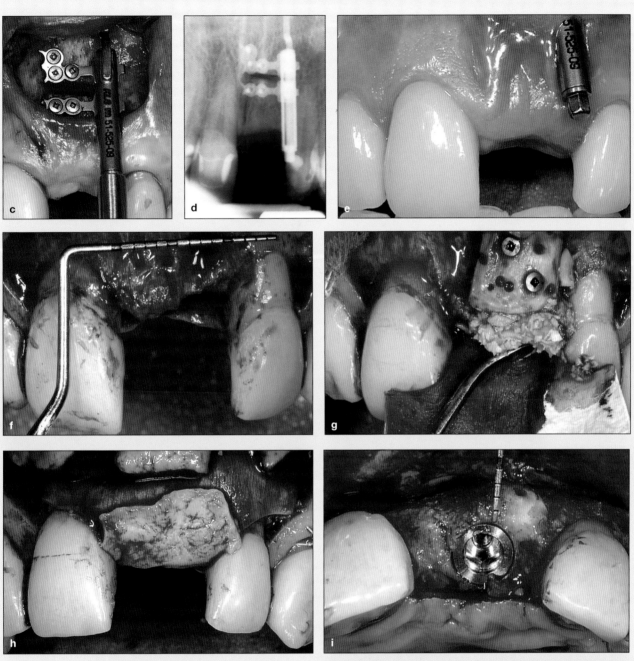

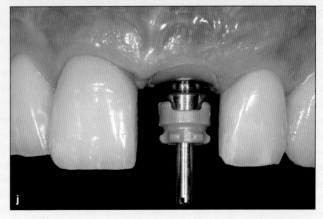

Fig 9-23 *cont.* / *(c)* The distractor for vertical bone augmentation in situ. *(d)* Radiograph after placement of the distractor. A gap must remain between the local bone and the loosened segment. This is where the callus will take shape. *(e)* Situation after the distraction phase. The defect is well compensated. *(f)* Clinical view after removal of the distractor. The segment was deliberately elongated excessively; horizontal augmentation is also required. *(g)* Horizontal bone augmentation is performed with a bone block, particulate bone, and xenogeneic material. A collagen membrane is placed before the final adaptation. *(h)* A soft tissue graft was additionally placed over the collagen membrane. *(i)* After 3 months of healing, a 4.5-mm-diameter implant was placed. *(j)* The impression was taken with a customized impression post, which was used to transfer the emergence profile of the provisional implant crown.

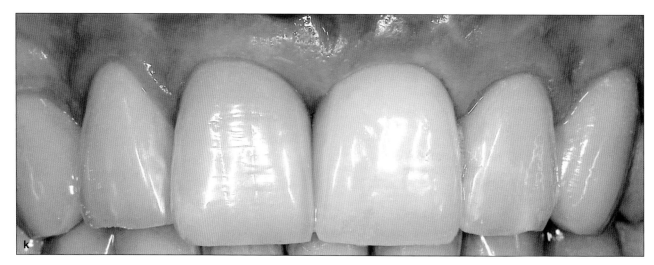

Fig 9-23 *cont.* / *(k)* Definitive restoration with all-ceramic restorations from canine to canine. (Surgery and prosthodontics performed by G. Körner; laboratory work performed by K. Müterthies.)

References

1. Herford AS, Nguyen K. Complex bone augmentation in alveolar ridge defects. Oral Maxillofac Surg Clin North Am 2015;27:227–244.

2. Kuchler U, von Arx T. Horizontal ridge augmentation in conjunction with or prior to implant placement in the anterior maxilla: A systematic review. Int J Oral Maxillofac Implants 2014;29(suppl):14–24.

3. Rocchietta I, Fontana F, Simion M. Clinical outcomes of vertical bone augmentation to enable dental implant placement: A systematic review. J Clin Periodontol 2008;35(8 suppl):203–215.

4. Al-Nawas B, Schiegnitz E. Augmentation procedures using bone substitute materials or autogenous bone: A systematic review and meta-analysis. Eur J Oral Implantol 2014;7(suppl 2):S219–S234.

5. Benic GI, Hämmerle CH. Horizontal bone augmentation by means of guided bone regeneration. Periodontol 2000 2014;66:13–40.

6. Esposito M, Grusovin MG, Coulthard P, Worthington HV. The efficacy of various bone augmentation procedures for dental implants: A Cochrane systematic review of randomized controlled clinical trials. Int J Oral Maxillofac Implants 2006;21:696–710.

7. Schliephake H, Neukam FW, Wichmann M. Survival analysis of endosseous implants in bone grafts used for the treatment of severe alveolar ridge atrophy. J Oral Maxillofac Surg 1997;55:1227–1233.

8. Garg AK. The use of a bone harvest system for autogenous bone grafts during implant procedures. Dent Implantol Update 1998;9:81–83.

9. Garg AK, Morales MJ, Navarro I, Duarte F. Autogenous mandibular bone grafts in the treatment of the resorbed maxillary anterior alveolar ridge: Rationale and approach. Implant Dent 1998;7:169–176.

10. Khoury F, Happe A. Zur Diagnostik und Methodik von intraoralen Knochenentnahmen. Zeitschrift für Zahnärztliche Implantologie 1999:167–176.

11. Proussaefs P. Clinical and histologic evaluation of the use of mandibular tori as donor site for mandibular block autografts: Report of three cases. Int J Periodontics Restorative Dent 2006;26:43–51.

12. Chiapasco M, Abati S, Romeo E, Vogel G. Clinical outcome of autogenous bone blocks or guided bone regeneration with e-PTFE membranes for the reconstruction of narrow edentulous ridges. Clin Oral Implants Res 1999;10:278–288.

13. Tinti C, Parma-Benfenati S, Polizzi G. Vertical ridge augmentation: What is the limit? Int J Periodontics Restorative Dent 1996;16:220–229.

14. von Arx T, Buser D. Horizontal ridge augmentation using autogenous block grafts and the guided bone regeneration technique with collagen membranes: A clinical study with 42 patients. Clin Oral Implants Res 2006;17:359–366.

15. Kon K, Shiota M, Ozeki M, Yamashita Y, Kasugai S. Bone augmentation ability of autogenous bone graft particles with different sizes: A histological and micro-computed tomography study. Clin Oral Implants Res 2009;20:1240–1246.

16. Khoury F, Khoury C. Mandibular bone block grafts: Diagnosis, instrumentation, harvesting techniques, and surgical procedures. In: Khoury F, Antoun H, Missika P (eds). Bone Augmentation in Oral Implantology. Chicago: Quintessence, 2007:115–212.

17. Khoury F, Antoun H, Missika P (eds). Bone Augmentation in Oral Implantology. Chicago: Quintessence, 2007.

18. Stimmelmayr M, Gernet W, Edelhoff D, Güth JF, Happe A, Beuer F. Two-stage horizontal bone grafting with the modified shell technique for subsequent implant placement: A case series. Int J Periodontics Restorative Dent 2014;34:269–276.

19. Cricchio G, Lundgren S. Donor site morbidity in two different approaches to anterior iliac crest bone harvesting. Clin Implant Dent Relat Res 2003;5:161–169.

20. Silva FM, Cortez AL, Moreira RW, Mazzonetto R. Complications of intraoral donor site for bone grafting prior to implant placement. Implant Dent 2006;15:420–426.

21. Misch CM. Comparison of intraoral donor sites for onlay grafting prior to implant placement. Int J Oral Maxillofac Implants 1997;12:767–776.

22. Happe A. Use of a piezoelectric surgical device to harvest bone grafts from the mandibular ramus: Report of 40 cases. Int J Periodontics Restorative Dent 2007;27:241–249.

23. Rajchel J, Ellis E 3rd, Fonseca RJ. The anatomical location of the mandibular canal: its relationship to the sagittal ramus osteotomy. Int J Adult Orthodon Orthognath Surg 1986;1:37–47.

24. Nkenke E, Radespiel-Tröger M, Wiltfang J, Schultze-Mosgau S, Winkler G, Neukam FW. Morbidity of harvesting of retromolar bone grafts: A prospective study. Clin Oral Implants Res 2002;13:514–521.

25. Montazem A, Valauri DV, St-Hilaire H, Buchbinder D. The mandibular symphysis as a donor site in maxillofacial bone grafting: A quantitative anatomic study. J Oral Maxillofac Surg 2000;58:1368–1371.

26. Happe A, Khoury F. Complications and risk factors in bone grafting procedures. In: Khoury F, Antoun H, Missika P (eds). Bone Augmentation in Oral Implantology. Chicago: Quintessence, 2007:405–429.

27. Raghoebar GM, Louwerse C, Kalk WW, Vissink A. Morbidity of chin bone harvesting. Clin Oral Implants Res 2001;12:503–507.

28. Joshi A. An investigation of post-operative morbidity following chin graft surgery. Br Dent J 2004;196:215–218.

29. Clavero J, Lundgren S. Ramus or chin grafts for maxillary sinus inlay and local onlay augmentation: Comparison of donor site morbidity and complications. Clin Implant Dent Relat Res 2003;5:154–160.

30. Kessler P, Thorwarth M, Bloch-Birkholz A, Nkenke E, Neukam FW. Harvesting of bone from the iliac crest: Comparison of the anterior and posterior sites. Br J Oral Maxillofac Surg 2005;43:51–56.

31. Wallace SS, Froum SJ. Effect of maxillary sinus augmentation on the survival of endosseous dental implants. A systematic review. Ann Periodontol 2003;8:328–343.

32. Esposito M, Grusovin MG, Rees J, et al. Interventions for replacing missing teeth: Augmentation procedures of the maxillary sinus. Cochrane Database Syst Rev 2010:CD008397.

33. Dahlin C, Linde A, Gottlow J, Nyman S. Healing of bone defects by guided tissue regeneration. Plast Reconstr Surg 1988;81:672–676.

34. Jovanovic SA, Nevins M. Bone formation utilizing titanium-reinforced barrier membranes. Int J Periodontics Restorative Dent 1995;15:56–69.

35. Zitzmann NU, Naef R, Schärer P. Resorbable versus nonresorbable membranes in combination with Bio-Oss for guided bone regeneration. Int J Oral Maxillofac Implants 1997;12:844–852.

36. Jung RE, Fenner N, Hämmerle CH, Zitzmann NU. Long-term outcome of implants placed with guided bone regeneration (GBR) using resorbable and non-resorbable membranes after 12-14 years. Clin Oral Implants Res 2013;24:1065–1073.

37. Canullo L, Trisi P, Simion M. Vertical ridge augmentation around implants using e-PTFE titanium-reinforced membrane and deproteinized bovine bone mineral (bio-oss): A case report. Int J Periodontics Restorative Dent 2006;26:355–361.

38. Rothamel D, Schwarz F, Sager M, Herten M, Sculean A, Becker J. Biodegradation of differently cross-linked collagen membranes: An experimental study in the rat. Clin Oral Implants Res 2005;16:369–378.

39. Becker J, Al-Nawas B, Klein MO, Schliephake H, Terheyden H, Schwarz F. Use of a new cross-linked collagen membrane for the treatment of dehiscence-type defects at titanium implants: A prospective, randomized-controlled double-blinded clinical multicenter study. Clin Oral Implants Res 2009;20:742–749.

40. Friedmann A, Strietzel FP, Maretzki B, Pitaru S, Bernimoulin JP. Observations on a new collagen barrier membrane in 16 consecutively treated patients. Clinical and histological findings. J Periodontol 2001;72:1616–1623.

41. Kozlovsky A, Aboodi G, Moses O, et al. Bio-degradation of a resorbable collagen membrane (Bio-Gide) applied in a double-layer technique in rats. Clin Oral Implants Res 2009;20:1116–1123.

42. Rothamel D, Schwarz F, Fienitz T, et al. Biocompatibility and biodegradation of a native porcine pericardium membrane: Results of in vitro and in vivo examinations. Int J Oral Maxillofac Implants 2012;27:146–154.

43. Troeltzsch M, Troeltzsch M, Kauffmann P, et al. Clinical efficacy of grafting materials in alveolar ridge augmentation: A systematic review. J Craniomaxillofac Surg 2016;44:1618–1629.

44. Crespi R, Capparé P, Romanos GE, Mariani E, Benasciutti E, Gherlone E. Corticocancellous porcine bone in the healing of human extraction sockets: Combining histomorphometry with osteoblast gene expression profiles in vivo. Int J Oral Maxillofac Implants 2011;26:866–872.

45. Barone A, Crespi R, Aldini NN, Fini M, Giardino R, Covani U. Maxillary sinus augmentation: Histologic and histomorphometric analysis. Int J Oral Maxillofac Implants 2005;20:519–525.

46. Hsu FY, Chueh SC, Wang YJ. Microspheres of hydroxyapatite/reconstituted collagen as supports for osteoblast cell growth. Biomaterials 1999;20:1931–1936.

47. Salasznyk RM, Williams WA, Boskey A, Batorsky A, Plopper GE. Adhesion to vitronectin and collagen I promotes osteogenic differentiation of human mesenchymal stem cells. J Biomed Biotechnol 2004;2004:24–34.

48. Trubiani O, Scarano A, Orsini G, et al. The performance of human periodontal ligament mesenchymal stem cells on xenogenic biomaterials. Int J Immunopathol Pharmacol 2007;20(1 suppl 1):87–91.

49. Wachtel H, Fickl S, Zuhr O, Hürzeler MB. The double-sling suture: A modified technique for primary wound closure. Eur J Esthet Dent 2006;1:314–324.

50. Burkhardt R, Lang NP. Coverage of localized gingival recessions: Comparison of micro- and macrosurgical techniques. J Clin Periodontol 2005;32:287–293.

51. Keith JD Jr, Petrungaro P, Leonetti JA, et al. Clinical and histologic evaluation of a mineralized block allograft: Results from the developmental period (2001-2004). Int J Periodontics Restorative Dent 2006;26:321–327.

52. Lyford RH, Mills MP, Knapp CI, Scheyer ET, Mellonig JT. Clinical evaluation of freeze-dried block allografts for alveolar ridge augmentation: A case series. Int J Periodontics Restorative Dent 2003;23:417–425.

53. Jacotti M. Simplified onlay grafting with a 3-dimensional block technique: A technical note. Int J Oral Maxillofac Implants 2006;21:635–639.

54. Schlee M, Rothamel D. Ridge augmentation using customized allogenic bone blocks: Proof of concept and histological findings. Implant Dent 2013;22:212–218.

55. Ilizarov G. Basic principles of transosseous compression and distraction osteosythesis [in Russian]. Orthop Travmatol Protez 1971;32(11):7–15.

56. Aghaloo TL, Moy PK. Which hard tissue augmentation techniques are the most successful in furnishing bony support for implant placement? Int J Oral Maxillofac Implants 2007;22(suppl):49–70.

57. Chiapasco M, Consolo U, Bianchi A, Ronchi P. Alveolar distraction osteogenesis for the correction of vertically deficient edentulous ridges: A multicenter prospective study on humans. Int J Oral Maxillofac Implants 2004;19:399–407.

58. Zöller JE, Lazar F, Neugebauer J. Clinical and sicientific background of tissue regeneration by alveolar callus distraction. In: Khoury F, Antoun H, Missika P (eds). Bone Augmentation in Oral Implantology. Chicago: Quintessence, 2007:279–298.

59. Chiapasco M, Romeo E, Casentini P, Rimondini L. Alveolar distraction osteogenesis vs. vertical guided bone regeneration for the correction of vertically deficient edentulous ridges: A 1-3-year prospective study on humans. Clin Oral Implants Res 2004;15:82–95.

211

"There is more to life than increasing its speed."

MAHATMA GANDHI

10

Implant Exposure Techniques

/ Arndt Happe, Gerd Körner

214

Depending on the timing of implant placement and the anatomical circumstances, augmentation is frequently performed in conjunction with implant placement in the esthetic zone.[1,2] These techniques often require primary mucosal coverage and therefore a second procedure to uncover the implant.

The decision regarding which technique to choose to uncover the implants depends on the anatomical circumstances before exposure as well as the surgical objectives. Is the only purpose of exposure to gain access to the implant, or will further corrections to the tissue be required? Exposure must not be underestimated as a surgical procedure: Decisive corrections can still be made at this stage. In cases of augmentation, the soft tissue flap often has to be mobilized to adequately cover the augmentation material. This sometimes means displacing the mucogingival junction, which can lead to esthetic and functional compromises. Exposure provides an opportunity to correct these compromises by apical displacement of the tissue. The importance of adequately keratinized mucosa around implants has been stressed in various clinical trials.[3]

Tissue thickening with connective tissue or connective tissue substitutes can still be done at the time of exposure. This chapter briefly outlines the relevant techniques for uncovering implants in the esthetic zone. Note that no destructive techniques (eg, electrotome, lasers) should be used. The appropriate exposure methods are also illustrated by clinical case studies in other chapters (eg, see Figs 9-20 to 9-22 in chapter 9).

Split-Finger Technique

This technique is suitable for uncovering one or more implants at the same time as papilla reconstruction. An intrasulcular incision is made in the area of the adjacent teeth and then runs palatally in the region of the planned interdental spaces. Depending on how much the tissue needs to be shifted in the buccal direction, the incision passes directly over the center of the implant or moves palatally at the palatal edge of the implant shoulder. This produces the typical W-shaped incision design (Fig 10-1).

The technique is also ideally suited to adjacent implants (Figs 10-2 and 10-3). Because of the specific incision technique and the excess parts of tissue palatal to the implants, the tissue can be spread around the gingiva formers so that no bone is exposed and an adequate tissue thickness is maintained all around the implants. At the same time, the tissue can easily be moved buccally so that a convexity is formed in the sense of an alveolar jugum.

Split-finger with CTG

After several surgical interventions, the soft tissue situation may be compromised and require improvement with a connective tissue graft (CTG). Figure 10-4 demonstrates this kind of case. When endodontic microsurgery was attempted, a vertical fracture became visible at the root of the maxillary right lateral incisor. Therefore, the tooth was first extracted. Bone augmentation of the site was completed 6 weeks later, then implants were placed after another 4 months. These different interventions led to a soft tissue deficiency in the region of the papillae (see Fig 10-4a). Papilla height is markedly reduced, especially in the area visible from the vestibular aspect. With the aid of a CTG combined with a split-finger technique according to Misch et al,[4] tissue is transferred interproximally from the palatal aspect to the vestibular aspect, and the apex of the palatal papilla is therefore moved in the vestibular direction (see the CTG at Exposure section in chapter 8).

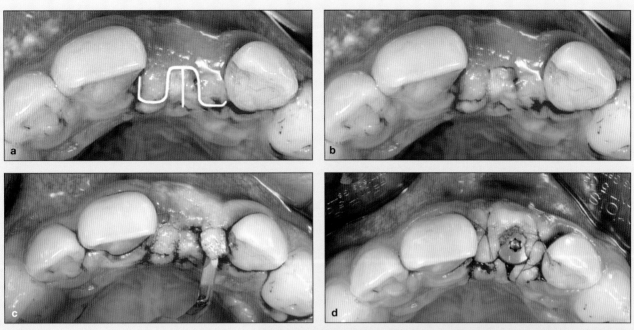

Fig 10-1 / *(a)* Planned incision path for the split-finger technique. *(b)* The incision is made along the planned path. *(c)* The papillary flaps can be readily dissected free with an angled micro scalpel. *(d)* Tissue adaptation around the gingiva former. *(e)* Condition after healing 2 weeks postoperatively.

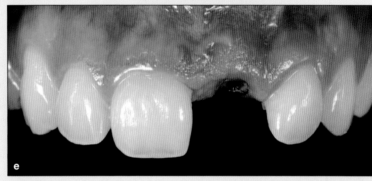

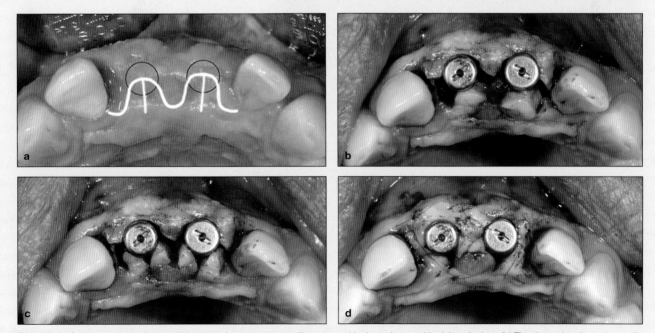

Fig 10-2 / *(a)* Locations of the adjacent implants at the maxillary central incisor sites and incision design. *(b)* The tissue has been buccally displaced after placement of the gingiva formers. *(c)* The palatal tissue excesses have been divided. *(d)* The soft tissue is adapted and sutured around the gingiva formers with 7-0 sutures.

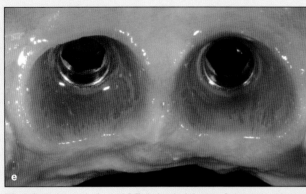 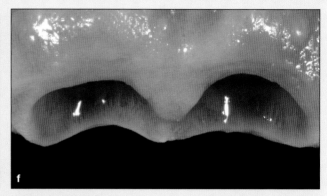

Fig 10-2 *cont.* / *(e and f)* Fully healed tissue after contouring with provisional restorations.

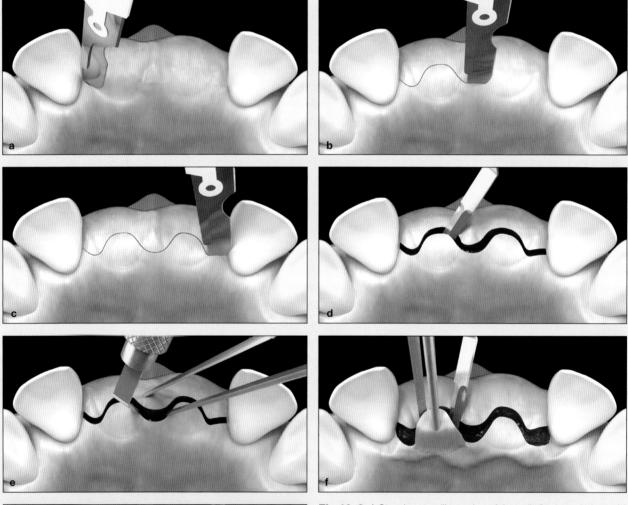

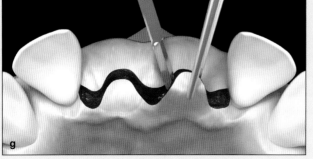

Fig 10-3 / Step-by-step illustration of the split-finger technique. *(a)* The incision begins at the adjacent tooth clearly palatal to the future papilla. *(b and c)* The incision is made in a wave pattern over the center of the implant, ending clearly palatally again at the other adjacent tooth. *(d to g)* The flaps are dissected (split) away from the bone with an angled microblade. →

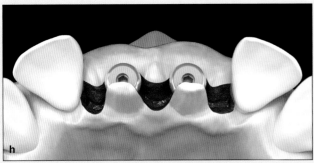

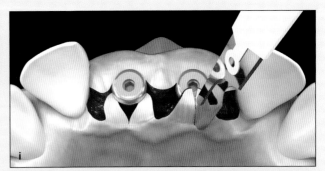

Fig 10-3 *cont.* / *(h)* The gingiva former pushes the buccal flap in the buccal direction, and the palatal flaps are propped up. *(i)* The palatal flaps are split. *(j)* The flaps are closed with 6-0 or 7-0 sutures.

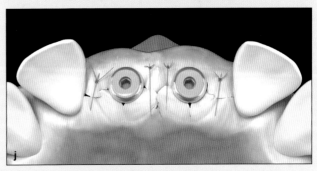

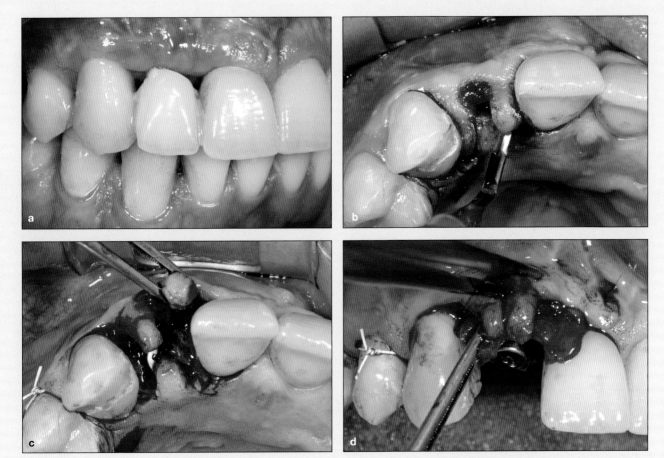

Fig 10-4 / *(a)* Loss of papillae after various surgical interventions at the maxillary right lateral incisor. The bonded partial denture is in place. *(b)* Dissection of the papillae with a microblade or micro scalpel. *(c)* The flap is prepared according to the split-finger design. *(d)* A CTG is introduced for relining.

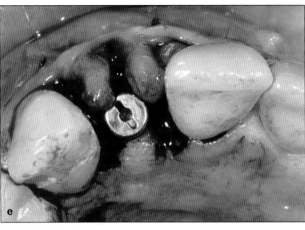
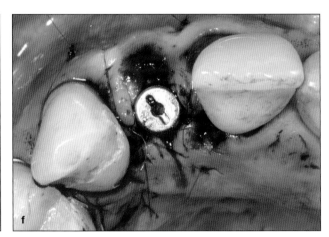

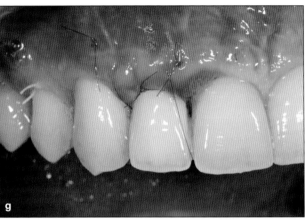
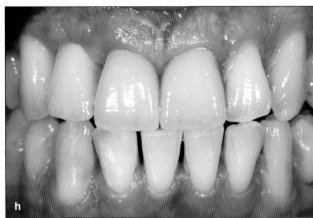

Fig 10-4 *cont.* / *(e and f)* The CTG is fixed with 7-0 sutures, and the soft tissues are apposed with 7-0 sutures. *(g)* Situation 1 week postoperatively: The tissue is coronally fixed with a holding suture over the provisional bonded partial denture. *(h)* Final appearance: The interproximal tissue in the region of the right lateral incisor has now moved buccally and is therefore visible.

Roll-Flap Technique

In the roll-flap technique, the papillae are not detached. The mucosa over the implant is deepithelialized so that a connective tissue flap is formed after incision and flap preparation. A small CTG can then be pedicled palatally to the connective tissue flap. The CTG is folded inward buccally and tucked into a supraperiosteal pocket prepared for the purpose (Fig 10-5). The clinical example depicted in Fig 10-6 shows how the vestibular tissue is thickened so that an alveolar jugum is reconstructed. The roll-flap technique can also be combined with the split-finger technique if the clinician also wants to exert an influence on the papillary area (Fig 10-7).

The technique can also be used in the premolar and molar region for several implants. This involves making an incision palatal to the implants, not perpendicular to the bone but in a tunneling fashion to ensure portions of connective tissue are pedicled palatal to the flap (Fig 10-8). The example in Fig 10-9 shows how keratinized tissue can be moved from the palatal aspect to the buccal aspect with this method. Furthermore, connective tissue is transferred from palatal to buccal. Therefore, implant exposure can contribute to additional reconstruction of the alveolar process. The interimplant areas can be covered with small rotation flaps from the palatal area (ie, modified Palacci technique[5]) or with free soft tissue grafts from the retromolar region (inlay grafts).[6]

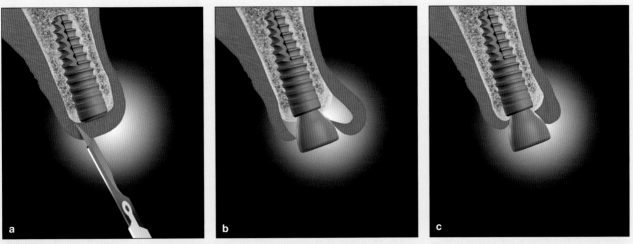

Fig 10-5 / Illustration of the roll-flap principle. *(a)* The incision is made palatal to the implant. The tissue over the implant has been deepithelialized. *(b)* After the implant is uncovered, the deepithelialized tissue is transferred in the buccal direction. *(c)* The transferred tissue is rolled inward buccal to the gingival former, which leads to soft tissue thickening.

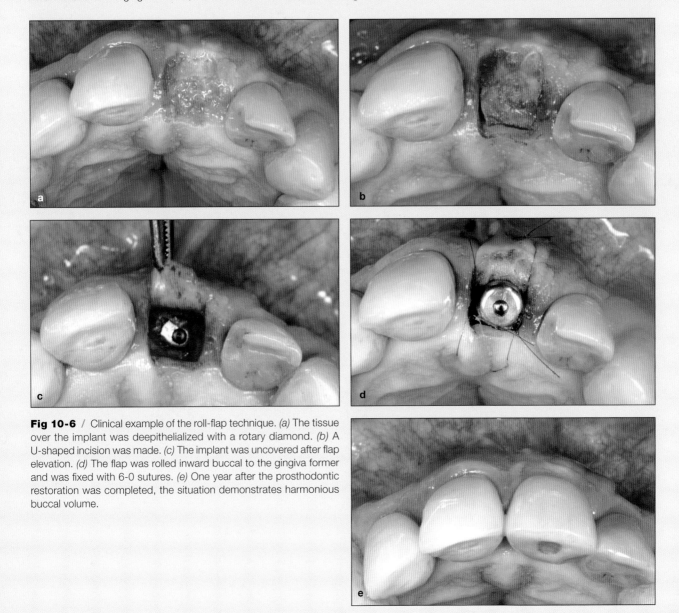

Fig 10-6 / Clinical example of the roll-flap technique. *(a)* The tissue over the implant was deepithelialized with a rotary diamond. *(b)* A U-shaped incision was made. *(c)* The implant was uncovered after flap elevation. *(d)* The flap was rolled inward buccal to the gingiva former and was fixed with 6-0 sutures. *(e)* One year after the prosthodontic restoration was completed, the situation demonstrates harmonious buccal volume.

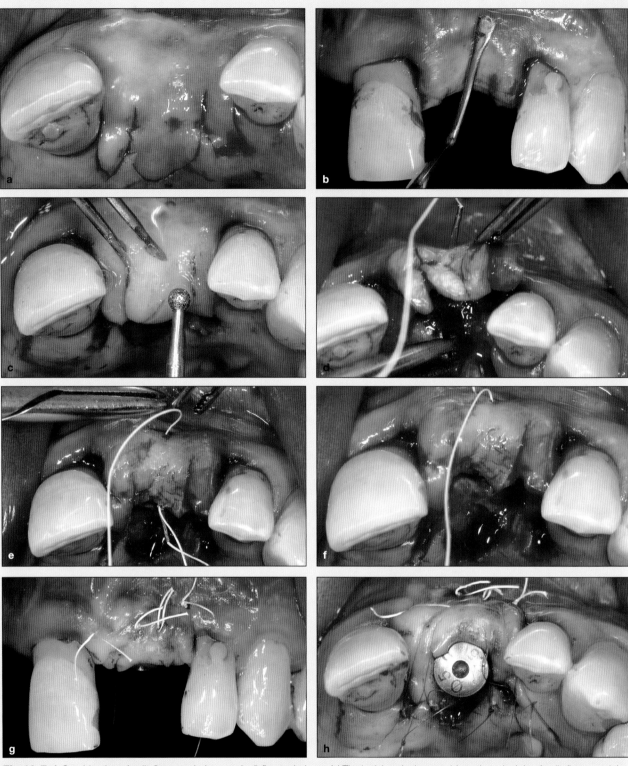

Fig 10-7 / Combination of split-finger technique and roll-flap technique. *(a)* The incision design combines the principle of split-finger and the roll-flap techniques. *(b)* A tunneling instrument is used to detach the area buccal to the implant. *(c)* The site of the roll flap is deepithelialized. *(d)* The suture technique starts from the buccal aspect. *(e and f)* The connective tissue flap is snared and pulled into the buccal pocket using a vertical mattress suture. *(g and h)* Buccal and occlusal views after surgery.

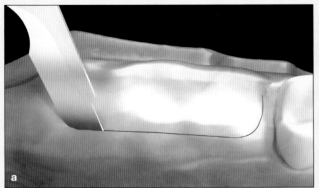

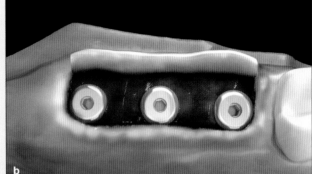

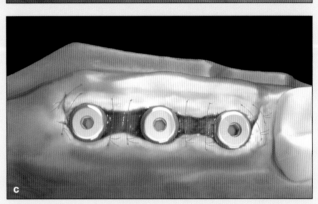

Fig 10-8 / Illustration of the roll-flap technique in the posterior dentition. *(a)* A transverse undermining palatal incision is made at stage-two surgery so that as much connective tissue as possible from the palate remains on the flap. *(b)* Once the gingiva formers are placed, the flap is transferred buccally. *(c)* Connective tissue is rolled inward buccally, and the interimplant areas are filled with grafts and sutured.

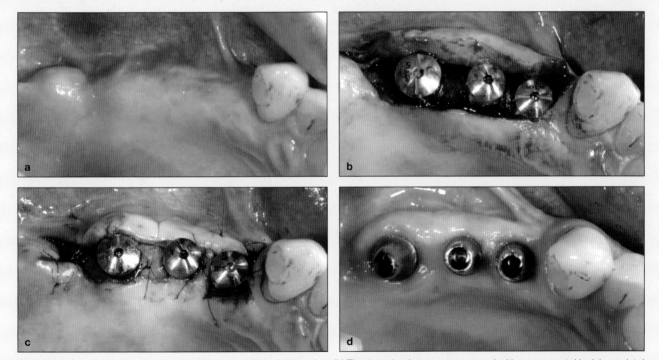

Fig 10-9 / *(a)* Free-end situation distal to the maxillary right canine. *(b)* The three implants are uncovered with a paracrestal incision palatal to the implants; connective tissue parts are visible on the flap. *(c)* Connective tissue is rolled inward after transfer in the buccal direction. A flap is folded inward from the palatal aspect between the premolar implants, and a free CTG is placed between the second premolar and first molar implants. *(d)* Healed alveolar process with abutment components in situ.

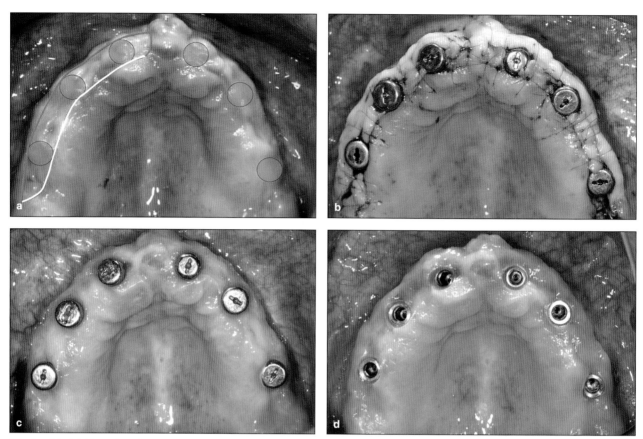

Fig 10-10 / *(a)* Location of implants and path of planned incision. The incision is made palatal to the implants *(white line)* and then turns to the buccal and runs buccal to the implants *(gray line)*. *(b)* Situation after the exposure operation is completed and inlay grafts are placed. *(c)* Healed ridge with gingiva formers in place. *(d)* Healed ridge after gingiva formers have been removed.

Inlay Grafts

It is a basic principle during implant exposure in the maxilla to transfer keratinized tissue from the palatal aspect to the buccal aspect. However, this leads to deficiencies between implants. If several implants are exposed with a crestal or paracrestal incision, as during apical displacement, this will result in interimplant tissue defects. These defects are then filled with full-thickness mucosal grafts or CTGs[6] (Fig 10-10). If the areas are not covered but left to granulate freely, defects might remain between implants, leading to esthetic and functional problems caused by inadequate papillae. Furthermore, this has an adverse effect on crestal bone remodeling, leading to increased peri-implant bone resorption.[7] Adequate soft tissue between implants or in pontic areas is necessary for sufficient soft tissue contouring.

Meander Technique

The meander technique may also be used to solve the problem of deficient tissue between implants when moving the flap from palatal to buccal. This technique involves raising a mucosal flap that merges palatally into parallel mucosal flaps that lie in the interproximal areas after buccal displacement (Fig 10-11). The technique is complex and must first be practiced on a suitable model (eg, an animal model) before it is used on patients. Figure 10-12 depicts a clinical case.[8]

Fig 10-11 / *(a)* Design of the incision for the meander technique. *(b)* The mucosal flap is displaced buccally; the finger-like flaps slide past each other, and the *brown* areas heal by secondary intention.

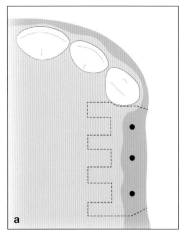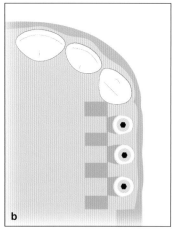

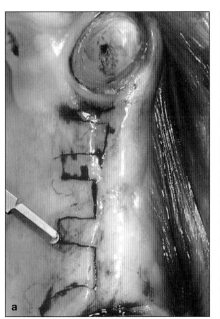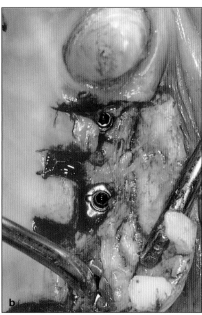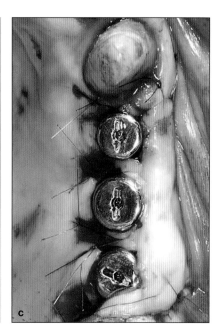

Fig 10-12 / *(a)* Implants at the sites of the maxillary left first premolar to first molar are uncovered by the meander method according to Körner (as demonstrated in Wachtel et al[8]). Note the displacement of the keratinized mucosa for simultaneous widening of the relevant structures buccal to the implants and interproximal to the canine. *(b and c)* Preparation of a split-skin flap by the meander method to uncover the implants and for apical displacement of the keratinized mucosa to improve the buccal and interproximal peri-implant situation.

Keyhole Access Expansion Technique

If the alveolar process is already anatomically shaped and the only requirement is to expose an implant, minimally invasive exposure can be completed with a stab incision and dilatation of the tissue. This technique, also known as *keyhole access expansion*, therefore works by displacement[9] (Fig 10-13). Because the surgeon only creates a small opening over the implant and has reduced-diameter access, the prefabricated gingiva former immediately exerts pressure on the interproximal tissue, which ideally rises up slightly as a result. The tissue can then be further contoured with provisional restorations. The advantage of this technique is that the peri-implant bone is not exposed and there is no scarring. Furthermore, no tissue is sacrificed. However, it leaves the surgeon with no possible means of further influencing the contouring of peri-implant tissue (see Chapter 8, Figs 8-10t to 8-10y).

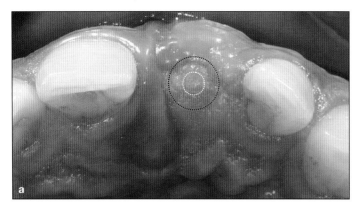
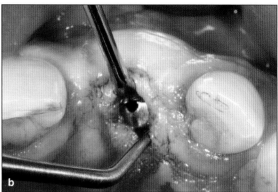
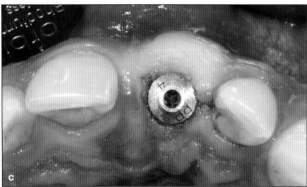
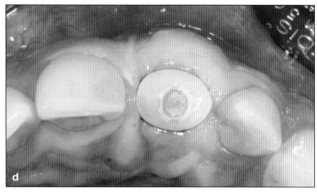
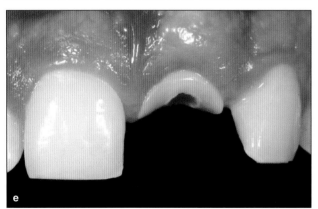

224

Fig 10-13 / *(a)* View after implant placement and augmentation (the implant position and diameter is indicated by the *black line*; the planned excision access is indicated by the *white line*). *(b)* Dilatation of the access opening with papilla dissector or tunneling knife. *(c)* Ischemia of the tissue is noticeable after the gingiva former is placed. *(d)* After a few days, further dilatation and contouring can be completed with a customized gingiva former. *(e)* Contoured peri-implant soft tissue.

References

1. Grunder U, Wenz B, Schupbach P. Guided bone regeneration around single-tooth implants in the esthetic zone: A case series. Int J Periodontics Restorative Dent 2011;31:613–620.
2. Buser D, Wittneben J, Bornstein MM, Grütter L, Chappuis V, Belser UC. Stability of contour augmentation and esthetic outcomes of implant-supported single crowns in the esthetic zone: 3-year results of a prospective study with early implant placement postextraction. J Periodontol 2011;82:342–349.
3. Brito C, Tenenbaum HC, Wong BK, Schmitt C, Nogueira-Filho G. Is keratinized mucosa indispensable to maintain peri-implant health? A systematic review of the literature. J Biomed Mater Res B Appl Biomater 2014;102:643–650.
4. Misch CE, Al-Shammari KF, Wang HL. Creation of interimplant papillae through a split-finger technique. Implant Dent 2004;13:20–27.
5. Palacci P. Aesthetic treatment of the anterior maxilla: Soft and hard tissue considerations. Oral Maxillofac Surg Clin North Am 2004;16:127–137.
6. Grunder U. The inlay-graft technique to create papillae between implants. J Esthet Dent 1997;9:165–168.
7. Berglundh T, Lindhe J. Dimension of the periimplant mucosa. Biological width revisited. J Clin Periodontol 1996;23:971–973.
8. Wachtel H, Schlee M, Körner G. ZMK - Live Sonderedition – DGP Frühjahrstagung. Berlin: Quintessence, 2004.
9. Happe A, Körner G, Nolte A. The keyhole access expansion technique for flapless implant stage-two surgery: Technical note. Int J Periodontics Restorative Dent 2010;30:97–101.

*"The greater our knowledge increases,
the more our ignorance unfolds."*

JOHN F. KENNEDY

11

Implant Abutments

/ Anja Zembic, Arndt Happe

226

W
hen missing teeth are replaced with implant reconstructions, the main aim is to replicate the natural teeth and create an esthetic appearance (Fig 11-1). Other aims include successful biologic integration and mechanical performance over a period of at least 5 years. Implant treatment is a therapy with good and successful predictability and high survival rates. Nevertheless, mechanical and biologic complications are not uncommon, and only about 66.4% of patients are entirely free of complications after 5 years.[1] For long-term success, the peri-implant tissue must be kept healthy, and the implant-abutment connection should be biologically and mechanically stable.

Implant-Abutment Connection

The implant abutment joins the implant to the oral cavity and plays a key role in the transition from bone to soft tissue. For this reason, the biocompatibility of the abutment is extremely important. Many different types of implants are currently available, but they all use two fundamental types of implant-abutment connection: external or internal. The external connection uses an external hex and a butt-joint connection (Fig 11-2). Internal connections can be further classified into conical Morse taper connections (Fig 11-3) or nonconical "tube in tube" connections. The results of in vitro experiments prove significantly higher resistance to bending for internal conical and nonconical connections than for external butt-joint connections.[2,3]

It is reasonable to assume that an internal implant-abutment connection might have a positive impact on clinical performance in terms of less frequent mechanical complications (eg, loosening or fracture of the components). A systematic review article that included 15 studies on implants with external connections and 9 studies on implants with internal connections partly supports this assumption and reports abutment screw fractures (0.2%) solely with externally anchored metal abutments.[4] On the other hand, no significant differences were found between externally and internally anchored abutments with regard to the incidence of abutment fractures and abutment screw loosening or their clinical performance.[4,5] However, biologic complications around implants were twice as frequent with external abutment connections as with internal abutment connections.[4]

Metallic bases

Internally connected zirconia abutments with a metallic base showed the highest fracture load in vitro compared with internally connected single-piece and externally connected zirconia abutments.[6] Zirconia is a more brittle material than titanium. If zirconia abutments are in contact with titanium implants and micromotion occurs around the joining surfaces, abrasive wear of the titanium ensues, and the abraded titanium particles become visible as a slightly blackish discoloration of the zirconia abutment (known as *fretting wear*)[7] (Fig 11-4). Zirconia abutments with an incorporated metallic base bring metal instead of zirconia into direct contact with titanium implants (Fig 11-5). In this way, the titanium wear around the implant-abutment connection can be reduced. The repercussions of wear for clinical performance are not known. It is likely that wear on the joining surfaces of implant and abutment contributes to greater rotational freedom. This might lead to mechanical complications (eg, screw loosening or fracture) in the case of implant-supported restorations that have already been functioning for several years. Laboratory findings confirm this assumption and show less rotational misfit for all-ceramic abutments with a metallic base than those without a metallic base.[8] Furthermore, internally connected single-piece zirconia abutments caused greater wear of titanium implants than internally connected single-piece

Fig 11-1 / *(a and b)* Five years after implant placement with a cement-retained all-ceramic crown on a zirconia abutment at the site of the right lateral incisor, the crown has a natural appearance with healthy and stable peri-implant mucosa.

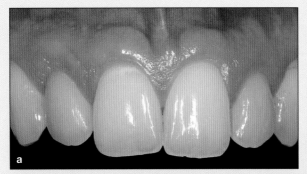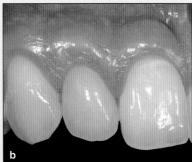

Fig 11-2 / *(a)* Externally connected zirconia abutment with butt joint and implant with external hex. (Courtesy of Dr Urs Brodbeck, Zürich, Switzerland.) *(b)* Radiograph of externally connected zirconia abutment with horizontal joining surfaces.

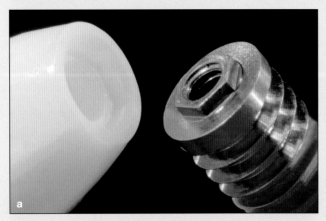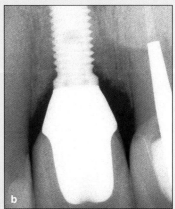

Fig 11-3 / *(a)* All-ceramic implant-supported crown cemented onto a single-piece zirconia abutment with an internal conical connection. *(b)* Radiograph of an internally connected zirconia abutment with a conical connection.

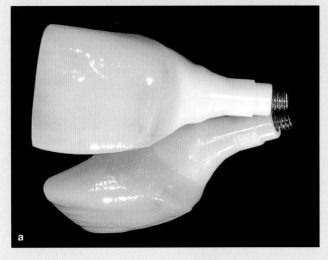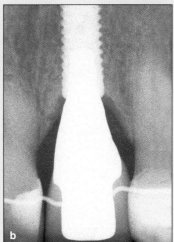

Fig 11-4 / Metallic particles demonstrating abrasive wear on the internal part of an externally connected zirconia abutment with a butt-joint connection. (Courtesy of Dr Urs Brodbeck, Zürich, Switzerland.)

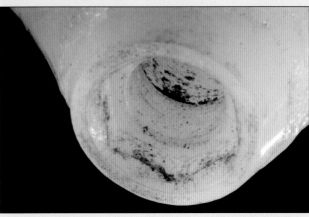

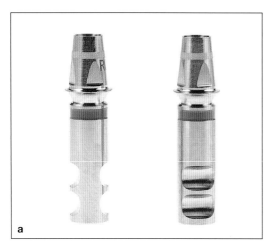
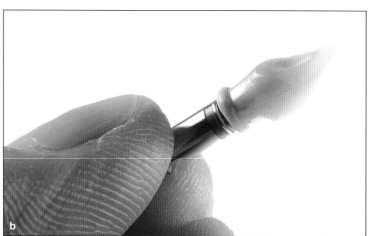
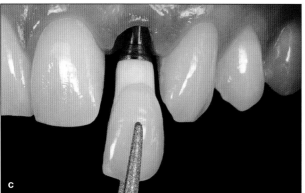
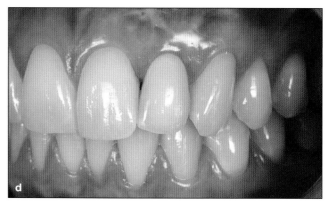

Fig 11-5 / *(a)* This metallic component forms the base for a zirconia abutment on a laboratory implant. *(b)* The crown is bonded to a titanium base. *(c)* The superstructure is tried in. *(d)* View of the restoration with the metallic base in place.

titanium abutments.[7,9] There is currently a lack of clinical trials on zirconia abutments with integrated metallic components. Therefore, the clinical value of metallic bases is not known. However, considering the superior in vitro results, internally connected zirconia abutments with metallic components should still be preferred to single-piece internally connected zirconia abutments. Furthermore, abutment fractures are easier to handle in practice if the zirconia does not impinge on the implant.

Microgap

Every type of implant-abutment connection also has some degree of bacterial leakage.[10,11] This microleakage is expressed as an increased number of inflammatory cells and an immune response, which stimulates resorption of the alveolar bone.[12–14] The area of microleakage (ie, microgap) is farther from the bone in internally connected abutments than externally connected abutments, which might prove advantageous for the stability of the peri-implant bone.

The microgap location may also explain the less frequent biologic complications of internally connected abutments noted previously.

Depending on the abutment configuration, different diameters of implant and abutment can be chosen for internally connected implants so that the abutment is narrower in the area of the connection. This is known as *platform switching*, a concept that has become relatively popular in implant therapy. This concept was recommended as a means of remedying the problem of adverse bone conditions between adjacent implants in the esthetic zone.[15,16] As a result of platform switching, the microgap shifts toward the center of the implant and away from the bone. In fact, there has been shown to be less bone resorption around implants with platform switching than those without platform switching (ie, with a flush implant-abutment connection).[17] Using platform switching is therefore advisable from a biologic perspective (see chapter 1, Fig 1-5b).

A study of internally connected single-piece zirconia abutments with and without platform switching revealed significantly higher bending moments for internally connected zirconia abutments with platform switching.[18] Nevertheless, it is important to bear in mind that a fracture of a zirconia abutment with platform switching occurs very deep in the implant (Fig 11-6), which makes abutment removal a difficult process that may damage the internal threads of the implant.

The extent of bacterial infiltration between implants and abutments also depends on how accurately the components fit together. The micromotion increases as fit accuracy diminishes, so the risk of complications also rises due to increased component wear. Abutments should be screwed to the torque recommended by the manufacturer. If the abutment screws do not reach the recommended torque, significantly larger micromotions occur at the joining surfaces of implant and abutment.[19] As a consequence, clinical performance might be impaired in the long term because of mechanical complications.

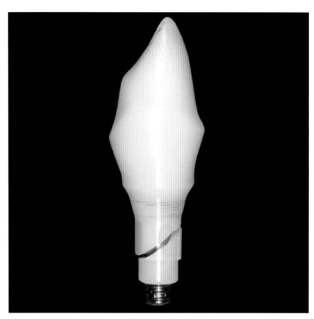

Fig 11-6 / Fracture pattern of a single-piece zirconia abutment with an internal conical connection.

Abutment Selection

When choosing an abutment, it is possible to use one from the same manufacturer as the implant or from a different manufacturer, and it is less expensive to use "generic" abutments. However, when the design and material are different between implant and abutment, the contact surfaces do not fit as accurately. An in vitro study showed some compromises in practical handling as well as higher rotational misfit rates for generic abutments than for abutments supplied from the implant manufacturer.[20] Mechanical failure may be a possible consequence.[20]

Misfits in the connection between abutment and implant may also occur if original zirconia abutments from one implant manufacturer (NobelProcera, Nobel Biocare) are used with implants from different manufacturers.[21] The use of components that match the implants from that particular manufacturer is therefore imperative for the successful biologic and mechanical performance of an implant restoration.

Abutment macrostructure

Dentists can choose between industrially manufactured standard abutments and custom abutments fabricated by a dental technician. The dimensions of prefabricated abutments are standardized, so the shape of the crown

has to compensate for the missing anatomical shape and hence the inadequate soft tissue support.

Customized abutments can be adapted to the individual clinical situation. They are therefore an ideal choice in cases where there is a wide discrepancy between implant and crown diameter. In addition, the position of the crown margin can be controlled, which is important for cemented reconstructions. Finally, the shape of the natural tooth can be imitated in the soft tissue emergence area. The main indication for custom abutments is to support a scalloped contour of the peri-implant mucosa and to create a natural emergence profile in the esthetic zone (Fig 11-7). At the same time, an unfavorable implant position can be compensated for with a custom abutment and a cemented reconstruction. Regardless of whether a prefabricated or a custom abutment is selected, the shape of the restoration should replicate the tooth being replaced and should ensure that it will be possible for the patient to be able to effectively clean the restoration.

In terms of shaping the abutment, a convex shape is usually preferable because it offers adequate soft tissue support and optimal cleanability. However, for the labial aspect, it may be advantageous to have a concave abutment shape to give space to the soft tissue and minimize pressure on the marginal mucosa (Fig 11-8). The emergence profile is important not only to the esthetic appearance but also to the development of a healthy vertical and horizontal biologic width.

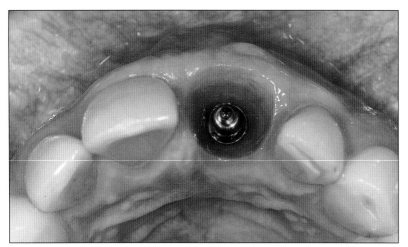

Fig 11-7 / The emergence profile is shaped to allow for the triangular shape of a central incisor, which gives the implant-supported crown a natural appearance.

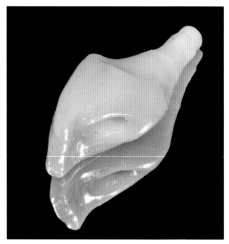

Fig 11-8 / Labially, a concave abutment shape may be advantageous to allow space for the soft tissue and minimize pressure on the marginal mucosa.

Abutments have close contact with the mucosa. To establish soft tissue adhesion, the abutment material must be biocompatible and must not cause adverse effects on the peri-implant hard and soft tissues. Under healthy conditions, a mucosal seal is formed, which consists of a barrier epithelium that adheres to the titanium surface with hemidesmosomes and underlying connective tissue, with fibers running parallel to the implant.[22] The connective tissue of the mucosa is poorer in blood vessels and fibroblasts but richer in collagen fibers than the connective tissue around teeth. The mucosal attachment therefore resembles scar tissue with a potentially reduced immune response.[23] As soon as the abutments are exposed to the oral cavity, they become contaminated with bacteria. A submucosal microflora similar to the teeth becomes established within a few weeks.[24]

Various preclinical and clinical trials have studied the formation of soft tissue attachment to different abutment materials. The soft tissue around titanium abutments consists of a junctional epithelium and underlying connective tissue, which attaches firmly to the abutment surface.[25] A comparable attachment can be seen around alumina and zirconia abutments.[25,26] By contrast, earlier animal studies with gold abutments showed increased peri-implant soft tissue inflammation and bone resorption where the attachment was apical to the implant-abutment connection.[25,27] More recent clinical trials support these results but indicate comparable clinical results for titanium and gold abutments.[28,29] Clinical comparison of zirconia and titanium abutments after 5 years showed better biologic results

for zirconia abutments with regard to peri-implant bone loss, probing depths, bleeding on probing, and plaque accumulation.[30]

Abutment microstructure: Surface roughness and surface free energy

Bacterial adhesion depends on the biocompatibility, surface free energy, and surface roughness of a material.[31] Formation of the biofilm is promoted by increasing surface free energy and surface roughness. A clinical trial found significantly less surface free energy at zirconia abutments than at titanium abutments.[32] This explains the less pronounced adhesion of plaque to zirconia test specimens compared with titanium specimens that had comparable surface roughness.[33]

With regard to abutment design, however, surface roughness (Ra) is a more important factor than surface free energy for plaque accumulation. Roughness is determined by the nature of the surface treatment. An Ra value of 0.2 μm was estimated as the optimal mean abutment roughness to reduce plaque adhesion and to enable establishment of a mucosal seal.[34] There was a positive effect on the composition of the microflora when the Ra value of 0.2 μm was reduced.

By contrast, a highly glazed finished zirconia surface led to increased probing depths and induced soft tissue recession.[35] Therefore, highly glazed finished zirconia abutments are not advantageous (Fig 11-9). A study on

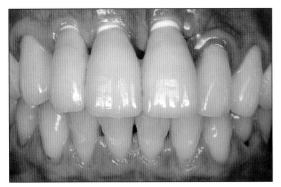

Fig 11-9 / Vestibular recessions at highly glazed zirconia abutments.

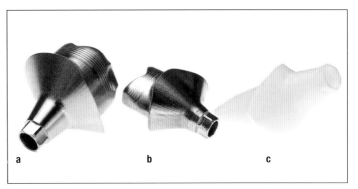

Fig 11-10 / CAD/CAM-fabricated custom abutments made of titanium *(a)*, an alloy with a high gold content *(b)*, and zirconia *(c)*.

231

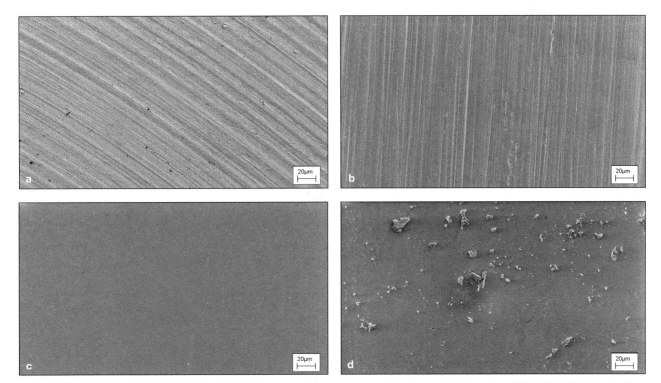

Fig 11-11 / Scanning electron microscope (SEM) images of various surfaces. Original magnification ×333. *(a)* Machined titanium surface. *(b)* Zirconia surface polished with a rubber polisher with diamond grit according to the polishing protocol described in chapter 12. *(c)* Highly glazed finished zirconia surface. *(d)* Smear layer after polishing zirconia with abrasive rubber polisher. (Courtesy of Dr Andreas Schäfer, Münster, Germany.)

the long-term clinical performance of zirconia abutments reported few recessions around implant crowns.[36] The abutments were polished before use in the mouth so the strength of the material would not be influenced. (A rough zirconia surface increases the probability of an abutment fracture in the long term.[37]) Generally speaking, a higher incidence of recessions was found around ceramic abutments than around metallic ones.[38]

The fabrication technique clearly influences the roughness of an abutment: The roughness of milled abutments

(29 μm) is below that of cast (98 μm) and sintered (115 μm) abutments.[39] Most abutments are currently milled using computer-aided design/computer-assisted manufacturing (CAD/CAM) technology (Fig 11-10).

An in vitro study showed that polishing zirconia with standard abrasive rubber polishers produces the desired roughness of 0.2 μm (comparable to milled titanium), whereas the high-glaze finishing renders the surfaces too smooth (0.07 μm)[40] (Fig 11-11). The polished surfaces have to be cleaned meticulously to clear them of polisher

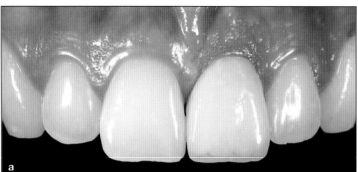
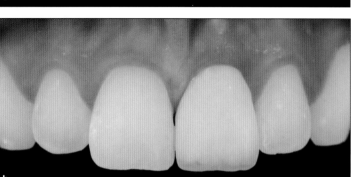

Fig 11-12 / *(a)* Implant restoration of the left central incisor with typical gray discoloration of the soft tissue. *(b)* Same image with a polarizing filter.

232

residue as much as possible. Unfortunately, the roughness of prefabricated abutments is often not specified by the various implant manufacturers.

Color and Esthetics

Patients have increased awareness and demands when it comes to esthetics—both for the "white esthetics" of the crown but also the "pink esthetics" of the peri-implant soft tissue. Factors that influence the color of the peri-implant soft tissue include the abutment material, soft tissue thickness, and restorative material (translucency and brightness).[41] While metal abutments combined with porcelain-fused-to-metal (PFM) crowns can cause a gray discoloration of the mucosa (Fig 11-12), ceramic abutments with all-ceramic crowns have the esthetic advantage of causing significantly less mucosal discoloration than metallic abutments.[42] A randomized controlled clinical trial compared the influence of titanium and zirconia on discoloration of the peri-implant mucosa.[43] A clinically visible color change to the peri-implant mucosa was observed with both materials. These results coincide with those of a study in which titanium, gold, and zirconia abutments in combination with all-ceramic

crowns caused a comparable visible color difference.[44] Mucosal thickness in these studies was roughly 2 mm. With increasing mucosal thickness (ie, > 2 mm), the influence of the abutment material on the esthetic outcome diminishes. Therefore, the esthetic advantage of ceramic abutments becomes more apparent in situations with a thin mucosa.

In a test on the effect of different color strips on peri-implant mucosa, no color difference was observed for the test colors light pink and light orange, which match the colors of soft tissue and dentin.[45] Yet, the results of a clinical trial showed that zirconia abutments veneered with pink ceramic had no effect on the peri-implant mucosal color compared with nonveneered white zirconia abutments.[41]

The human eye perceives differences in color brightness more subtly than shade. One study investigated the effect of fluorescent veneered zirconia abutments on the color of peri-implant mucosa.[46] A light orange veneering ceramic was used, and the results showed no color difference in the soft tissue versus the natural reference teeth in 42% of patients and markedly less color variation than in trials with conventional zirconia abutments. Monolithic high-performance ceramics with different optical properties are now available for abutment manufacture (Fig 11-13).

Fig 11-13 / *(a)* Different abutment materials with different colors. *(b)* Appearance of the materials under ultraviolet light. Only the fluorescent stained zirconia and lithium disilicate exhibit fluorescent properties.

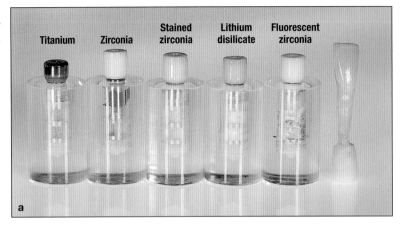

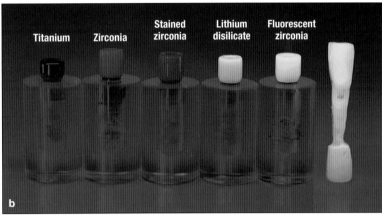

All the quoted studies compare the peri-implant mucosa with the gingiva of natural teeth. However, it should be noted that vascularization of the soft tissue has a decisive influence on its color.[47] Peri-implant mucosa resembles scar tissue and contains more collagen fibers but fewer blood vessels than gingiva. Therefore, the effect of the differing makeup of mucosa and gingiva on soft tissue color might explain the reported differences.

Ceramic Implant Abutments

The first generation of ceramic abutments was manufactured from alumina. Clinical trials documented fracture rates ranging from 1.9% to 7% after 1 to 5 years.[48–50] Subsequently, in 1995 zirconia was introduced as an abutment material: another high-performance ceramic with the highest fracture toughness and flexural strength. Zirconia rapidly developed into the first-choice ceramic abutment material. A special feature of zirconia is its resistance to crack propagation; this so-called transformation tough-

ening leads to better fracture toughness of the material.[51] However, this property can become weaker as the material ages. Laboratory data demonstrated a decrease in fracture toughness of 50% when zirconia was subjected to a simulated 10-year aging process in a humid environment.[52] In vitro data are difficult to apply to clinical situations, and a current prospective study shows excellent performance and survival rates for zirconia abutments after more than 10 years in function.[36] Other prospective studies on different types of zirconia abutments demonstrate survival rates of 100% after up to 5 years of functional loading.[30,53–56]

Accordingly, aging of zirconia abutments in the oral cavity will not necessarily lead to complete failure. On the other hand, two prospective studies report fractures after 1 and 3 years of clinical functioning in 18% of internally connected single-piece zirconia abutments.[57,58] Another retrospective study reported zirconia abutment fractures in 10% of cases after 12 years.[59] Different abutment types and implant systems were used in this trial. Externally connected abutments with horizontal butt joints showed higher survival rates over a period of up to 5 years than abutments with an internal connection. This highlights the fracture risk of internally connected single-piece abutments and justifies the use of zirconia abutments with a metallic component.

Additional long-term data are required to more accurately analyze the effects of aging on the survival of different types of zirconia abutments. A comparison of zirconia and titanium abutments revealed similar results after 5 years in terms of survival rates as well as technical and biologic complications.[30] However, zirconia abutments tended to show better esthetic results than titanium abutments after 1 year.[57] The fact that the stability of zirconia abutments is influenced by variables such as the fabrication method or the abutment wall thickness has been well studied. For an abutment to prove clinically successful, the wall thickness should not be less than 0.5 mm. As yet there is no standardized protocol for handling zirconia abutments in the laboratory or practice setting. Future studies should therefore specify in more detail the fabrication method, surface roughness, and wall thickness of zirconia abutments.

Conclusion

When selecting the abutment type, it is important to note that internally and externally connected abutments perform equally well, although there is more scientific information currently available about external abutment connections. In esthetically sensitive areas, bone-level implants—with inherent internal connections—are recommended for an esthetically attractive result. If a zirconia abutment is used in these cases, it is advisable to choose an abutment with an integrated metallic component to avoid direct contact between the zirconia and the implant. When making their choice, dentists should bear in mind that single-piece internally connected zirconia abutments entail a risk of fractures that are difficult to resolve and can cause damage to the internal threads of the implant. Regardless of the connection type, all abutments should be tightened with the predefined torque recommended by the manufacturer. The use of abutments and components made by the implant manufacturer is strongly recommended to avoid unforeseen mechanical complications. Custom abutments are the preferred choice in the esthetic zone for cemented reconstructions. This is especially true for cases with a wide discrepancy between implant and crown diameter and in situations where the implant position differs from the planned, ideal prosthetic position. Otherwise, standard abutments can also be chosen.

In the esthetically sensitive and visible areas with a thin mucosa, zirconia is the abutment material of choice to avoid mucosal discoloration. Metallic abutments can be used in esthetically irrelevant areas and for thick soft tissue biotypes. The wall thickness of zirconia abutments should be no less than 0.5 mm, and the abutments should be fabricated according to a standardized protocol. The surface should not be polished to a high-glaze finish. The ideal roughness of the abutment surface is approximately 0.2 μm.

References

1. Pjetursson BE, Thoma D, Jung R, Zwahlen M, Zembic A. A systematic review of the survival and complication rates of implant supported fixed dental prostheses (FDPs) after a mean observation period of at least 5 years. Clin Oral Implants Res 2012;23(suppl 6):22–38.
2. Norton MR. An in vitro evaluation of the strength of an internal conical interface compared to a butt joint interface in implant design. Clin Oral Implants Res 1997;8:290–298.
3. Truninger TC, Stawarczyk B, Leutert CR, Sailer TR, Hämmerle CH, Sailer I. Bending moments of zirconia and titanium abutments with internal and external implant-abutment connections after aging and chewing simulation. Clin Oral Implants Res 2012;23:12–18.
4. Zembic A, Kim S, Zwahlen M, Kelly JR. Systematic review of the survival rate and incidence of biologic, technical, and esthetic complications of single implant abutments supporting fixed prostheses. Int J Oral Maxillofac Implants 2014;29(suppl):99–116.
5. Theoharidou A, Petridis HP, Tzannas K, Garefis P. Abutment screw loosening in single-implant restorations: A systematic review. Int J Oral Maxillofac Implants 2008;23:681–690.
6. Sailer I, Sailer T, Stawarczyk B, Jung RE, Hämmerle CH. In vitro study of the influence of the type of connection on the fracture load of zirconia abutments with internal and external implant-abutment connections. Int J Oral Maxillofac Implants 2009;24:850–858.
7. Stimmelmayr M, Edelhoff D, Güth JF, Erdelt K, Happe A, Beyer F. Wear at the titanium-titanium and the titanium-zirconia implant-abutment interface: A comparative in vitro study. Dent Mater 2012;28:1215–1220.
8. Garine WN, Funkenbusch PD, Ercoli C, Wodenscheck J, Murphy WC. Measurement of the rotational misfit and implant-abutment gap of all-ceramic abutments. Int J Oral Maxillofac Implants 2007;22:928–938.
9. Klotz MW, Taylor TD, Goldberg AJ. Wear at the titanium-zirconia implant-abutment interface: A pilot study. Int J Oral Maxillofac Implants 2011;26:970–975.
10. Harder S, Dimaczek B, Açil Y, Terheyden H, Freitag-Wolf S, Kern M. Molecular leakage at implant-abutment connection: In vitro investigation of tightness of internal conical implant-abutment connections against endotoxin penetration. Clin Oral Investig 2010;14:427–432.
11. Romanos GE, Biltucci MT, Kokaras A, Paster BJ. Bacterial composition at the implant-abutment connection under loading in vivo. Clin Implant Dent Relat Res 2016;18:138–145.

12. Ericsson I, Persson LG, Berglundh T, Marinello CP, Lindhe J, Klinge B. Different types of inflammatory reactions in peri-implant soft tissues. J Clin Periodontol 1995;22:255–261.

13. Hermann JS, Buser D, Schenk RK, Schoolfield JD, Cochran DL. Biologic width around one- and two-piece titanium implants. Clin Oral Implants Res 2001;12:559–571.

14. Broggini N, McManus LM, Hermann JS, et al. Persistent acute inflammation at the implant-abutment interface. J Dent Res 2003;82:232–237.

15. Lazzara RJ, Porter SS. Platform switching: A new concept in implant dentistry for controlling postrestorative crestal bone levels. Int J Periodontics Restorative Dent 2006;26:9–17.

16. Grunder U, Gracis S, Capelli M. Influence of the 3-D bone-to-implant relationship on esthetics. Int J Periodontics Restorative Dent 2005;25:113–119.

17. Chrcanovic BR, Albrektsson T, Wennerberg A. Platform switch and dental implants: A meta-analysis. J Dent 2015;43:629–646.

18. Leutert CR, Stawarczyk B, Truninger TC, Hämmerle CH, Sailer I. Bending moments and types of failure of zirconia and titanium abutments with internal implant-abutment connections: A laboratory study. Int J Oral Maxillofac Implants 2012;27:505–512.

19. Gratton DG, Aquilino SA, Stanford CM. Micromotion and dynamic fatigue properties of the dental implant-abutment interface. J Prosthet Dent 2001;85:47–52.

20. Gigandet M, Bigolin G, Faoro F, Bürgin W, Brägger U. Implants with original and non-original abutment connections. Clin Implant Dent Relat Res 2014;16:303–311.

21. de Morais Alves da Cunha T, de Araújo RP, da Rocha PV, Amoedo RM. Comparison of fit accuracy between Procera custom abutments and three implant systems. Clin Implant Dent Relat Res 2012;14:890–895.

22. Berglundh T, Lindhe J, Ericsson I, Marinello CP, Liljenberg B, Thomsen P. The soft tissue barrier at implants and teeth. Clin Oral Implants Res 1991;2:81–90.

23. Berglundh T, Lindhe J, Jonsson K, Ericsson I. The topography of the vascular systems in the periodontal and peri-implant tissues in the dog. J Clin Periodontol 1994;21:189–193.

24. Salvi GE, Fürst MM, Lang NP, Persson GR. One-year bacterial colonization patterns of Staphylococcus aureus and other bacteria at implants and adjacent teeth. Clin Oral Implants Res 2008;19:242–248.

25. Abrahamsson I, Berglundh T, Glantz PO, Lindhe J. The mucosal attachment at different abutments. An experimental study in dogs. J Clin Periodontol 1998;25:721–727.

26. Nakamura K, Kanno T, Milleding P, Örtengren U. Zirconia as a dental implant abutment material: A systematic review. Int J Prosthodont 2010;23:299–309.

27. Welander M, Abrahamsson I, Berglundh T. The mucosal barrier at implant abutments of different materials. Clin Oral Implants Res 2008;19:635–641.

28. Linkevicius T, Apse P. Influence of abutment material on stability of peri-implant tissues: A systematic review. Int J Oral Maxillofac Implants 2008;26:449–456.

29. Vigolo P, Givani A, Majzoub Z, Cordioli G. A 4-year prospective study to assess peri-implant hard and soft tissues adjacent to titanium versus gold-alloy abutments in cemented single implant crowns. Int J Prosthodont 2006;15:250–256.

30. Zembic A, Bösch A, Jung RE, Hämmerle CH, Sailer I. Five-year results of a randomized controlled clinical trial comparing zirconia and titanium abutments supporting single-implant crowns in canine and posterior regions. Clin Oral Implants Res 2013;24:384–390.

31. Teughels W, Van Assche N, Sliepen I, Quirynen M. Effect of material characteristics and/or surface topography on biofilm development. Clin Oral Implants Res 2006;17(suppl):68–81.

32. Salihoglu U, Boynuegri D, Engin D, Duman AN, Gökalp P, Balos K. Bacterial adhesion and colonization differences between zirconium oxide and titanium alloys: An in vivo human study. Int J Oral Maxillofac Implants 2011;26:101–107.

33. Rimondini L, Cerroni L, Carrassi A, Torricelli P. Bacterial colonization of zirconia ceramic surfaces: An in vitro and in vivo study. Int J Oral Maxillofac Implants 2002;17:793–798.

34. Quirynen M, Bollen CM, Papaioannou W, Van Eldere J, van Steenberghe D. The influence of titanium abutment surface roughness on plaque accumulation and gingivitis: Short-term observations. Int J Oral Maxillofac Implants 1996;11:169–178.

35. Bollen CM, Papaioanno W, Van Eldere J, Schepers E, Quirynen M, van Steenberghe D. The influence of abutment surface roughness on plaque accumulation and peri-implant mucositis. Clin Oral Implants Res 1996;7:201–211.

36. Zembic A, Philipp AO, Hämmerle CHF, Wohlwend A, Sailer I. Eleven-year follow-up of a prospective study of zirconia implant abutments supporting single all-ceramic crowns in anterior and premolar regions. Clin Implant Dent Relat Res 2015;17(suppl 2):e417–e426.

37. Luthardt RG, Holzhüter MS, Rudolph H, Herold V, Walter MH. CAD/CAM-machining effects on Y-TZP zirconia. Dent Mater 2004;20:655–662.

38. Sailer I, Philipp A, Zembic A, Pjetursson BE, Hammerle CH, Zwahlen M. A systematic review of the performance of ceramic and metal implant abutments supporting fixed implant reconstructions. Clin Oral Implants Res 2009;20(suppl 4):4–31.

39. Fernández M, Delgado L, Molmeneu M, Garcia D, Rodríguez D. Analysis of the misfit of dental implant-supported prostheses made with three manufacturing processes. J Prosthet Dent 2014;111:116–123.

40. Happe A, Röling N, Schäfer A, Rothamel D. Effects of different polishing protocols on the surface roughness of Y-TZP surfaces used for custom-made implant abutments: A controlled morphologic SEM and profilometric pilot study. J Prosthet Dent 2015;113:440–447.

41. Büchi DL, Sailer I, Fehmer V, Hämmerle CHF, Thoma DS. All-ceramic single-tooth implant reconstructions using modified zirconia abutments: A prospective randomized controlled clinical trial of the effect of pink veneering ceramic on the esthetic outcomes. Int J Periodontics Restorative Dent 2014;34:29–37.

42. Jung RE, Holderegger C, Sailer I, Khraisat A, Suter A, Hämmerle CH. The effect of all-ceramic and porcelain-fused-to-metal restorations on marginal peri-implant soft tissue color: A randomized controlled clinical trial. Int J Periodontics Restorative Dent 2008;28:357–365.

43. Zembic A, Sailer I, Jung RE, Hämmerle CH. Randomized-controlled clinical trial of customized zirconia and titanium implant abutments for single-tooth implants in canine and posterior regions: 3-year results. Clin Oral Implants Res 2009;20:802–808.

44. Bressan E, Paniz G, Lops D, Corazza B, Romeo E, Favero G. Influence of abutment material on the gingival color of implant-supported all-ceramic restorations: A prospective multicenter study. Clin Oral Implants Res 2001;22:631–637.

45. Ishikawa-Nagai S, Da Silva JD, Weber HP, Park SE. Optical phenomenon of peri-implant soft tissue. Part II. Preferred implant neck color to improve soft tissue esthetics. Clin Oral Implants Res 2007;18:575–580.

46. Happe A, Schulte-Mattler V, Fickl S, Naumann M, Zöller JE, Rothamel D. Spectrophotometric assessment of peri-implant mucosa after resoration with zirconia abutments veneered with fluorescent ceramic: A controlled, retrospective clinical study. Clin Oral Implants Res 2013;24(suppl A100):28–33.

47. Kleinheinz J, Büchter A, Fillies T, Joos U. Vascular basis of mucosal color. Head Face Med 2005;1:4.

48. Andersson B, Glauser R, Maglione M, Taylor A. Ceramic implant abutments for shortspan FPDs: A prospective 5-year multicenter study. Int J Prosthodont 2003;16:640–646.

49. Andersson B, Taylor A, Lang BR, et al. Alumina ceramic implant abutments used for single-tooth replacement: A prospective 1- to 3-year multicenter study. Int J Prosthodont 2001;14:432–438.

50. Henriksson K, Jemt T. Evaluation of custom-made procera ceramic abutments for single-implant tooth replacement: A prospective 1-year follow-up study. Int J Prosthodont 2003;16:626–630.

51. Piconi C, Maccauro G. Zirconia as a ceramic biomaterial. Biomaterials 1999;20:1–25.

52. Studart AR, Filser F, Kocher P, Gauckler LJ. Fatigue of zirconia under cyclic loading in water and its implications for the design of dental bridges. Dent Materials 2007;23:106–114.

53. Canullo L. Clinical outcome study of customized zirconia abutments for single-implant restorations. Int J Prosthodont 2007;20:489–493.

54. Hosseini M, Worsaae N, Schiødt M, Gotfredsen K. A 3-year prospective study of implant-supported, single-tooth restorations of all-ceramic and metal-ceramic materials in patients with tooth agenesis. Clin Oral Implants Res 2013;24:1078–1087.

55. Lops D, Bressan E, Chiapasco M, Rossi A, Romeo E. Zirconia and titanium implant abutments for single-tooth implant prostheses after 5 years of function in posterior regions. Int J Oral Maxillofac Implants 2013;28:281–287.

56. Cooper LF, Stanford C, Feine J, McGuire M. Prospective assessment of CAD/CAM zirconia abutment and lithium disilicate crown restorations: 2.4 year results. J Prosthet Dent 2016;116:33–39.

57. Carrillo de Albornoz A, Vignoletti F, Ferrantino L, Cárdenas E, De Sanctis M, Sanz M. A randomized trial on the aesthetic outcomes of implant-supported restorations with zirconia or titanium abutments. J Clin Periodontol 2014;41:1161–1169.

58. Ferrari F, Tricarico MG, Cagidiaco MC, et al. 3-year randomized controlled prospective clinical trial on different CAD-CAM implant abutments. Clin Implant Dent Relat Res 2016;18:1134–1141.

59. Passos SP, Linke B, Larjava H, French D. Performance of zirconia abutments for implant-supported single-tooth crowns in esthetic areas: A retrospective study up to 12-year follow-up. Clin Oral Implants Res 2016;27:47–54.

236

"A smile is the prettiest thing you can wear."

COCO CHANEL

12

Superstructure and Peri-Implant/ Restorative Interface

/ Arndt Happe, Pascal Holthaus

F or dental implants to function, they must penetrate the oral mucosa and be in contact with the oral cavity. This results in a transmucosal connection between the external environment and the internal parts of the implant. To prevent bacterial invasion, which might jeopardize either the initial incorporation phase or the long-term success of the implant, a crucial element of tissue integration is the formation of a barrier that will be effective in the long term. This will form an effective bond between vital tissue and the foreign body (ie, the implant). Therefore, soft tissue integration is a key factor in implant success just as osseointegration is (Fig 12-1).

The interface between the peri-implant soft tissue and the restoration is extremely important to this soft tissue integration. This is the area of the implant restoration where the abutment is joined to the implant in the case of two-part bone-level implants and where various implant components, materials, surfaces, and tissues come together. The design of this interface is extremely important to the long-term retention of implant restorations and to sustained esthetics. Even if the implant position is perfect and surgical preparation is meticulous, an unfavorable superstructure design can compromise the outcome. For instance, the example depicted in Fig 12-2 shows the typical gray discoloration of tissue in the case of thin soft tissue and a radiographically suboptimal abutment design.

Various factors have been identified that interact with the peri-implant tissue or influence the vertical position of the crestal bone and the dimension and position of the peri-implant soft tissues: individual biotype, quality of the peri-implant tissue, restorative environment, and abutment characteristics, including the implant-abutment connection[1-5] (see chapter 11). This chapter specifically discusses the fabrication of the superstructure.

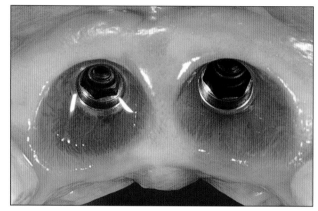

Fig 12-1 / This peri-implant tissue is free of irritation.

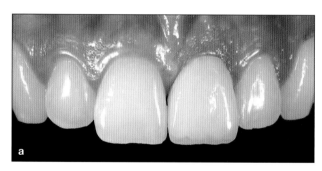

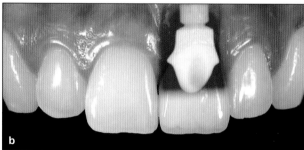

Fig 12-2 / *(a)* Typical gray discoloration of the tissue at the left central incisor site. *(b)* Superimposing the radiograph also reveals a very angular abutment design.

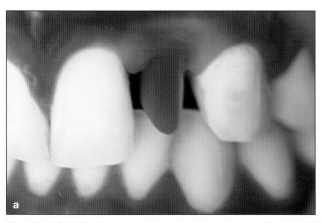 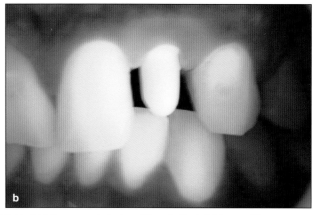

Fig 12-3 / *(a)* Nonfluorescent zirconia abutment under ultraviolet (UV) light. *(b)* A fluorescent abutment boosts the brightness of the mucosa.

Porcelain-Fused-to-Metal Versus All-Ceramic

All-ceramic restorations are now standard for tooth replacement treatments in the esthetic zone, and all-ceramic abutments made of zirconia have proven successful in clinical use. Nevertheless, many practitioners still like to use porcelain-fused-to-metal (PFM) restorations, which have been in use for decades. That is not a problem with thicker tissue types. A clinical trial by Bressan[6] showed that all abutment materials (eg, gold, titanium, zirconia) essentially cause visible discoloration of the soft tissue, although this is more pronounced with metals.

In a prospective randomized controlled trial involving 30 patients, PFM restorations were compared directly with all-ceramic restorations on implants.[7] The results showed that both materials cause color changes. However, the all-ceramic restorations performed markedly better. Some research results with fluorescent-dyed zirconia or with zirconia abutments veneered with fluorescent ceramic show that these measures lead to a further improvement in the optical qualities of the abutment[8,9] (Fig 12-3).

Regarding the biologic reaction, a systematic review[4] concluded that titanium and zirconia cause similar tissue reactions, and even cast gold abutments can be used because they entail no risk of crestal bone resorption or negative tissue reactions. Bonding a metallic base to the custom zirconia abutment combines the strength of metal with the esthetics of zirconia (see chapter 11).

Screw-Retained Versus Cement-Retained

239

Various authors have reported the relationship between cement remnants, which are pressed into the submucosal peri-implant tissue during cementation, and peri-implant inflammation.[10,11] A systematic review discussing whether implant superstructures should be cemented or screw-retained concludes that screw-retained restorations are associated with more technical complications, while cement-retained restorations have more (sometimes severe) biologic complications that can lead to implant loss.[12] It should be noted that most of the restorations studied were crowns cemented onto prefabricated abutments. When custom, anatomically shaped abutments are used, the cement margin can be placed so that cement remnants can easily be retrieved and the risk is markedly reduced.[11]

The authors recommend using a screw-retained crown, if possible (Fig 12-4), or choosing custom abutments for cement-retained crowns and completely removing all traces of submucosal luting cement.

For screw-retained restorations, a combination of a zirconia abutment and a fully anatomical crown made of lithium disilicate can be used as an alternative to layered crowns. This may be advisable for financial reasons or for esthetic reasons in the premolar region, which is often visible in the smile. Instead of cementing a conventional crown onto the abutment intraorally, a crown with occlusal screw access may be used. The crown can be joined to the

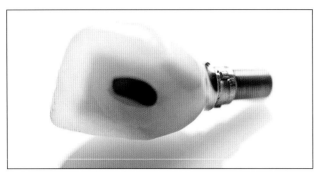

Fig 12-4 / Screw-retained central incisor crown with veneered zirconia framework. It has been bonded onto a titanium base.

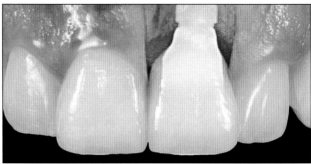

Fig 12-5 / Superimposing the radiograph over the clinical situation reveals a harmonious abutment design that is slim in the area of the deep connective tissue.

240

abutment in the laboratory to avoid intraoral cementation with excessive pressing of cement residue into submucosal areas. The advantage of using a fully anatomical pressed or milled lithium disilicate restoration is that it has better light-optical properties than zirconia as well as markedly higher fracture strength than conventionally veneered PFM crowns. As an alternative, a fully anatomical crown made of zirconia or lithium disilicate could also be fabricated directly on the titanium base.

Emergence Profile

The *emergence profile* denotes where the implant reconstruction emerges. The abutment serves as the three-dimensional (3D) transition from the geometric implant diameter to the anatomical emergence profile of the crown. Because the implant diameter is usually smaller than the emergence area of the restoration, the abutment needs to be tapered outward to guarantee correct morphology of the crown. In addition, the available soft tissue can be conditioned via the emergence profile, ie, the restoration exerts pressure on the soft tissue so that it is anatomically shaped (Fig 12-5).

Because any desired abutment shape can be achieved with a modern workflow, the question arises of what the ideal emergence profile of the abutment is. Assuming that there is only one correct position for the clinical crown (which ideally has been established beforehand by esthetic analysis or wax-up), the 3D position of the implant shoulder is pivotal to the macrogeometry of the abutment. The shape of the abutment results from the desired position of the crown and the position of the implant shoulder (see Fig 12-6).

The implant depth and the soft tissue thickness play a major role. If the soft tissue is very thin or the implant is not placed very deeply, there is little vertical space available to shape an emergence profile at all. If the implant is very deep, there is a lot of height available for the emergence profile, but the microgap is also very deep, which might lead to tissue destruction due to resorptive processes, resulting in recession. The force vector acting on the peri-implant soft tissue usually changes along with the insertion depth (Fig 12-6a).

If the implant occupies a far buccal position, the tissue can only be minimally conditioned buccally and the soft tissue can no longer be influenced via the restoration (Fig 12-6b). If it is positioned too far palatally, this can result in a balcony-type buccal shape that only presses the tissue in the apical direction and might present a site for plaque retention (Fig 12-6c). This effect is lessened when implant depth is greater.

Interproximally, it may be advisable to exert pressure with the abutment to support the interproximal soft tissue or even push it up into a papilla-type structure. The buccal situation is usually different. Concave shaping may be advantageous to avoid additional compression of the buccal soft tissue and therefore tissue thinning or an apical shift in the tissue[13] (Figs 12-6d and 12-6e).

It is sensible to start narrowly in the area of the soft tissue and only taper the abutment outward after 2 mm to reduce pressure on the connective tissue zone specifically and on the soft tissue in general upon insertion and to leave space for tissue and vessels[13] (Fig 12-7). An *O-ring* profile (ie, a circular groove or indentation at the abutment) has not been shown to have any influence on peri-implant soft tissue in clinical trials.[14,15]

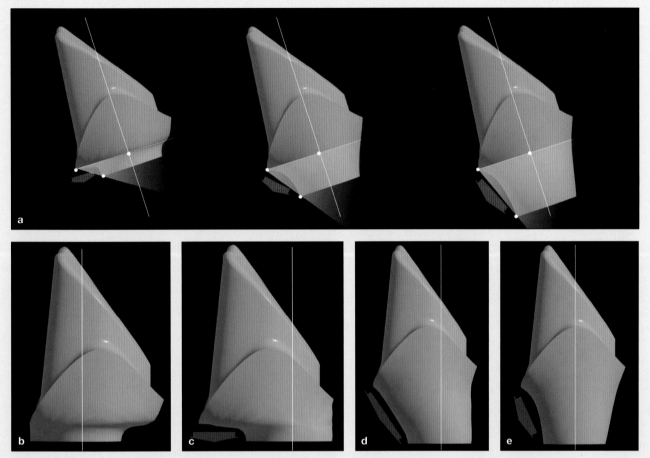

Fig 12-6 / (a) When the position of the crown is the same, differing implant depths result in different abutment designs and different pressure vectors on the soft tissue. (b) If the implant is positioned too deeply and too far buccally, the buccal soft tissue cannot be conditioned. (c) If it is placed not deeply enough and rather palatally, the result is a rectangular "balcony" and an apical force vector. (d) This abutment has a more convex shape buccally. (e) This abutment is more buccally concave, which leaves more space for soft tissue.

Fig 12-7 / (a) Cast with ground emergence profile. The emergence profile starts narrowly close to the implant shoulder and does not widen until it becomes more marginal to the anatomical emergence profile. (b) Emergence profile with titanium bonding base (Straumann Bone Level Implant).

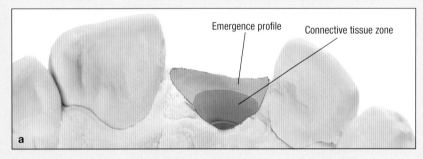

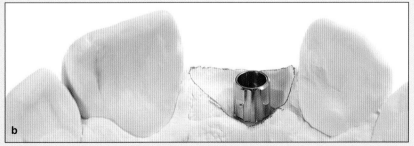

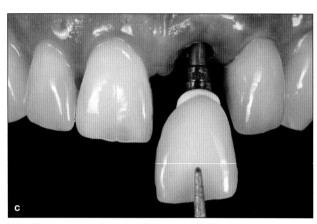

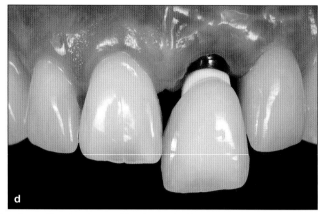

Fig 12-7 *cont.* / *(c and d)* Screw-retained implant crown on titanium base (Camlog Screw-Line implant). Once again, the abutment is narrowly shaped close to the shoulder area, then anatomically widened toward the margin.

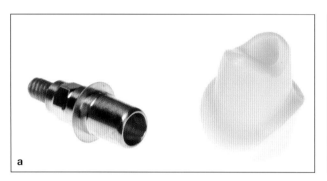

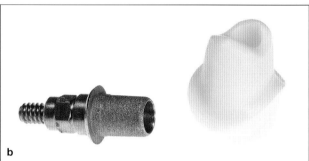

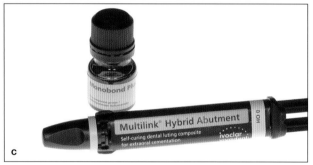

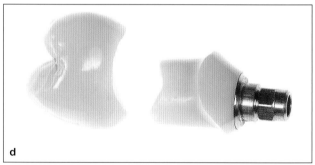

Fig 12-8 / *(a)* Titanium bonding base and computer-aided design/computer-assisted manufacturing (CAD/CAM) fabricated zirconia abutment (Xive, Dentsply Sirona). *(b)* The bonding surfaces on the titanium base and the zirconia part are airborne-particle abraded to ensure optimal adhesion. *(c)* Adhesive cementing material (Multilink Hybrid Abutment) with primer (Monobond Plus). *(d)* Finished hybrid abutment with lithium disilicate crown.

Developing the emergence profile and fabricating custom abutments

Nearly all implant systems currently offer metallic components that can be used as the bonding base for a zirconia abutment. Various adhesive bonding agents are available that have also been clinically tested. The authors have had several years' experience with Panavia 21 (Kuraray Dental) with the bonding agents Alloy Primer and Clearfil Ceramic Primer (Kuraray Dental) and Multilink Implant or Multilink Hybrid Abutment (Ivoclar Vivadent) with the primer Monobond Plus (Ivoclar Vivadent). A good fit of the

parts as well as airborne-particle abrasion of the bonding surfaces significantly increase the bond between the parts[16] (Fig 12-8).

Case 1: Screw-retained single crown

If an impression is taken of an implant with a prefabricated impression post, the geometric circular diameter of the impression post is transferred to the cast (Figs 12-9a and 12-9b). To obtain an anatomical emergence profile, it is

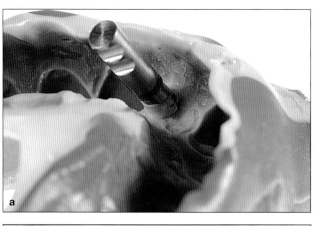
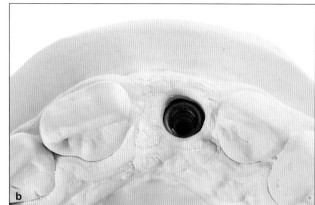
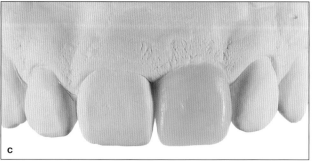
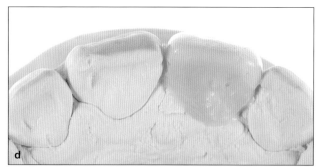
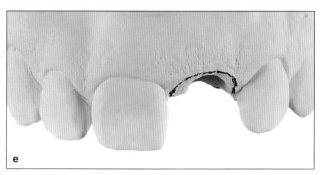
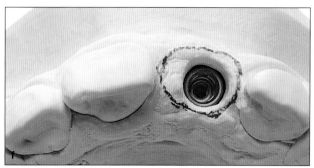

243

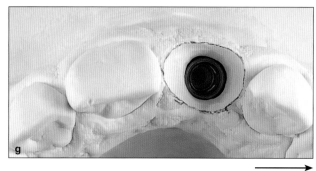

Fig 12-9 / *(a)* Impression with silicone. The laboratory implant has already been screwed onto the impression post. *(b)* The clinical implant position is transferred to the cast. The emergence profile is geometric and not anatomical. *(c and d)* Wax-up of the left central incisor. *(e and f)* The emergence profile is transferred to the cast with a pencil. *(g)* Ground emergence profile.

important to include a wax-up or setup during fabrication of an implant crown, as with all restorative measures. This is used to determine the correct dimensions and localization and helps in shaping the appropriate emergence profile. The anatomical shape of the tooth being replaced can be transferred to the cast with the aid of a sharp pencil or a scalpel blade (Figs 12-9c to 12-9f). Inside this contour, the funnel to the implant shoulder is then widened with a cutter

to produce an anatomically fitting profile (Fig 12-9g). The metallic bonding base is inserted, and a zirconia abutment is constructed that represents the reduced tooth shape (Figs 12-9h to 12-9n). The chosen abutment design and emergence profile are checked using various silicone keys (see Figs 12-9k and 12-9l).

Only after the abutment has been veneered and tried in is the structure bonded to the metallic base (Figs 12-9o

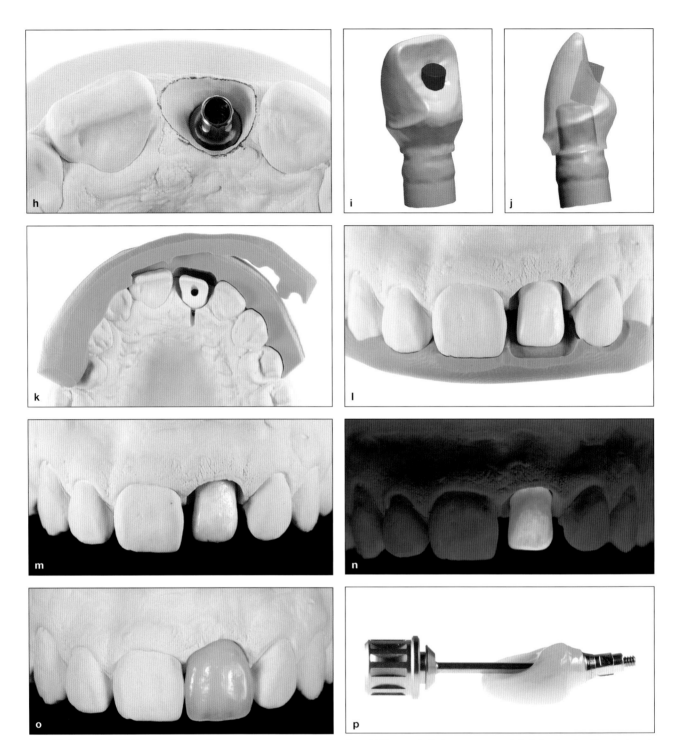

244

Fig 12-9 *cont.* / *(h)* Bonding base in the ground emergence profile. *(i and j)* Screenshots from process of digitally shaping the abutment. *(k and l)* The silicone key taken from the anatomical wax-up is used to check the dimensions of the zirconia abutment. *(m)* Dyed zirconia abutment. *(n)* The abutment exhibits fluorescent properties, which can be seen in UV light. *(o)* Completed restoration. Grinding the emergence profile produces a recession buccally on the cast, but clinically the tissue is pushed slightly in the buccal direction. *(p)* The screw-retained crown is joined to the metallic base using a screwdriver.

and 12-9p). For the intermediate firing and the unfired try-in, the abutment components are only joined using temporary cement so that the structure can be tried in the mouth. Multilink Hybrid Abutment is used to join the components. This provides a mechanically durable and highly esthetic screw-retained implant crown. There is no concern for cement residue and therefore no risk to the long-term prognosis.

Case 2: Screw-retained single crowns

This method (Fig 12-10) contains the same working steps as in case 1, although only about 3.5 to 4 mm of soft tissue height is to be expected between the implants, measured from the implant shoulder. This means that the interproximal contact surfaces of the teeth are usually closed up to this height in the area of the interproximal soft tissue. It may be advisable to first work with provisional restorations to give the tissues time to mature. After about 6 months, there are few if any additional changes to the tissues.

Case 3: Single-tooth implant and adjacent veneer

The combination of all-ceramic restorations on natural abutments and implants (Fig 12-11) is always a challenge because dental ceramics deliver different optical results on different substrates (eg, natural tooth versus abutment material). It can be advantageous to place the veneer first and only then record the shade for the implant crown.

In this case, a prefabricated bonding base was not used, but a prefabricated titanium abutment was customized to serve as the bonding base (see Figs 12-11g and 12-11h). The benefit of this approach is a markedly enlarged retentive area compared with prefabricated CAD/CAM bonding bases. However, this method precludes the use of abutment design software for a single construction because it is not possible to import individual bonding bases into the software. Only the ergonomic data for CAD/CAM bonding bases of the implant manufacturers are on file. The abutment design is transferred to the modified bonding base with contouring resin using the wax-up or setup information and, for a screw-retained anterior crown, it is constructed from the vestibular direction, similar to a veneer preparation, to achieve an anatomical abutment design. As much as possible, the screw accesses should not be prepared from PFM, but they should be shaped in zirconia because this avoids flaking when the screwdriver is tilted. For a cement-retained restoration, a classic die situation is created with contouring resin as the abutment design.

A double scan is used to pick up the digital construction. Only the individual bonding base is scanned in, and the zirconia structure modeled in acrylic resin is placed over it (see Figs 12-11i and 12-11j). The advantage of a mixture of analog and digital construction is that the emergence profile and the anatomical structures are easier to check on the plaster cast—particularly for anatomical design.

Before the sintering process, the zirconia structure is dyed fluorescent and tooth-colored. The fluorescent abutment base serves as a support, especially for thin tissue types, to intensify the brightness of the gingival color. For try-in, it has proved successful to screw the implant crown in place first, then try in the all-ceramic restoration of the adjacent tooth to simplify adjustment of the contact surfaces. Exactly the opposite principle applies to the definitive placement because the cement residue is easier to remove from the restoration on the natural abutment as long as the implant reconstruction is not yet in place.

Case 4: Supragingivally cemented implant restoration

Small implant diameters in particular are often difficult to restore with all-ceramic superstructures because most systems do not provide prefabricated all-ceramic abutments. The clinical case study illustrated in Fig 12-12, therefore, was completed with a prefabricated titanium abutment that was modified so it could serve as the bonding base for a substantial zirconia portion of the abutment. Because fabrication of a conventional zirconia abutment with a titanium base plus an all-ceramic crown could no longer have conformed to the material thicknesses (especially interproximally), a significant zirconia abutment portion was fabricated, and it was sealed with a veneer only on the vestibular aspect in the area of the screw access. After the sintering process, this large zirconia abutment was additionally veneered with a thin layer of highly fluorescent ceramic material (see Fig 12-12e). This serves the purpose of additional control of the basic color of the abutment and helps ensure a better adhesive bond on insertion because the glass phase of the fused porcelain is etchable, unlike zirconia. This type of construction permitted an all-ceramic restoration of the implant. In addition, the cement gap is entirely supragingival, which reliably prevents luting cement from being pressed into submucosal areas.

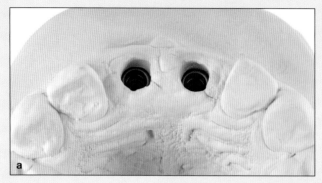

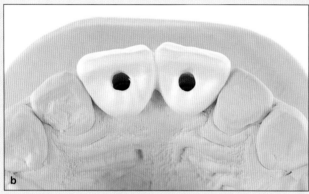

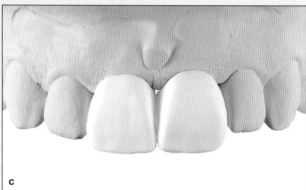

246

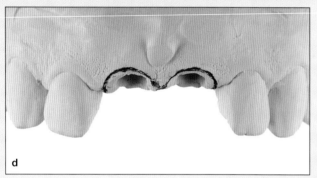

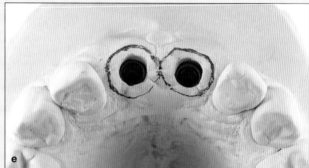

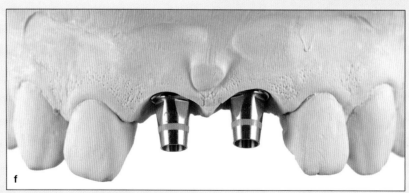

Fig 12-10 / *(a)* Cast with model implants in the sites of the maxillary central incisors. *(b and c)* Views of the milled setup. *(d and e)* Views of the transferred emergence profile. *(f)* Titanium bases on the cast. ⟶

Fig 12-10 *cont.* / *(g and h)* Screenshots from the digital abutment-shaping process. *(i)* Checking the dimensions of the abutments with a silicone key (transfer of the wax-up). *(j)* Fluorescent abutments in UV light. *(k)* Drawing the surface morphology. *(l)* A screwdriver is used to show the screw access holes on the palatal aspect. *(m)* Completed superstructures on the cast. *(n)* Clinical view of the implant crowns a few days after they were placed. (Surgery performed by A. Happe; prosthodontics performed by B. van den Bosch; laboratory work performed by P. Holthaus.)

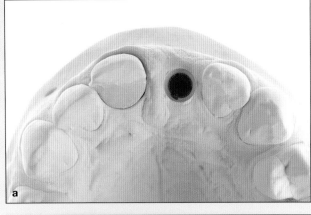

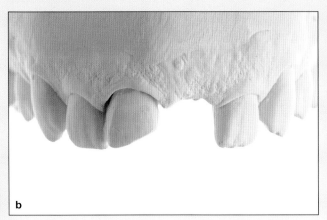

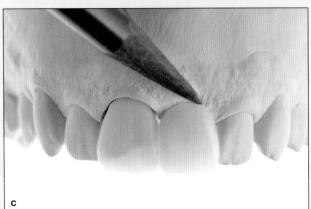

248

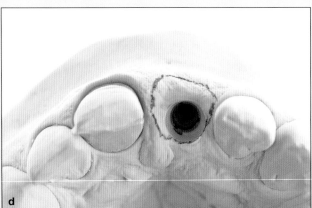

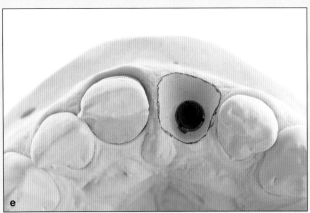

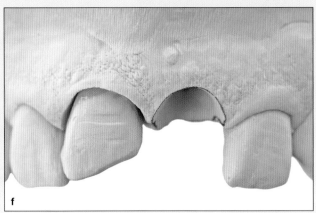

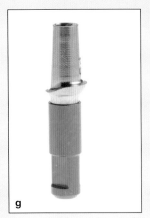

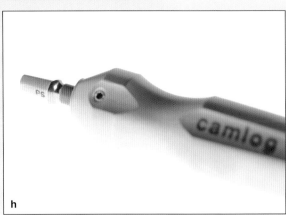

Fig 12-11 / *(a and b)* Cast with veneer preparation at the maxillary right central incisor and implant at the left central incisor. *(c)* Transferring the emergence profile using the wax-up. *(d)* Anatomical contour on the cast. *(e and f)* Ground emergence profile. The right central incisor die can be removed. *(g)* Prefabricated titanium abutment on analog. *(h)* Handle for machining the abutment. →

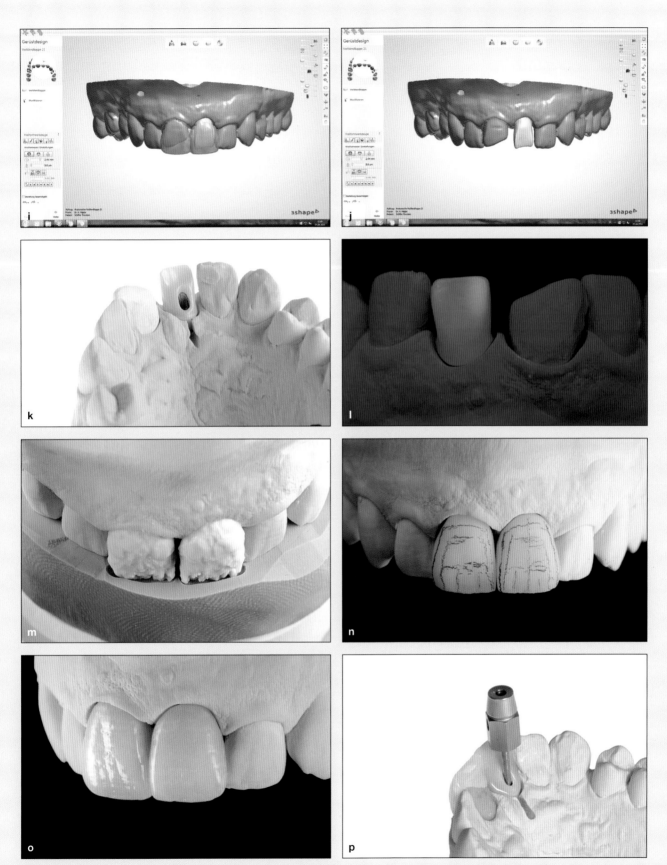

Fig 12-11 *cont.* / *(i and j)* Screenshots from the digital abutment-shaping process. *(k)* Finished zirconia abutment on adapted titanium abutment on the cast. *(l)* Fluorescent abutment in UV light. *(m)* As the ceramic is layered, the morphology is constantly checked with a silicone key taken from the wax-up. *(n)* Drawing the surface morphology. *(o)* The surfaces of the veneer and implant crown have been polished to a silk-matte high glaze. *(p)* Definitive restorations on the cast with screwdriver in the palatal screw access hole.

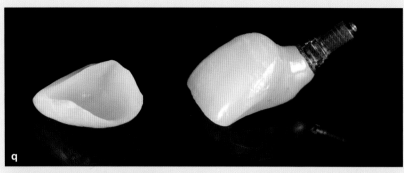

Fig 12-11 *cont.* / *(q)* Veneer and implant crown bonded onto the titanium abutment. *(r)* Implant crown on the cast. *(s and t)* Clinical view of the veneer and restoration without and with a polarizing filter to reveal the internal characteristics.

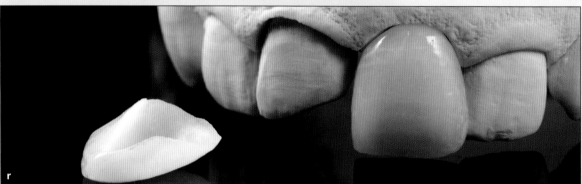

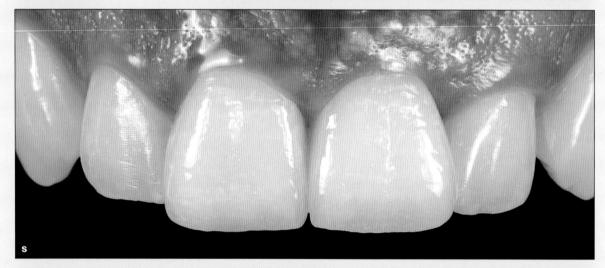

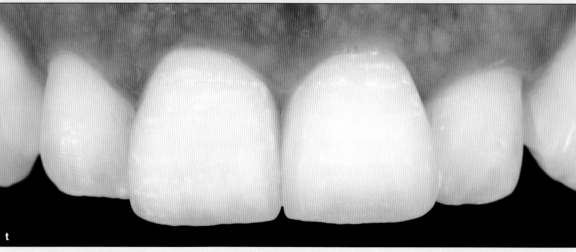

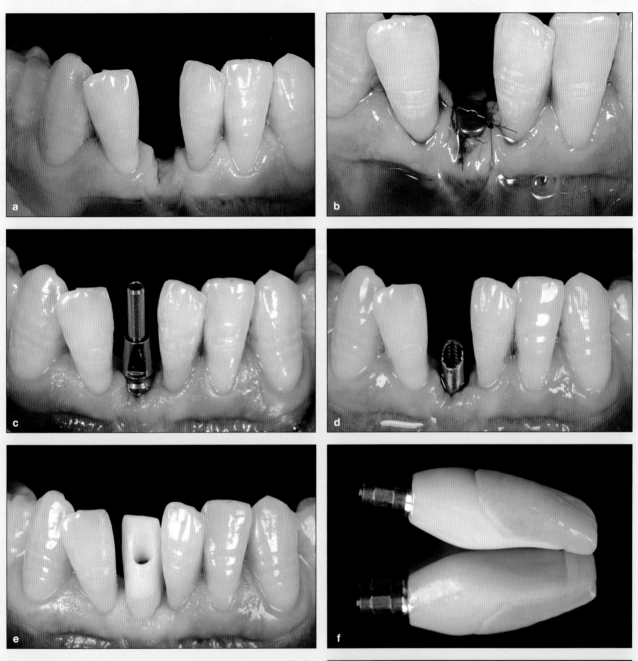

Fig 12-12 / *(a)* The single-tooth edentulous gap at the mandibular right central incisor. *(b)* Clinical view of the implant after exposure with gingiva former in situ. *(c)* Impression post in situ. *(d)* Custom titanium abutment in situ. *(e)* Zirconia abutment with vestibular screw fitting. The abutment was extraorally bonded to the titanium part by the laboratory. *(f)* Superstructure before placement. *(g)* The veneer seals the screw hole. All the margins of the veneer lie supragingivally.

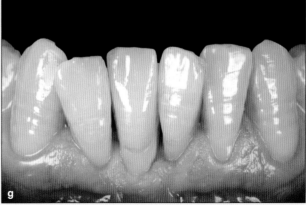

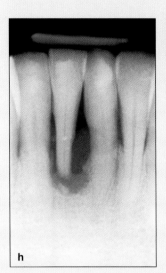
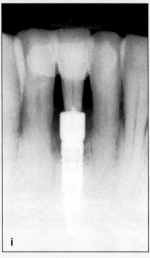
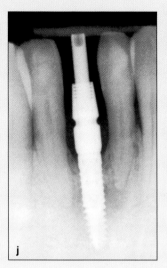
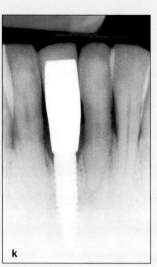

Fig 12-12 *cont.* / *(h to k)* Comparison of radiographs. *(h)* The radiograph shows that the mandibular right central incisor is not worth preserving. *(i)* Implant in situ. *(j)* Impression post in situ. *(k)* Completed superstructure in situ. (Surgery and prosthodontics performed by A. Happe; laboratory work performed by A. Nolte.)

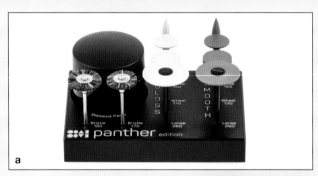
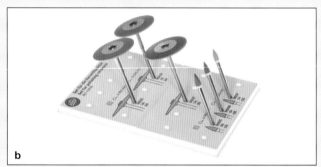
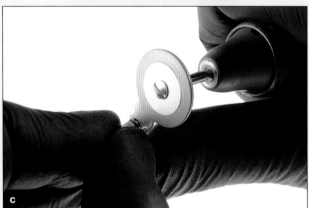
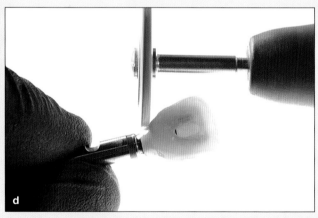

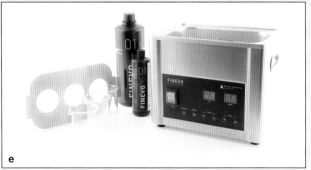

Fig 12-13 / *(a)* Polishing set for machining zirconia abutments. *(b)* Polishing set with rubber polishers for the handpiece. *(c and d)* All the subgingival areas of the abutment are only machined using the blue, red, and gray polishers and not brought to a high glaze with brushes and pastes. *(e)* Commercially available system for abutment cleaning (Finevo Reinigung, Sirius Ceramics).

Surface Treatment

The surface condition in the subgingival area is an important issue with CAD/CAM-fabricated abutments made of zirconia. The surface requires a certain roughness to achieve adequate adhesion with soft tissue. Surfaces with a highly glazed finish encourage deep growth of the epithelium but not adhesion of the connective tissue.[17,18] Clinically, highly glazed finished zirconia abutments exhibit greater probing depths and more bleeding on probing than machined titanium abutments.[19] To create a surface that resembles a machined titanium surface in terms of morphology and roughness, different rubber polishers with different roughness levels are used. Special polishing sets for abutments are now available that are intended to facilitate ideal surface treatment (Fig 12-13a). The authors use the porcelain polishing set 4326A.104 (Komet Dental, Brasseler) with diamond grit-interspersed rubber polishers (Figs 12-13b to 12-13d). If the polishers are used in succession (ie, blue, red, gray), the surface appears highly glazed but has a roughness of approximately 0.2 μm, which approximates to the roughness of machined titanium. To achieve this, a speed of 13,000 rpm and a pressure of approximately 1 N (equivalent to approximately 100 g) should be applied.[20]

After the polishing process, the abutment has to be cleared of the smear layer and contaminants from the polisher. To do this, the abutment is cleaned for 5 minutes in an ultrasonic bath, then with a steam blaster (at about a 5-cm distance) at approximately 600 kPa (equivalent to 6 bar) for 10 seconds.[20] Commercial systems are available for cleaning abutments (Fig 12-13e).

References

1. Kan JY, Rungcharassaeng K, Umezu K, Kois JC. Dimensions of peri-implant mucosa: An evaluation of maxillary anterior single implants in humans. J Periodontol 2003;74:557–562.
2. Bühler-Frey C, Burkhardt R. Evidenz für die Bedeutung mastikatorischer Mukosa um enossale Implantate – eine kritische Literaturübersicht. Implantologie 2008;16:155–159.
3. Salama H, Salama MA, Garber D, Adar P. The interproximal height of bone: A guidepost to predictable aesthetic strategies and soft tissue contours in anterior tooth replacement. Pract Periodontics Aesthet Dent 1998;10:1131–1141.
4. Linkevičius T, Apse P. Influence of abutment material on stability of peri-implant tissues: A systematic review. Int J Oral Maxillofac Implants 2008;26:449–456.
5. Steinebrunner L, Wolfart S, Bössmann K, Kern M. In vitro evaluation of bacterial leakage along the implant-abutment interface of different implant systems. Int J Oral Maxillofac Implants 2005;20:875–881.
6. Bressan E, Paniz G, Lops D, Corazza B, Romeo E, Favero G. Influence of abutment material on the gingival color of implant-supported all-ceramic restorations: A prospective multicenter study. Clin Oral Implants Res 2001;22:631–637.
7. Jung RE, Holderegger C, Sailer I, Khraisat A, Suter A, Hämmerle CH. The effect of all-ceramic and porcelain-fused-to-metal restorations on marginal peri-implant soft tissue color: A randomized controlled clinical trial. Int J Periodontics Restorative Dent 2008;28:357–365.
8. Happe A, Schulte-Mattler V, Fickl S, Naumann M, Zöller JE, Rothamel D. Spectrophotometric assessment of peri-implant mucosa after resoration with zirconia abutments veneered with fluorescent ceramic: A controlled, retrospective clinical study. Clin Oral Implants Res 2013;24(suppl A100):28–33.
9. Happe A, Schulte-Mattler V, Strassert C, et al. In vitro color changes of soft tissues caused by dyed fluorescent zirconia and non-dyed, nonfluorescent zirconia in thin mucosa. Int J Periodontics Restorative Dent 2013;33:e1–e8.
10. Wilson TG Jr. The positive relationship between excess cement and peri-implant disease: A prospective clinical endoscopic study. J Periodontol 2009;80(9):1388–1392.
11. Linkevicius T, Vindasiute E, Puisys A, Linkeviciene L, Maslova N, Puriene A. The influence of the cementation margin position on the amount of undetected cement. A prospective clinical study. Clin Oral Implants Res 2013;24:71–76.
12. Sailer I, Mühlemann S, Zwahlen M, Hämmerle C, Schneider D. Cemented and scew-retained implant reconstructions: A systematic review of the survival and complication rates. Clin Oral Implants Res 2012;23(suppl 6):163–201.
13. Rompen E, Raepsaet N, Domken O, Touati B, Van Dooren E. Soft tissue stability at the facial aspect of gingivally converging abutments in the esthetic zone: A pilot clinical study. J Prosthet Dent 2007;97(6 suppl):S119–S125.
14. Patil R, van Brakel R, Iyer K, Huddleston Slater J, de Putter C, Cune M. A comparative study to evaluate the effect of two different abutment designs on soft tissue healing and stability of mucosal margins. Clin Oral Implants Res 2013;24:336–341.
15. Weinländer M, Lekovic V, Spadijer-Gostovic S, Milicic B, Wegscheider WA, Piehslinger E. Soft tissue development around abutments with a circular macro-groove in healed sites of partially edentulous posterior maxillae and mandibles: A clinical pilot study. Clin Oral Implants Res 2011;22:743–752.
16. Ebert A, Hedderich J, Kern M. Retention of zirconia ceramic copings bonded to titanium abutments. Int J Oral Maxillofac Implants 2007;22:921–927.
17. Lindhe J, Berglundh T. The interface between the mucosa and the implant. Periodontol 2000 1998;17:47–54.
18. Meyle J. Cell adhesion and spreading on different implant surfaces. In: Lang NP, Karring T, Lindhe JT (eds). Proceedings of the 3rd European Workshop on Periodontology: Implant Dentistry. Berlin: Quintessence, 1999:55–72.
19. Bollen CM, Papaioanno W, Van Eldere J, Schepers E, Quirynen M, van Steenberghe D. The influence of abutment surface roughness on plaque accumulation and peri-implant mucositis. Clin Oral Implants Res 1996;7:201–211.
20. Happe AR, Beuer F, Schäfer A, Nickenig HJ, Rothamel D. How to establish a suitable surface roughness for zirconia implant abutments under laboratory conditions [abstract]. Clin Oral Implants Res 2012;23(suppl 7):44.

253

*"The greatest glory in living lies not in never falling,
but in rising every time we fall."*

NELSON MANDELA

13

Complications

/ Arndt Happe, Gerd Körner

Various complications can adversely affect both the esthetic appearance and the biologic and functional outcomes of an implant restoration in the anterior dentition. The following factors are keys to success, and a potential failure can occur if they are not taken into consideration:

- Correct three-dimensional (3D) implant position
- Appropriate bone architecture and stable bone volume
- Adequate thickness and quality of soft tissue
- Development and preservation of the soft tissue contour
- Transmucosal form, material, and surface of abutment and restoration

Problems can often be attributed equally to several of the key factors. In the case depicted in Fig 13-1, for example, the position of the implants is not correct because they were placed too far facially. The diameter of 5 mm is relatively thick, and both the bone volume as well as the soft tissue thickness and quality are inadequate. Figure 13-2 shows an esthetic failure caused by an uneven soft tissue contour and the implants showing through. Furthermore, implants were placed during the growth phase, which meant that the subsequent jaw growth led to a vertical discrepancy. The vestibular tissue is too thin, and the implants were placed too far facially.

Incorrectly Positioned Implants

A typical error is excessive vestibular angulation of the implant or positioning the implant too far facially. This is illustrated by the case depicted in Fig 13-3. Furthermore, the implant diameter of 5 mm used for the lateral incisor was far too large, which further exacerbates the problem. The implant body is clearly located outside the contour of the ridge. An excessively pronounced angulation often results from a poor bone supply. The implant axis is then adapted to the local bone rather than the prosthetically advisable position. The same is true of implants that are placed too deep (ie, the implant shoulder is too apical). Once again, a reduced amount of bone is often the cause (Figs 13-4 and 13-5). These disastrous results highlight the importance of using templates to plan and correctly implement the implant positions. They also illustrate, however, that correct positioning is often only achievable in conjunction with bone augmentation. These situations can frequently only be corrected by explantation and placement of a new implant. The biologic interrelations between biologic width, soft tissue, and implant position in the esthetic zone were first described by Grunder et al,[1] and correct positioning is also described in detail in his book.[2]

The case depicted in Fig 13-6 shows how important complete planning is when placing implants in the anterior region. After a cycling accident, the patient had been treated elsewhere with three implants in both maxillary left incisor sites and the right lateral incisor site. Less than 2 years later, she presented for treatment because she was very unhappy with the esthetic outcome. She said she did not want to go on living like this, which highlights how emotionally charged the mouth can be and the impact that esthetic appearance can have on people. It also makes us as clinicians aware of the huge responsibility we have in treating the anterior dentition.

Esthetic analysis reveals several obvious esthetic shortcomings: the soft tissue contour is unnatural; the natural anterior teeth (ie, canines and right central incisor) have recessions; the right lateral incisor implant is not positioned deeply enough, which means the shoulder lies too far coronally; and the interdental papilla is missing between the left incisor implants, where there is also too little tissue. Reconstruction of hard and soft tissues was not performed or was not successful. The superstructure does not imitate the natural teeth, and the shoulders of the tissue-level implants show through the cervical

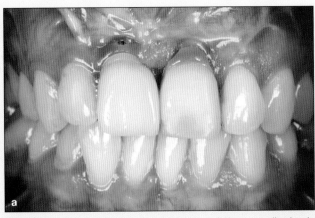 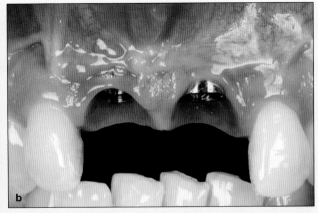

Fig 13-1 / *(a)* Esthetic failure due to poor soft tissue quality, inadequate augmentation, and suboptimal implant position with the titanium showing through. Prosthetic concealment of the implant shoulder at the left central incisor implant was attempted. *(b)* The situation with the superstructure removed. The shoulder of the left central incisor implant is exposed, and the soft tissue at the right central incisor implant is perforated.

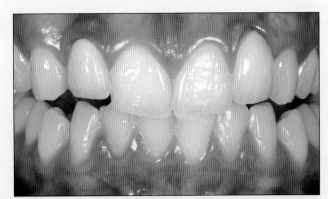

Fig 13-2 / Esthetic failure caused by implant placement during the growth phase.

257

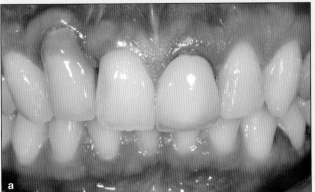

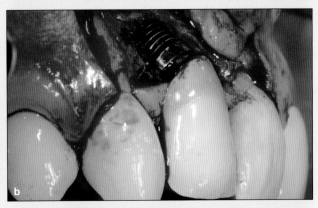

Fig 13-3 / *(a)* Esthetic failure with implant at the maxillary right lateral incisor. This will be treated with explantation. *(b)* After flap formation, the extreme discrepancy between tooth inclination and implant axis becomes apparent. *(c)* The impression post further illustrates the extreme angulation of the implant.

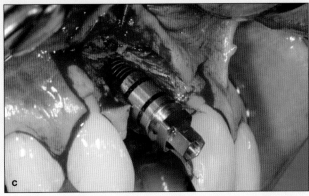

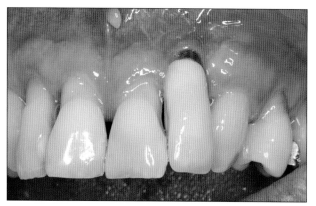

Fig 13-4 / Esthetic failure at the maxillary left lateral incisor due to incorrect implant position and excessive implant diameter.

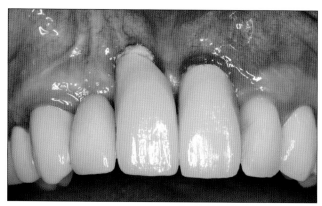

Fig 13-5 / Esthetic failure at the maxillary central incisors due to deficient ridge augmentation with resulting incorrect implant positions.

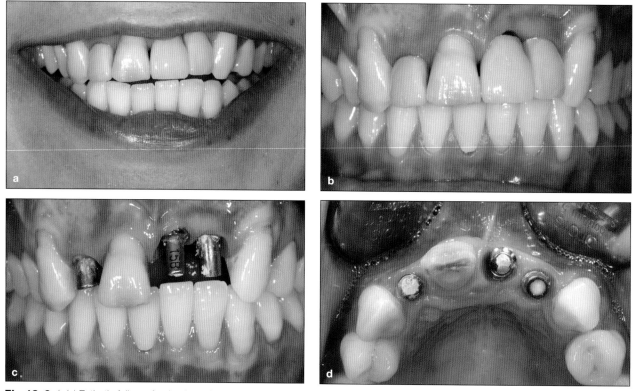

Fig 13-6 / (a) Esthetic failure after implant placement. The patient is dissatisfied with her smile. (b) Intraoral view with implants at the maxillary left central and lateral incisor and right lateral incisor sites and recessions at the canines and remaining right central incisor. (c and d) Condition after removal of the implant crowns.

peri-implant soft tissue. After the patient had been fully advised on treatment options, it was decided to remove the three implants and start a new treatment intended to cover the recessions around the natural anterior teeth and place new implants with reconstructive measures for the hard and soft tissues. The interimplant soft tissue situation between the left incisors was addressed first as a clear limitation. This was fully clarified with the patient because it is not possible to predictably reconstruct a satisfactory papilla between two implants when 3D bone augmentation needs to be performed.[3] After the revised treatment was completed, this area was still somewhat compromised; fortunately, the patient tolerates this because the overall situation is improved.

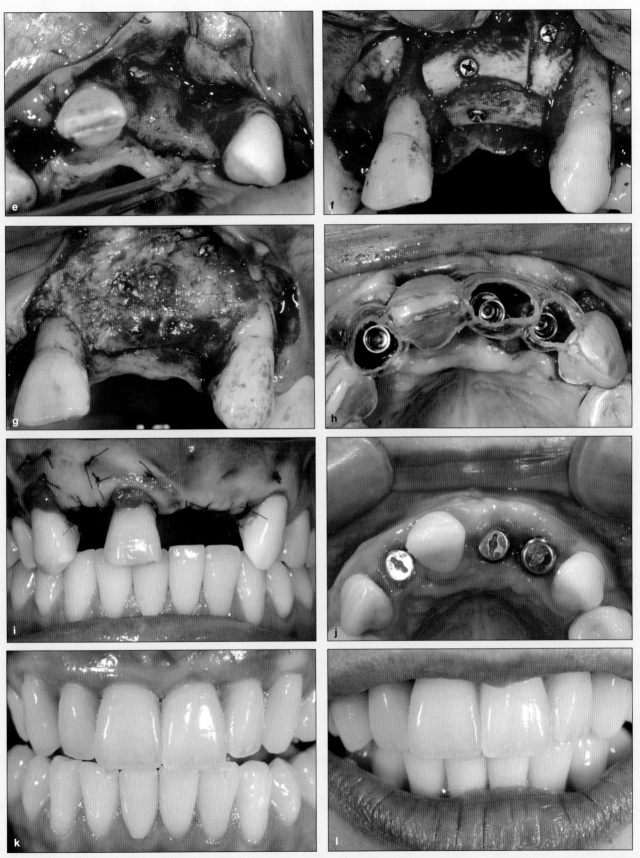

Fig 13-6 *cont.* / *(e)* Condition 6 weeks after explantation. A 3D bone defect is evident at the left incisors. *(f)* Augmentation in the area of the right incisors with bone grafts from the retromolar region. *(g)* Augmented area 4 months after bone buildup. The osteosynthesis screws will be removed. *(h)* Implants are placed according to prosthetic considerations with a template for orientation. *(i)* The soft tissue is augmented with subepithelial connective tissue grafts in a separate session. *(j)* Condition several weeks after exposure of the implants. *(k)* Clinical view of the outcome after prosthetic restoration. *(l)* Final smile. (Surgery and prosthodontics performed by A. Happe; laboratory work performed by A. Nolte.)

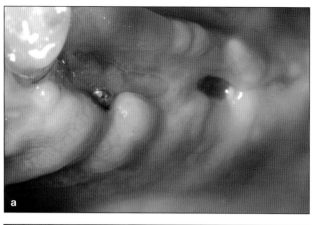
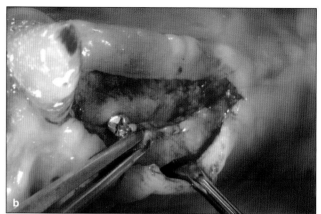

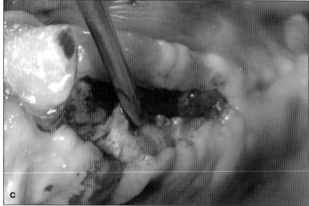
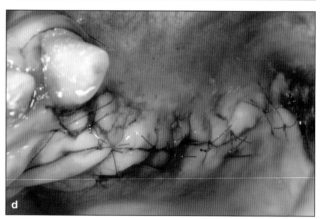

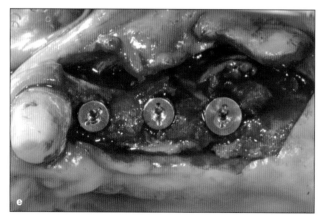

Fig 13-7 / *(a)* Dehiscence several weeks after bone augmentation with an autogenous bone graft. *(b)* The wound margins are excised, and the augmentation material is debrided. The connective tissue flap is prepared from the palatal aspect. *(c)* The connective tissue flap stretches to provide coverage from the palatal aspect. *(d)* In addition, a mucoperiosteal flap was formed from the buccal aspect, and the area was covered in two layers. *(e)* Implants were placed as planned into the healed bone.

Hard Tissue Complications

Dehiscence

A typical complication after bone augmentation is dehiscence or exposure of augmentation material. Because primary coverage of augmentation material is a basic requirement for the procedure to succeed, this can mean total or partial loss of that material. There can be many different types of causes, such as excessive tension on the flap, mechanical irritation caused by provisional res-

torations, or circulatory disturbances in the flap.[4,5] These dehiscences typically occur in the first 1 to 3 weeks after augmentation, while dehiscences caused by pressure from provisional restorations can also appear later.

Surgical intervention should not be performed immediately; it will not be successful before the wound margins have matured. Patients should be instructed to dab the area locally with chlorhexidine gel and wait until the soft tissue has matured enough to allow for renewed surgical coverage of the site. For this purpose, infected portions of any membranes or substitute material are removed,

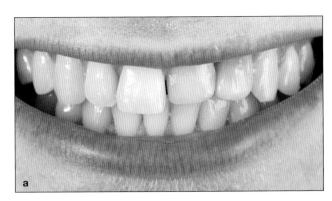
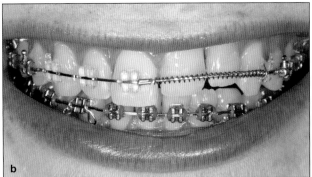
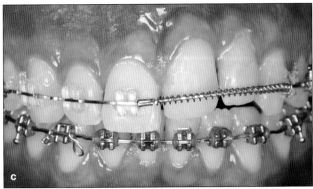
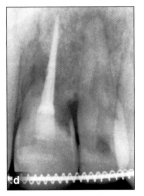

Fig 13-8 / *(a)* Initial smile before the start of any treatment. There had been prior anterior tooth trauma with ankylosis and retention of the maxillary left incisors. *(b and c)* Smile and intraoral situation at the start of treatment. *(d)* Radiograph at the start of treatment, with more pronounced external resorption at the central incisor and early resorption at the lateral incisor.

exposed bone is debrided, and the site is thoroughly irrigated with saline. Renewed soft tissue coverage can then be attempted in the decontaminated area with flap mobilization and additional connective tissue flaps (Fig 13-7). However, exposed areas of augmented bone or substitute material almost always result in partial loss of augmentation material and more severe resorption, so the bone volume achieved is usually insufficient.

Resorption

Even if postoperative healing of the soft tissue is uncomplicated, above-average resorption can occur. This can be induced by mechanical irritations such as pressure from provisional restorations, or by inflammatory processes or other tissue reactions with unknown causes. Figure 13-8 illustrates a more complex case that involved severe horizontal resorption of augmented bone. As a child, the patient had suffered an anterior tooth trauma in the region of the maxillary left incisors, which initially produced ankylosis and later external resorption around these teeth. The ankylosis during jaw growth led to the

typical retention of teeth so that an irregular contour of the marginal soft tissue developed, with a vertical deficit at the left incisors.

The implantology treatment was begun after the patient was fully grown. Orthodontic extrusion was performed for the maxillary left lateral incisor because an attachment was still detected at that site on the radiograph. The purpose was to move the crestal bone in a coronal direction. At the time of extraction, the socket seal technique was used to preserve as much tissue as possible. After complete healing of the alveolar process, 3D bone augmentation was performed using the Khoury technique. Despite uncomplicated healing, more severe bone resorption occurred during the incorporation phase. However, a vertical improvement in the bone supply was achieved by the first augmentation with autogenous bone, so it was possible to place two implants as planned. Nevertheless, an additional second augmentation had to performed to correct the horizontal deficit with guided bone regeneration. The end result is acceptable, but it still exhibits the typical situation with an inadequate papilla between adjacent implants.

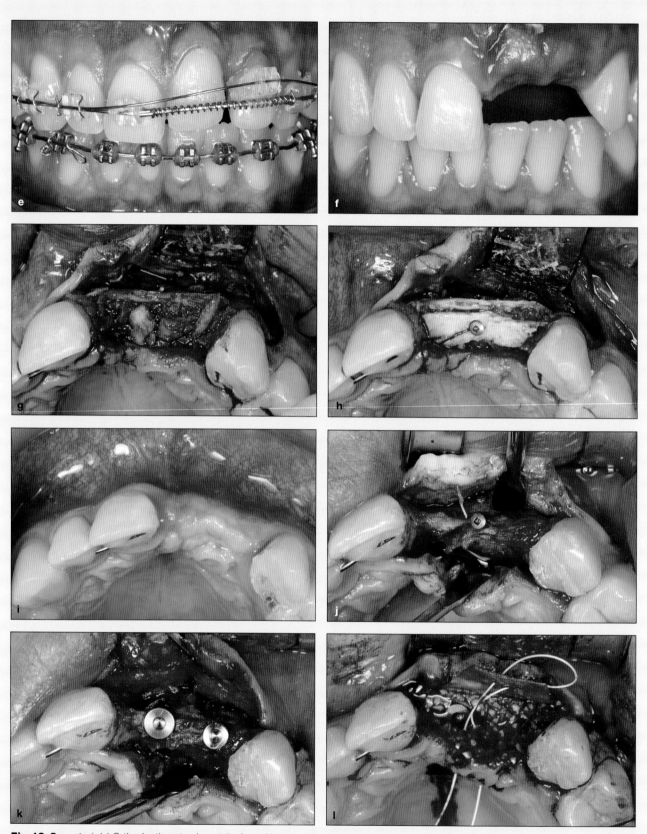

Fig 13-8 *cont.* / *(e)* Orthodontic extrusion at the lateral incisor to improve the vertical tissue supply. *(f)* Fully healed alveolar process after extrusion at the lateral incisor and soft tissue augmentation upon extraction of both incisors. Condition prior to augmentation. *(g)* 3D reconstruction of the alveolar process with autogenous bone grafts with a buccal bone plate and bone chips. *(h)* Occlusal sealing is completed with a thin bone plate and osteosynthesis screw. *(i)* Alveolar process 3 months after augmentation. There is pronounced horizontal volume loss. *(j)* After flap formation, it becomes clear that there has been excessive horizontal resorption. *(k)* Implants are placed at the sites of the central incisor (3.8-mm-diameter implant) and the lateral incisor (3.3-mm-diameter implant). *(l)* Horizontal augmentation is performed with a resorbable GBR membrane and bone substitute material.

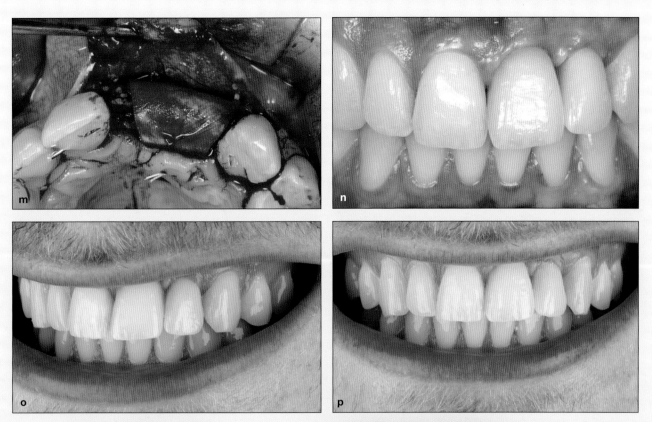

263

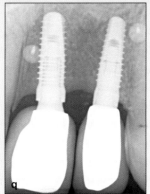

Fig 13-8 *cont.* / *(m)* The membrane is fixed buccally with two titanium pins and stabilized palatally with a suture. *(n)* Final intraoral image after reconstruction of tissue and finalized superstructure. *(o and p)* Frontal and semilateral views of smile after treatment. *(q)* Radiograph after completion of treatment (the implant system used for the lateral incisor does not permit platform switching). *(r)* Final portrait.

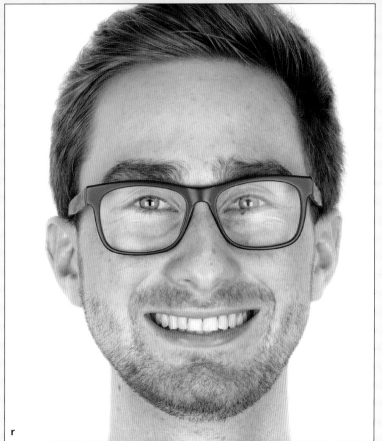

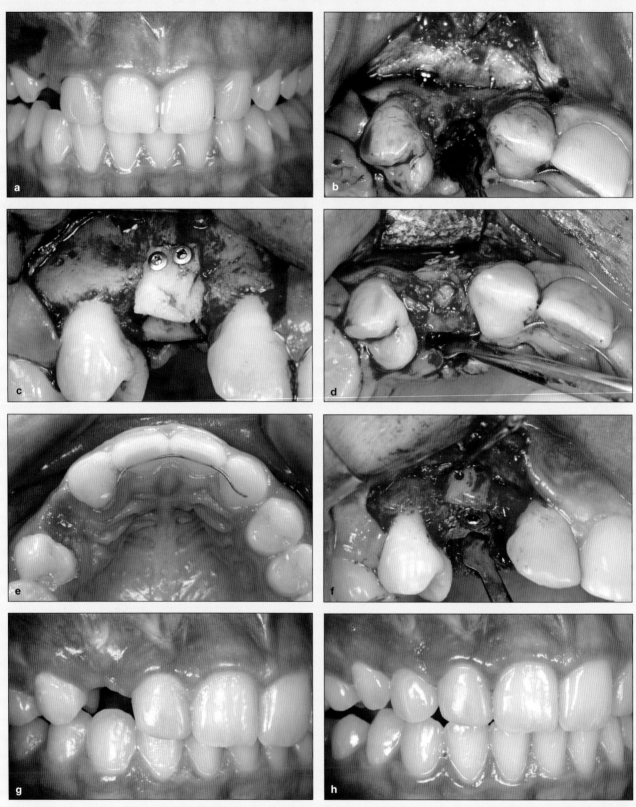

Fig 13-9 / *(a)* Condition after unsuccessful augmentation attempt at the maxillary right canine. *(b)* Bone defect at the canine. The remaining titanium pins can be seen. The buccal and palatal bone lamellae are absent. *(c)* Reconstruction of the buccal and palatal bone lamellae with autogenous bone plates. *(d)* The space between the bone plates is filled with particulate grafts. *(e)* Healed site 12 weeks after augmentation. *(f)* The bone grafts have incorporated well, allowing for a 3.8-mm implant to be successfully placed at the canine site. *(g)* Before exposure of the implant, the alveolar process has been successfully reconstructed. *(h)* Condition after prosthetic restoration. ⟶

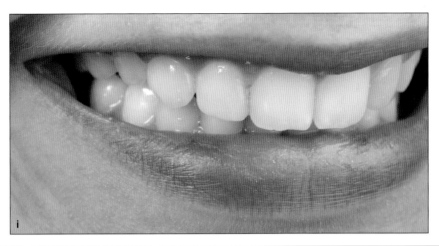

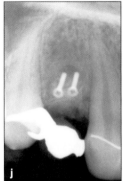
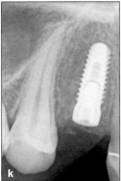

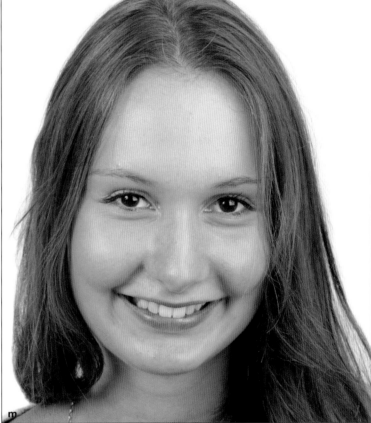

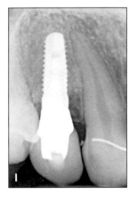

Fig 13-9 *cont.* / *(i)* Smile after completion of the treatment. *(j)* Radiograph after augmentation. *(k)* Radiograph after implant placement. *(l)* Radiograph 6 months after completion of the prosthodontics. *(m)* Final portrait.

Failed augmentation attempts

Augmentation can fail for a variety of reasons. Aside from the previously mentioned soft tissue complications and resorptions caused by irritation or inflammation, the potential of bone substitute materials is often overestimated, or the indications for the material are not properly observed.[6] The limitations of the different techniques are described in chapter 9. The case illustrated in Fig 13-9 shows the condition after an unsuccessful augmentation attempt in the region of the maxillary right canine using bovine bone substitute and collagen membrane. However, because the buccal and palatal lamella were absent and this case involved a 3D ridge defect with a pronounced vertical component, the defect could only have been successfully treated with autogenous bone grafts. In this case, the defect was reconstructed with Khoury's bone plate technique.[7]

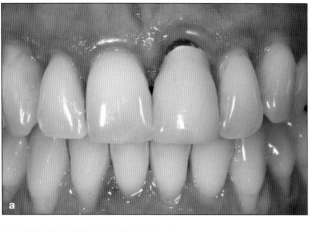
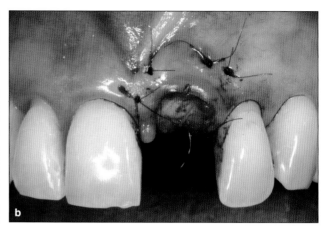
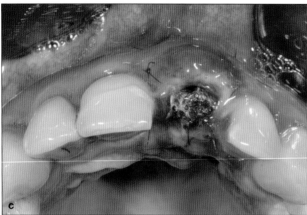
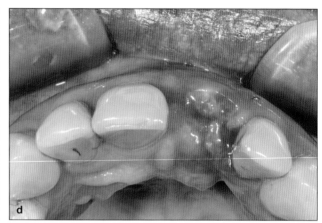

Fig 13-10 / *(a)* Preoperative situation with the maxillary left central incisor not worth preserving. Because of the recession, immediate implant placement was not considered. *(b)* Extraction and alveolar sealing by socket seal surgery with a connective tissue graft (CTG) from the palate. *(c)* After 1 week, there was superficial necrosis of the graft with inflammation of the surrounding tissue. *(d)* Healing of the site 2 weeks postoperatively.

⟶

Soft Tissue Complications

Complications associated with ridge preservation

Free or pedicle soft tissue grafts are used in the surgical techniques of ridge preservation. Volume stability, however, seems rather better with pedicle grafts.[8] With both techniques, it is rare for a wound healing disorder to occur with complete necrosis of the graft.[9,10] When a wound healing disorder results, there is usually only partial necrosis; the superficial portions of the graft become necrotic, while the basal portions increase and are later epithelialized by the adjacent tissue. Figure 13-10 shows this kind of case: Superficial necrosis occurred, but this complication hardly impaired the end result because there was no appreciable tissue loss.

When there is total loss of the graft, the outcome is different (Fig 13-11). This case involved total loss caused by necrosis of a pedicle graft, so the situation was far worse after the complication than before the intervention. The patient could only be successfully treated after renewed augmentation and periodontal plastic surgery had been performed.

Risk factors for soft tissue complications are nicotine abuse, traumatic treatment of the tissue, excessively thin biotype, excessively thin shaping of the graft, and pressure on the graft during the postoperative healing phase.

Complications associated with immediate implant placement

Tissue defects arising from soft tissue complications prior to implant placement can still be surgically compensated before or at the time of implant placement. By contrast, complications arising from immediate implant placement are much more serious. Surgical measures to manage

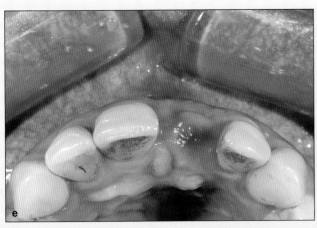

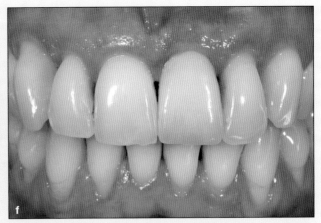

Fig 13-10 *cont.* / *(e)* Fully healed site 6 weeks after extraction. *(f)* Completion of the treatment with single-tooth implant at the left central incisor.

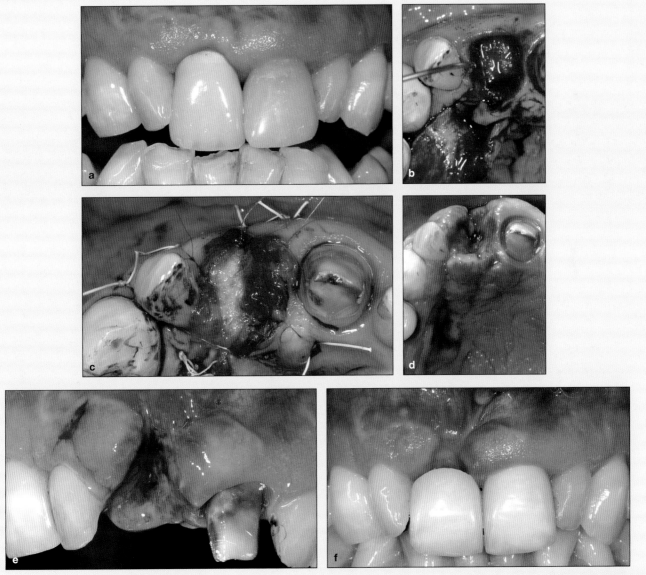

Fig 13-11 / *(a)* The maxillary right central incisor is not worth preserving. Recession can be seen prior to extraction. *(b)* The socket is filled with substitute material, and a palatally pedicled CTG is prepared. *(c)* The socket is sealed with a pedicle CTG from the right central incisor to the right first premolar. *(d and e)* After 10 days, necrosis of the flap in the area of the socket has occurred with resulting tissue defects from the occlusal aspect. *(f)* Appearance of the tissue defect 12 weeks postoperatively.

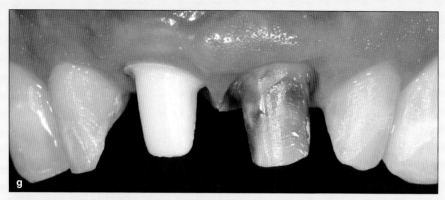

Fig 13-11 *cont.* / *(g)* Condition after reconstruction of the alveolar process with hard and soft tissue augmentation and implant placement at the right central incisor. *(h)* Completion of the treatment with all-ceramic reconstruction of the maxillary anterior dentition. (Surgery and prosthodontics performed by G. Körner; laboratory work performed by K. Müterthies.)

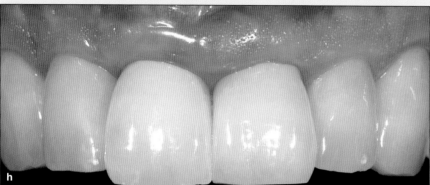

268

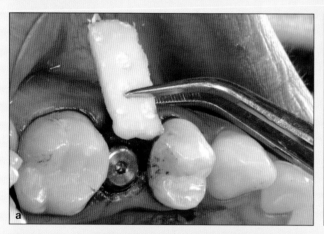

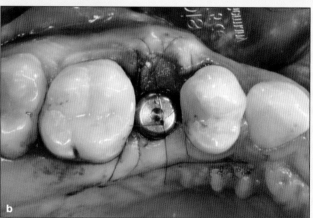

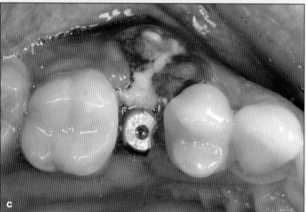

Fig 13-12 / *(a)* Porcine dermal matrix for augmentation in the case of immediate implant placement at the maxillary right second premolar site. *(b)* Completion of immediate implant placement. *(c)* After 1 week, there is impaired wound healing and necrosis of the covering soft tissue.

Fig 13-13 / Implant at the right central incisor with distal papilla made of porcelain. The loss of the papilla can be explained by loss of the mesial attachment at the right lateral incisor.

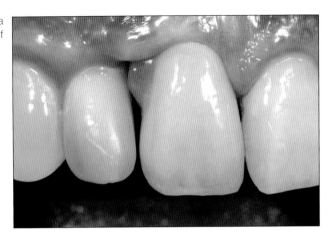

269

these complications are more difficult because the implant has already been placed. Figure 13-12 shows flap necrosis over a soft tissue augmentation material with porcine dermis. Presumably, the material was not sufficiently rehydrated, leading to a lack of tissue integration. Soft tissue recession may result. Furthermore, inflammatory processes may also lead to a loss of attachment at the adjacent tooth so that papilla loss may ensue (Fig 13-13). Figure 13-14 shows another case in which a wound healing disorder occurred after immediate implant placement and soft tissue augmentation with substitute material. Only 1 week postoperatively, superficial necrosis of the covering soft tissue was clinically apparent. Nevertheless, the substitute material was incorporated, and the implant could be restored without further corrective surgical measures. One year after the procedure, the only evidence of the complication was slight scarring.

Complications after augmentation

Soft tissue complications are the primary complications associated with more extensive bone augmentation. If flap necrosis occurs due to circulatory disorders, the augmentation material is exposed, and the microorganisms of the oral cavity will become infected. Flap dehiscences,

which are caused by too much tension on the flap or inadequate suturing technique, also lead to this outcome. See the previous section on dehiscences for treatment of this complication.

Complications after prosthodontics

Soft tissue recessions are a common problem in the esthetic region. They are typical of immediate implants if an inappropriate case selection or unsuitable technique was chosen.[11] However, soft tissue recessions can still occur even after delayed or late implant placement. This can have various causes. If insufficient keratinized mucosa is available around the implants or if the soft tissue is not fixed, tissue stability is frequently inadequate for a long-term esthetic outcome (Fig 13-15). In other cases, the augmented bone volume is sometimes not stable, and a loss of volume ensues over a prolonged time period because of the bone remodeling processes. If this is associated with crestal bone loss, it may be expressed as recession of the covering soft tissue. Sometimes the etiology of the recession is unknown and one can only speculate on potential causes based on the patient's history and local findings.

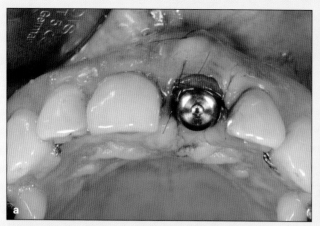

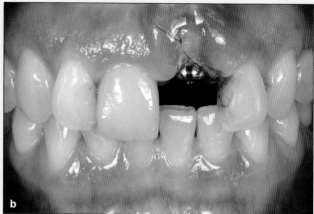

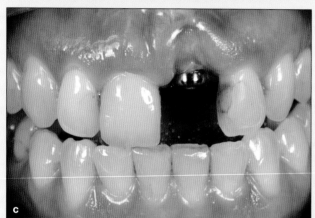

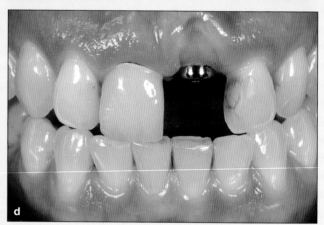

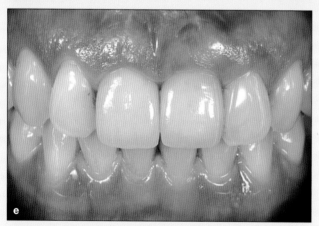

Fig 13-14 / *(a)* Immediate implant placement with buccal interposition of an acellular dermal matrix. *(b)* Condition after 1 week with superficial necrosis. *(c)* Condition after 4 weeks. *(d)* Condition after 12 weeks. *(e)* Final image 1 year postoperatively with superstructure in place. The soft tissue esthetics have apparently not suffered from the complication.

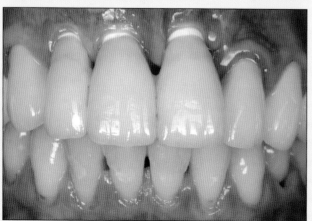

Fig 13-15 / Soft tissue recession at the implants from the maxillary right lateral incisor to the left central incisor. There is insufficient tissue quality and stability in this area.

Fig 13-16 / Fractured zirconia abutment at the maxillary right canine. This was part of a zirconia partial denture from the canine to the right central incisor.

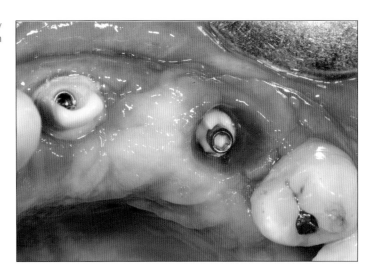

Inadequate Form, Material, and Surface of Abutment and Restoration

Abutment fracture

Correct abutment design has been discussed in previous chapters. Although zirconia abutments yield very good clinical results, fractures of all-ceramic abutments were a commonly reported complication in the past[12] (Fig 13-16). These fractures mainly arise from screw loosening followed by incorrect loading of the abutment. Screw loosening can be a consequence of wear around the implant-abutment interface. Using a metallic base reduces this wear and substantially increases the strength of zirconia abutments and therefore resistance to fracture.[13,14]

Excess cement

Excessive amounts of cement are another typical problem of restorations cemented onto implants[15] (Fig 13-17). The excess cement is pressed under the mucosa when the prosthesis is attached, resulting in inflammatory processes. A review article on screw-retained versus cemented superstructures concluded that screw-retained restorations have more technical complications, while cemented restorations have more serious biologic complications such as crestal bone loss and implant loss.[16] Crown margins placed deeply below the tissue do not allow cement residue to

be removed.[17,18] To avoid this problem, screw retention should be preferred to cementation, if possible, or the crown margins should be shaped in a way that allows easy access for removal of cement remnants. For this purpose, custom zirconia abutments should be used that allow adequate cement removal. The removability of the particular cement also plays a role: Acrylic-resin-based flowable cements usually cause more problems because cement remnants are not visible or are difficult to clean. Glass ionomer cements are frequently more suitable, but these do not provide genuine adhesive cementation.

Chipping and fractures

Implant restorations are associated with more ceramic chipping because the threshold of tactile sensitivity of implants is roughly eight times higher than for natural teeth, and higher forces are at work due to the ankylotic connection between the implant and the bone itself.[19] Hyperbalance contacts frequently play a role in dynamic occlusion (Figs 13-18 and 13-19). The patient in Fig 13-19 suffered a complete fracture of a relatively thick, adhesively cemented, fully anatomical lithium disilicate crown; the zirconia abutment remained intact. The reasons for this might be mechanical overloading due to bruxism, implant as antagonist, or excessively strong contacts. A careful risk analysis, choice of material, and an appropriate occlusal concept are important prognostic factors in these circumstances.

271

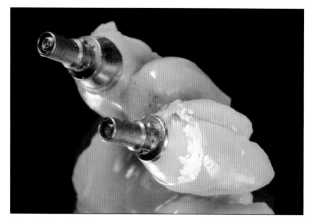

Fig 13-17 / This implant-supported partial denture had to be removed after a ceramic fracture. After removal, it became clear how much excessive cement was present during restoration placement and was pressing on the mucosa.

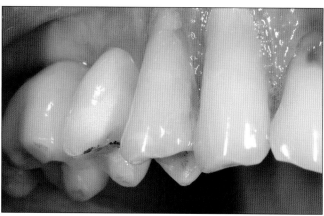

Fig 13-18 / Ceramic fracture at the maxillary right second molar caused by hyperbalance contacts in dynamic occlusion.

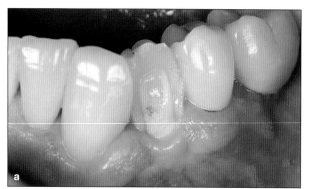

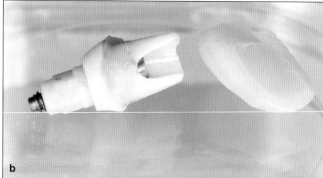

Fig 13-19 / (a) Complete fracture of the all-ceramic implant crown at the mandibular left first premolar. (b) The zirconia abutment with buccal fragment. The abutment is intact.

Accessibility for oral hygiene

The ability to access the superstructure for oral hygiene is a very important prognostic factor. If the patient is not able to perform adequate oral hygiene measures, there will inevitably be peri-implant inflammatory reactions that will subsequently result in tissue loss and cause an esthetic complication. Figure 13-20 shows a dramatic situation; the patient had been treated with implants and a full-arch restoration elsewhere 2 years previously and presented with massive peri-implant inflammatory reactions. The cause lay in the overcontoured superstructure. An attempt was made to use pink ceramic to compensate for a tissue deficit and the exposed necks of tissue-level implants. However, because the pink ceramic was applied in the form of a labial plate, the implants were no longer accessible for oral hygiene.

Inadequate Development and Preservation of Soft Tissue Contour

After exposure, the tissue still undergoes a lengthy period of maturation, which can lead to soft tissue recessions. Therefore, it is important to wait at least 3 months after exposure in the esthetic zone before placing the definitive restoration.[20] Otherwise, tissue deficits around the superstructure may occur, which will impair the esthetics (Fig 13-21). However, it is not only premature restoration that can cause an inadequate emergence profile. Soft tissue that is too thin or insufficient implant depth can also result in too little tissue height becoming available for a suitable emergence profile to develop. The correlations between placement depth and emergence profile are explored in chapters 5 and 12. Thickening soft tissue with connective tissue grafts or substitute material is almost always advisable in the esthetic zone (see chapter 8).

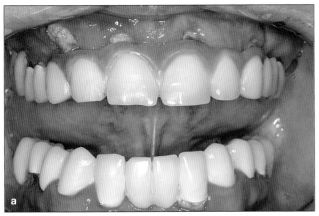 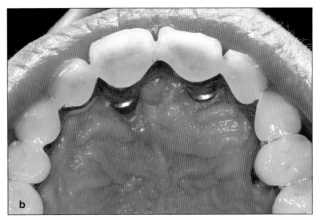

Fig 13-20 / *(a)* Fixed implant denture in the maxilla. There was massive tissue loss resulting from peri-implantitis because the patient was unable to access the restoration for oral hygiene. *(b)* The shoulders of the tissue-level implants lie in a supramucosal position; the implant positions are not ideal.

Fig 13-21 / *(a)* The emergence profile is suboptimal mesial to the left central incisor because the soft tissue is insufficient. This can result in impaction of food. The papilla distal to the right central incisor is slightly inflamed due to poor cleaning. *(b)* After crestal bone resorption, there is inadequate space available to develop the emergence profile. This is why it had to be given a partly rectangular shape.

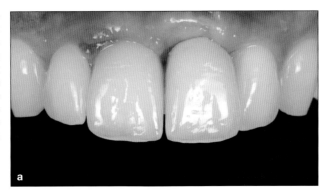 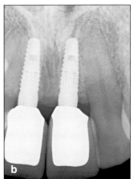

273

References

1. Grunder U, Gracis S, Capelli M. Influence of the 3-D bone-to-implant relationship on esthetics. Int J Periodontics Restorative Dent 2005;25:113–119.
2. Grunder U. Implants in the Esthetic Zone: A Step-by-Step Treatment Strategy. Berlin: Quintessence, 2016.
3. Tymstra N, Meijer HJ, Stellingsma K, Raghoebar GM, Vissink A. Treatment outcome and patient satisfaction with two adjacent implant-supported restorations in the esthetic zone. Int J Periodontics Restorative Dent 2010;30:307–316.
4. Happe A, Khoury F. Complications and risk factors in bone grafting procedures. In: Khoury F, Antoun H, Missika P (eds). Bone Augmentation in Oral Implantology. Chicago: Quintessence, 2007:405–429.
5. Kleinheinz J, Büchter A, Kruse-Lösler B, Weingart D, Joos U. Incision design in implant dentistry based on vascularization of the mucosa. Clin Oral Implants Res 2005;16:518–523.
6. Al-Nawas B, Schiegnitz E. Augmentation procedures using bone substitute materials or autogenous bone: A systematic review and meta-analysis. Eur J Oral Implantol 2014;7(suppl 2):S219–S234.
7. Khoury F, Antoun H, Missika P (eds). Bone Augmentation in Oral Implantology. Chicago: Quintessence, 2007.
8. Akcalı A, Schneider D, Ünlü F, Bıcakcı N, Köse T, Hämmerle CH. Soft tissue augmentation of ridge defects in the maxillary anterior area using two different methods: A randomized controlled clinical trial. Clin Oral Implants Res 2015;26:688–695.
9. Khoury F, Happe A. The palatal subepithelial connective tissue flap method for soft tissue management to cover maxillary defects: A clinical report. Int J Oral Maxillofac Implants 2000;15:415–418.
10. Jung RE, Siegenthaler DW, Hämmerle CH. Postextraction tissue management: A soft tissue punch technique. Int J Periodontics Restorative Dent 2004;24:545–553.
11. Chen ST, Buser D. Clinical and esthetic outcomes of implants placed in postextraction sites. Int J Oral Maxillofac Implants 2009;24(suppl):186–217.
12. Sailer I, Zembic A, Jung RE, Siegenthaler D, Holderegger C, Hämmerle CH. Randomized controlled clinical trial of customized zirconia and titanium implant abutments for canine and posterior single-tooth implant reconstructions: Preliminary results at 1 year of function. Clin Oral Implants Res 2009;20:219–225.

13. Stimmelmayr M, Edelhoff D, Güth JF, Erdelt K, Happe A, Beyer F. Wear at the titanium-titanium and the titanium-zirconia implant-abutment interface: A comparative in vitro study. Dent Mater 2012;28:1215–1220.

14. Truninger TC, Stawarczyk B, Leutert CR, Sailer TR, Hämmerle CH, Sailer I. Bending moments of zirconia and titanium abutments with internal and external implant-abutment connections after aging and chewing simulation. Clin Oral Implants Res 2012;23:12–18.

15. Wilson TG Jr. The positive relationship between excess cement and peri-implant disease: A prospective clinical endoscopic study. J Periodontol 2009;80:1388–1392.

16. Sailer I, Mühlemann S, Zwahlen M, Hämmerle C, Schneider D. Cemented and scew-retained implant reconstructions: A systematic review of the survival and complication rates. Clin Oral Implants Res 2012;23(suppl 6):163–201.

17. Linkevičius T, Vindašiūtė E, Puišys A, Pečiuliené V. The influence of margin location on the amount of undetected cement excess after delivery of cement-retained implant restorations. Clin Oral Implants Res 2011;22:1379–1384.

18. Linkevičius T, Vindašiūtė E, Puišys A, Linkevičiené L, Maslova N, Puriene A. The influence of the cementation margin position on the amount of undetected cement. A prospective clinical study. Clin Oral Implants Res 2013;24:71–76.

19. Hämmerle CH, Wagner D, Braägger U, et al. Threshold of tactile sensitivity perceived with dental endosseous implants and natural teeth. Clin Oral Implants Res 1995;6:83–90.

20. Small PN, Tarnow DP. Gingival recession around implants: A 1-year longitudinal prospective study. Int J Oral Maxillofac Implants 2000;15:527–532.

*"Life is not a matter of holding good cards,
but of playing a poor hand well."*

ROBERT LOUIS STEVENSON

14

Complex Cases

/ Tomohiro Ishikawa, Gerd Körner, Arndt Happe

Many patients present with complex problems requiring a comprehensive therapeutic approach. This chapter is dedicated to cases that can only be solved by this kind of comprehensive approach: patients with highly problematic anatomy in the esthetic zone or other complicated dental requirements. The decision-making process and key success factors are explained in detail in each particular case study.

A typical problem of complex cases is severe tissue loss caused by advanced periodontal disease, trauma, or an endodontic infection. In complex cases, dentists often treat more than simply tooth loss and tissue loss caused by infection or trauma: Because tissue or tooth loss can also lead to pathologic migration of the remaining teeth, dentists are frequently confronted with space problems. Patients may also exhibit congenital malocclusion, tooth agenesis, or malformed teeth. Considering these added complications, an even more important role in treatment planning is attributed to space management (ie, dealing with the available space) for long-term esthetic and functional results.

This chapter examines the two most difficult aspects of complex cases: space management and tissue reconstruction where there is substantial destruction of alveolar ridges.

The following key success factors should be considered in complex cases:

- Interdisciplinary approach with treatment by specialists
- Appropriate space management
- Reconstruction of deficient crestal segments
- Ideal three-dimensional (3D) implant position from a prosthetic perspective

Orthodontic Cases and Space Management

Possibly the most difficult aspect of gap or space management is making an accurate assessment of the implant and tooth positions. The decisions on these positions are normally made with the aid of an orthodontic setup and a diagnostic wax-up in a collaboration between the orthodontist, prosthodontist, and surgeon.[1,2]

The schedule of orthodontic and implant therapy can be divided into three basic sequences: orthodontics, implant therapy, restoration (OI); implant therapy, provisional restoration, orthodontics (IO); or a more complex combination of orthodontic and implantology sequences in which several steps are repeated (combination) (Table 14-1).

These schedules are considered for definitive implants. Another option is to use temporary implants as anchoring points. These temporary anchorage devices (TADs) can be used to create the necessary spaces to facilitate optimal implant positioning before definitive implant placement.

Tooth movements do not always follow the orthodontic setup. A second or third correction (setup model) can sometimes become necessary during the course of the orthodontic treatment. Therefore, it is more reliable to place implants only after the orthodontics are completed or as late as possible during the orthodontic treatment phase.

If treatment necessitates one or more implants as a vertical stop, or if an anchorage device is required, the preferred treatment procedure follows the IO sequence. The risk with this sequence is that the ideal implant locations will change after orthodontic treatment, resulting in incorrectly positioned implants. Following the three rules listed in Box 14-1 will help to minimize this risk (Fig 14-1).

During the treatment process, the team needs to cooperate continuously to ensure successful space management, establish a stable posterior occlusion, and achieve satisfactory esthetics with appropriate anterior guidance. Building a cooperative relationship within the treatment and planning team for orthodontic and implantology treatment

Table 14-1 Time sequence of orthodontics and implant therapy

Name	Sequence	Indications
OI	1. Orthodontics 2. Implant surgery 3. Provisional restoration	Existing teeth offer reciprocal anchorage and a vertical stop. Normally used when tooth loss is minimal.
IO	1. Implant surgery 2. Provisional restoration 3. Orthodontics	Lack of reciprocal anchorage. Lack of vertical stop.
Combination	Combination sequence	Tooth movements are difficult to predict. Temporary anchorage devices can be used. An initial implant provides anchorage, and a gap is orthodontically created for a subsequent implant.

Fig 14-1 / Example of application of the three rules listed in Box 14-1.

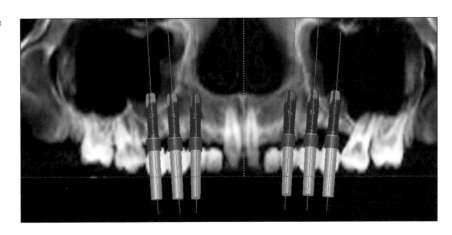

277

Box 14-1 Three basic rules for implant placement in complex cases

1. Small teeth (eg, lateral incisors) or teeth in esthetically sensitive areas should be replaced by pontics and without using implants. This is particularly relevant to restorations done before orthodontic treatment is completed.
2. If possible, a pontic should lie between natural residual teeth and implants.
3. Platform switching should be used to preserve tissue and gain space.

can involve some effort, but the results arising from good communication between dentists with an awareness of the biologic and clinical limitations of the individual case are undoubtedly worth this effort.

All team members should bear responsibility for their own particular discipline, but also for their function within the overall treatment plan. Furthermore, the long-term follow-up and aftercare need to be planned and set up with a view to lifelong craniofacial growth. This applies particularly to very young patients (see case 2).[3]

Case 1

The following were key factors for therapeutic success in this case:

- Space management
- OI sequence
- Orthodontics for patients with periodontal damage
- Esthetic implant therapy for patients with periodontal damage

A 38-year-old patient presented with severe generalized chronic periodontitis combined with an Angle Class II, division 2 malocclusion with a deep bite. In addition, pathologic tooth movements of several teeth disrupted the occlusion. Orthodontic correction with reciprocal anchorage on the existing teeth was planned (Figs 14-2a to 14-2f).

Radiographs confirmed moderate-to-severe chronic periodontitis and pathologic tooth movements[4] (Figs 14-2g and 14-4h). Both mandibular first molars had already been

278

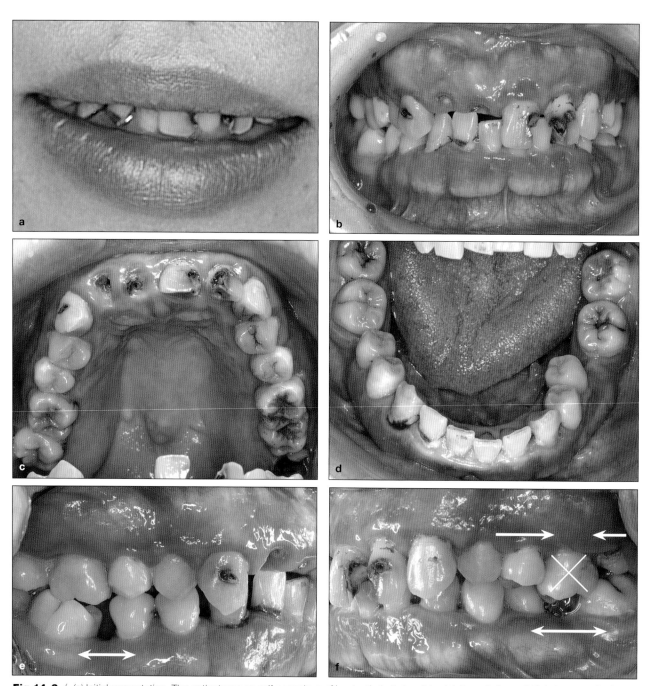

Fig 14-2 / *(a)* Initial presentation. The patient was so self-conscious of her teeth that she did not fully smile for an initial photograph. *(b to f)* The intraoral situation shows severe inflammation. *White arrows* indicate planned orthodontic movement, *white x* indicates tooth to be extracted.

extracted, and extraction was also planned for all maxillary incisors and the maxillary left first molar because of advanced caries and bone resorption. Before the orthodontic treatment or implant surgery could begin, all the inflammation had to be completely resolved.[5,6] In this case, the orthodontic treatment was performed before implant therapy was started (Figs 14-2i to 14-2m). Although the inflammation at the maxillary left incisors was difficult

to control, these teeth were retained as space-holders and anchors for the orthodontic wire. The maxillary left incisors were extracted after the orthodontic treatment. Four months later, 2D and 3D radiographic examination revealed horizontal and vertical bone defects that would have impaired the esthetic result. As part of the preoperative planning, the position of the future incisal edges and the visibility of the incisors were tested with the aid

Fig 14-2 *cont.* / *(g and h)* Radiographs at initial presentation. *(i to l)* Situation 1 month before the orthodontic treatment was completed.

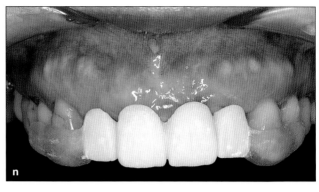

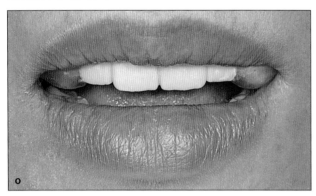

Fig 14-2 *cont.* / *(m)* Frontal view near the end of orthodonic treatment. *(n and o)* The visibility of the incisors was tested using a mock-up.

→

of the radiographic template (Figs 14-2n to 14-2s). In this instance, the template served as a virtual mock-up. The maxillary right central incisor and left lateral incisor were selected as implant sites. The implants were alternated with pontics to avoid esthetic problems caused by adjacent implants. After the extraction wounds had healed, the result was a highly pronounced 3D crestal defect (Figs 14-2t and 14-2u). This was successfully reconstructed with guided bone regeneration (GBR) with titanium mesh and a collagen membrane. Two implants with platform switching were placed into the prosthetically ideal 3D positions at the sites of the right central incisor and left lateral incisor. To check the implant positions as well as the volume and shape of the regenerated tissue, the surgical template was also used intraoperatively during the augmentation[7,8] (Figs 14-2v and 14-2w). There were two separate rounds of soft tissue conditioning, as follows:

1. At the start of conditioning, the pontic base is typically built up deep into the soft tissue and up to the palatal border of the gingiva former or the cover screw. Material is then gradually applied toward the vestibular aspect[9] (Figs 14-2x to 14-2aa).

2. Adaptation by further application of acrylic resin was continued for 1 to 2 months until the very thin covering soft tissue was removed with a simple noninvasive procedure (Figs 14-2bb to 14-2ee). The superstructure was then created, in this case a computer-aided design/computer-assisted manufacturing (CAD/CAM) screw-retained partial denture. Screw-retained restorations avoid the risk of peri-implantitis caused by excess cement. Furthermore, the implant is readily accessible in the event of problems.[10-13]

The interdisciplinary approach involving periodontal treatment, orthodontic correction, and implant therapy produced a satisfactory esthetic outcome (Figs 14-2ff to 14-2ii). A smile with natural dentofacial esthetics was restored after the treatment. This outcome would not have been possible without 3D tissue regeneration and modeling with the aid of a diagnostic template. It should again be noted at this point that, after treatment, all patients should receive oral hygiene instruction matched to their risk of periodontitis and should regularly be recalled for oral hygiene appointments (Figs 14-2kk and 14-2ll). This patient attended supportive periodontal therapy (SPT) once a month for professional teeth cleaning and care of restorations (Figs 14-2mm abnd 14-2nn).

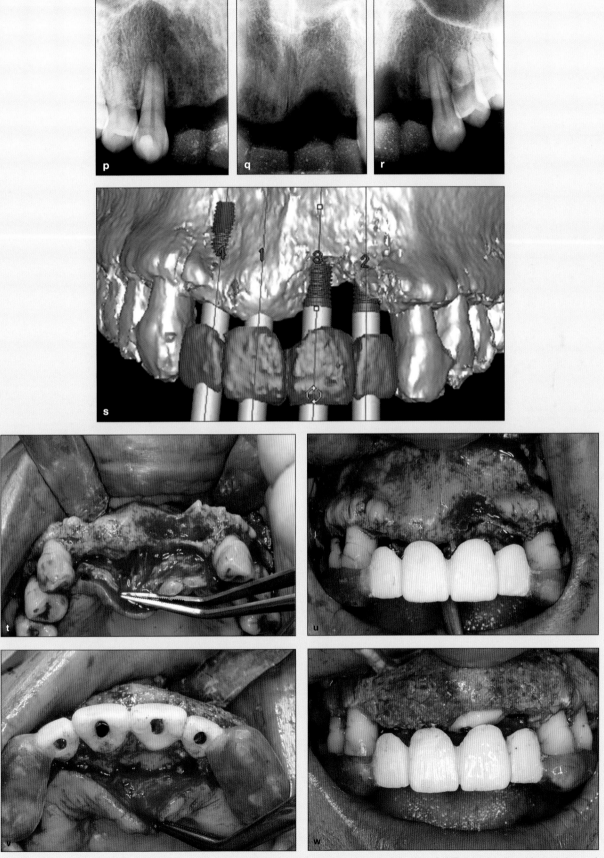

Fig 14-2 *cont.* / *(p to s)* Radiographs and digital planning using the diagnostic template. *(t and u)* The occlusal and frontal views of the bone defect show that the interdental bone height was inadequate. *(v and w)* The occlusal and frontal view of the augmented ridge with implants in situ at the sites of the maxillary right central incisor and left lateral incisor.

282

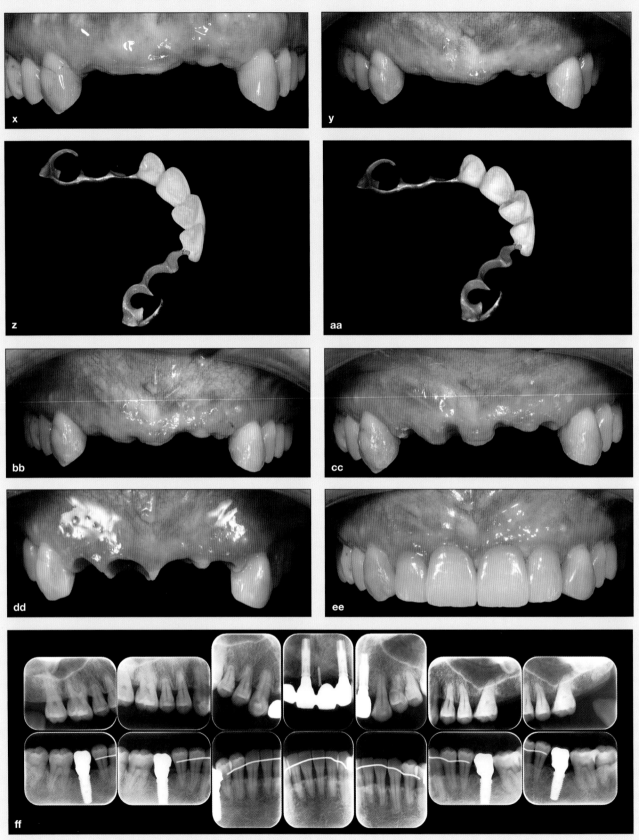

Fig 14-2 *cont.* / *(x and y)* Comparison of before and after GBR. Note the significant improvement of the papillae morphology. *(z and aa)* At the start of the remodeling procedure, the ovate pontic is typically expanded deep into the soft tissue to the palatal edge of the submerged healing abutment or the cover screw. The material is then gradually expanded toward the buccal aspect. *(bb and cc)* Comparison of the first adjustment of the pontic base and 2 weeks later. The volume should not be increased by more than 1 to 1.5 mm per week, and the ischemia should disappear within a few minutes. *(dd)* Final soft tissue contour 10 months after the start of remodeling. *(ee)* Final result. *(ff)* Radiographs after treatment.

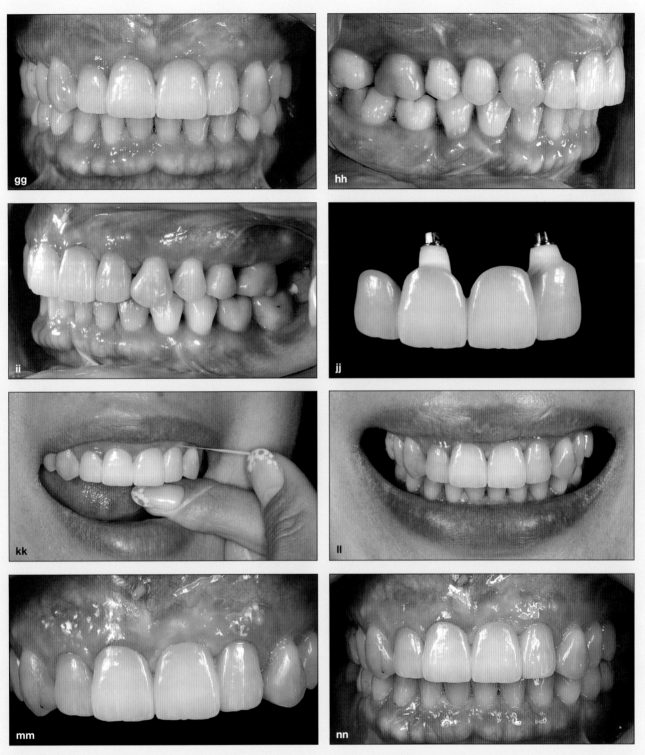

Fig 14-2 *cont.* / *(gg)* Final appearance from frontal view. *(hh and ii)* Lateral views of the final situation. A correct canine relationship and stable occlusion were established with the treatment, facilitating care and maintenance and ensuring long-term success. *(jj)* The CAD/CAM-fabricated screw-retained definitive restoration. *(kk)* The patient was instructed on the use of dental floss at home. *(ll)* The patient smiling with the new definitive restorations. *(mm and nn)* The reconstructed function and esthetics are maintained 6 years after treatment. (Surgery and prosthodontics performed by T. Ishikawa; orthodontics performed by K. Kida; laboratory work performed by K. Nakajima.)

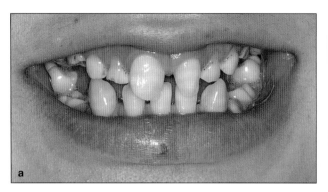
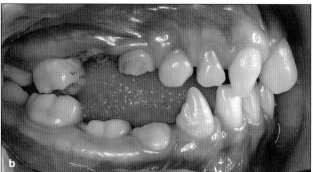
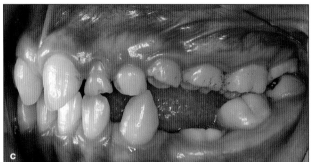
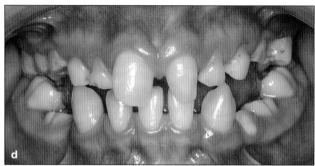

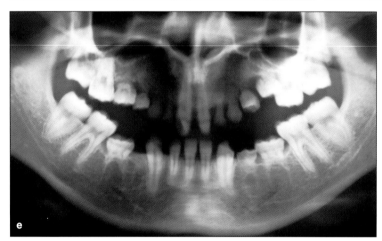

Fig 14-3 / *(a)* The patient has a high smile line. *(b to d)* A total of 13 teeth were absent. The remaining anterior teeth were malformed, and several posterior teeth were in infraocclusion. *(e)* Panoramic radiograph of the initial situation. ⟶

Case 2

The following were key factors for therapeutic success in this case:

- Space management
- IO sequence in the maxilla
- Combination sequence in the mandible
- Anticipating the implant position

A 19-year-old patient with agenesis of 13 teeth and various hypoplasias was referred by another dentist (Fig 14-3a). The maxillary premolars to lateral incisors were absent, as well as all mandibular premolars and the mandibular left lateral incisor. The maxillary central incisors and mandibular canines were malformed (Figs 14-3b to 14-3f).

The persistent primary teeth were ankylosed with pronounced infraocclusion. The patient has a high smile line. A setup was developed by the orthodontist (Fig 14-3g). Orthodontists are generally inclined to avoid molar movements, but the possibility of anchorage on implants should be taken into consideration. This provides an opportunity to reconstruct the entire occlusion. Using silicone keys, the orthodontic setup was transferred to a radiographic template made of radiopaque acrylic resin to allow for a clinical try-in (Figs 14-3h to 14-3o).[14–17] Therefore, the

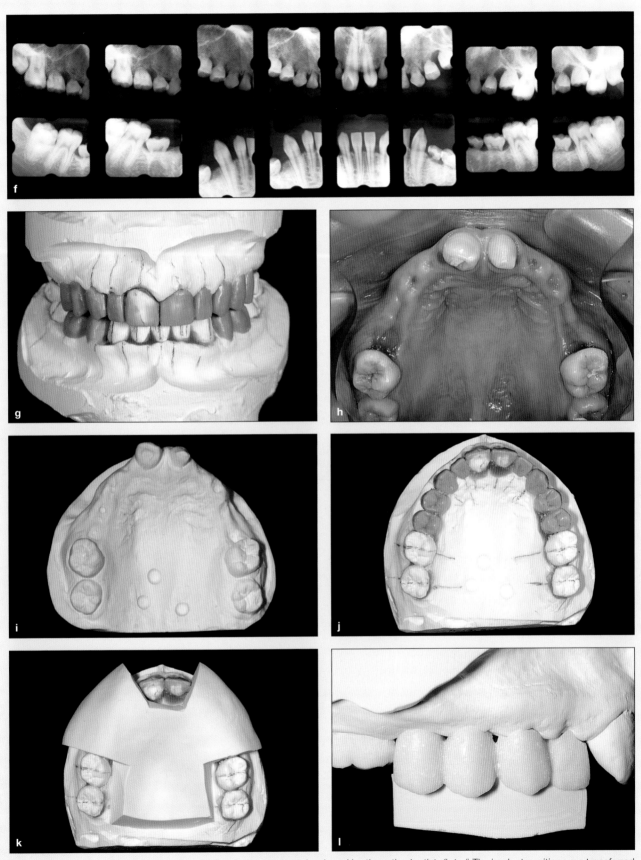

Fig 14-3 *cont.* / *(f)* Apical radiographs. *(g)* The first setup cast developed by the orthodontist. *(h to j)* The implant positions are transferred from the setup cast to the original working cast. First, an orthodontic setup is made for the diagnostic wax-up. The working cast for the diagnostic template is fabricated with artificial reference structures (three depressions in the palate) and copied for the orthodontic setup and the diagnostic wax-up. *(k and l)* The positions of the wax-up are then transferred to the cast. →

Fig 14-3 *cont.* / *(m to o)* After the wax-up positions are transferred to the working cast, the future implant positions are anticipated and transferred as well.[14–17] *(p to u)* The proportions are analyzed. The diagnostic template fabricated according to the orthodontic setup model conveys an idea of the ideal future shape of the alveolar ridge.

orthodontic proposal to the patient could be tested for plausibility and the anatomical conditions could be analyzed with cone beam computed tomography (CBCT) (Figs 14-3p to 14-3u).

Based on strategic considerations, the maxillary sites selected for implant placement were the canine and premolar sites (Figs 14-3v to 14-3aa; see Box 14-1). A strategically advantageous choice of implant positions is particularly important in cases that also necessitate orthodontic treatment. Orthodontic treatment began as soon as the implants were functioning. In the maxilla, the treatment procedure followed the IO sequence.

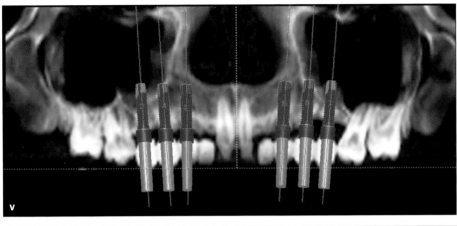

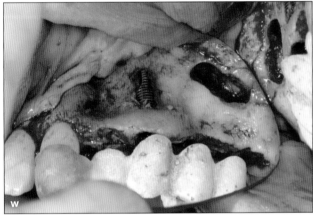
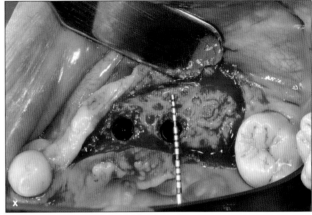

287

Fig 14-3 *cont.* / *(v)* The implant sites are strategically chosen (see Box 14-1). *(w and x)* Implant placement begins. ⟶

After the success of the first orthodontic treatment, a second orthodontic setup was prepared (Fig 14-3bb). The planned definitive tooth positions can be altered during the course of the orthodontic treatment. In this case, a second setup cast was fabricated and the changes were taken into account.[18] Thanks to extensions mesial to the positions of the lateral incisors, it was possible to react to the changes resulting from the orthodontic treatment by adapting the pontic form.

In the mandible, the treatment followed an IOI combination sequence. The space in the gap at the premolar region was assessed as being too small for two adjacent implants, so the canine was to be orthodontically moved away from the planned implant position (Figs 14-3cc to 14-3ee). The first step was implant placement in the site of the second premolar. Using this implant as an anchor, the canine was moved mesially to free up space at the first premolar site for another implant. After adequate space was formed at the first premolar site, the implant was to be placed.

When the 4-mm-diameter implant at the premolar site was restored with a 7-mm-wide crown, there was not enough space to maintain the necessary 3-mm distance from the adjacent implant and 1.5-mm distance from the adjacent tooth (Figs 14-3ff and 14-3gg). The treatment team (ie, orthodontist, dental technician, surgeon, and prosthodontist) must fully absorb these rules and always bear in mind that they apply on both sides of the implant. All team members need to make sure from the start of treatment that, in an IOI sequence, each step is planned not as an individual event but in the context of the overall treatment.

The end result achieved was esthetically and functionally satisfactory (Figs 14-3hh to 14-3rr). However, an even better occlusal relationship could have been created if it had been planned to move the molars as well when using the implant anchors.

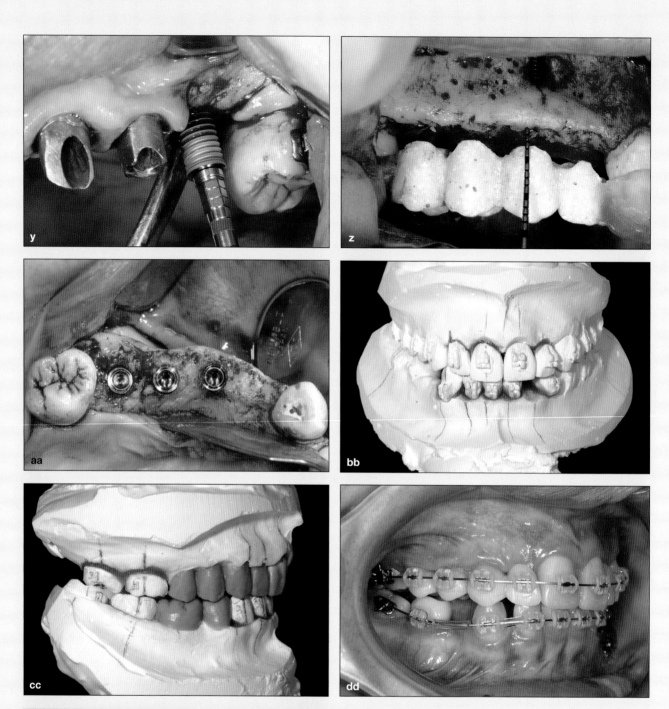

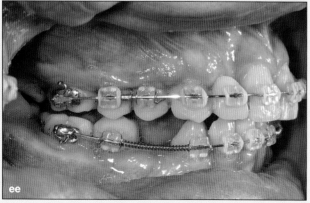

Fig 14-3 *cont.* / *(y to aa)* The implants are placed as precisely and accurately as possible in the planned positions. *(bb)* The second orthodontic setup cast. *(cc)* When planning for the mandible, the problem was the lack of space for two implants and the existing canine. *(dd and ee)* IOI sequence in the mandible. →

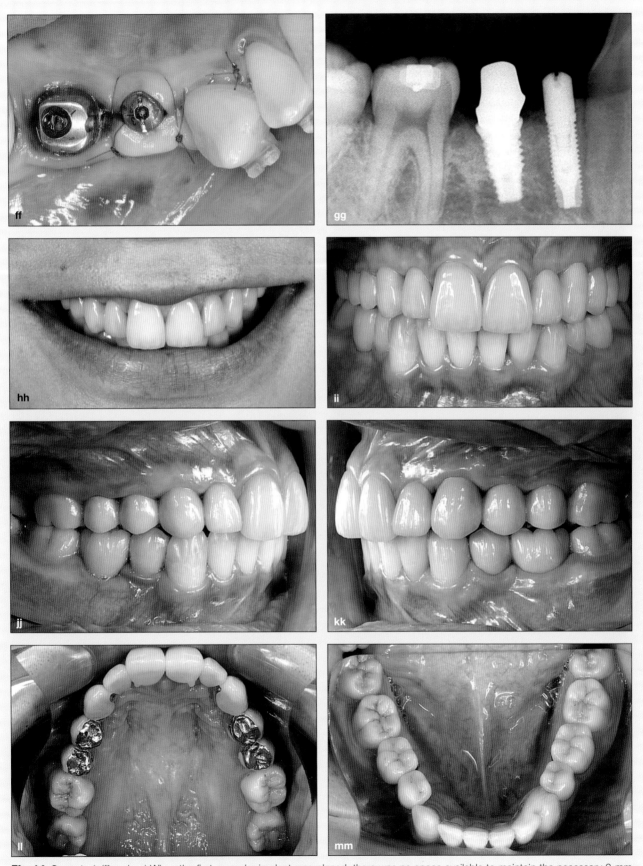

Fig 14-3 *cont.* / *(ff and gg)* When the first premolar implant was placed, there was no space available to maintain the necessary 3-mm distance from the adjacent second premolar implant and 1.5-mm distance from the adjacent natural canine. *(hh)* The patient smiling after completion of the treatment. *(ii to mm)* Frontal, lateral, and occlusal views of the end result. If the treatment plan had included implant anchors to move the molars, a better occlusal relationship could have been established. →

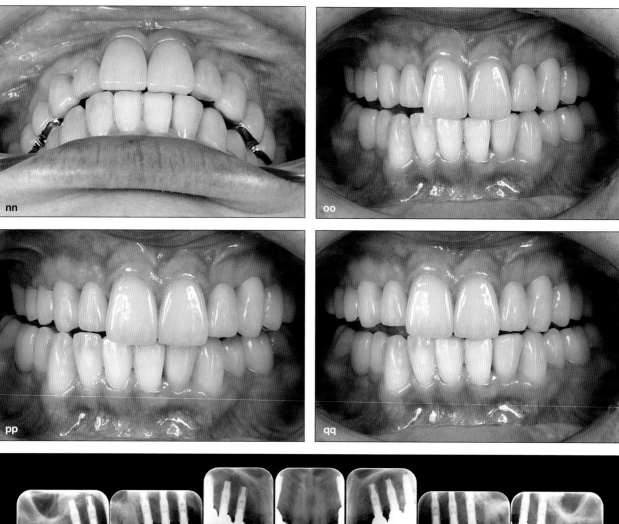

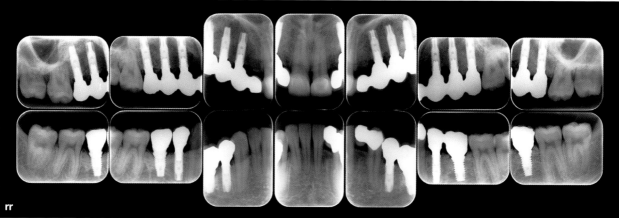

Fig 14-3 *cont.* / *(nn to qq)* Acceptable anterior guidance. The shape of the mandibular anterior teeth was adapted to create correct anterior guidance by using direct composite restorations. *(rr)* Radiographs after completion of treatment. (Surgery and prosthodontics performed by T. Ishikawa; orthodontics performed by K. Kida; laboratory work performed by K. Nakajima.)

Extensive Tissue Reconstruction

The most common factors causing severe alveolar ridge defects include the following pathologic changes:

- Trauma
- Advanced periodontal diseases
- Sizeable endodontic lesions
- Infections after root fracture
- Neoplasias and malignancies

Esthetic implant therapy can be more complicated when there is severe tissue loss. The design of the definitive restoration is influenced by several factors, including the functional and esthetic demands as well as financial constraints of patients, the smile line and visibility of the interdental papillae, the degree of severity of the tissue reconstruction, and level of oral hygiene. The patient as well as the dentist must be aware of the biologic limitations of implant therapy and develop realistic objectives for the individual situation.

A wide variety of techniques are reported in the literature for vertical and horizontal augmentation of the bony ridge (eg, GBR, lateral and onlay grafts, distraction osteogenesis; see chapter 9). Even with advanced methods, vertical augmentation always remains a greater problem than horizontal augmentation, and the necessity of vertical augmentation is one of the features that characterize a complex case.[19,20]

Forced orthodontic extrusion is one predictable technique for vertical augmentation of hard and soft tissue.[21,22] Orthodontic extrusion has therefore proved to be a very useful measure in complex cases where genuine vertical tissue loss is often present together with generalized bone resorption resulting from advanced periodontal disease.[23]

The combination of orthodontic extrusion and the root submergence technique has particular potential for esthetic and functional results in patients with severe preexisting periodontal damage.[24] More predictable results can be achieved in this situation with relatively few invasive measures than can be achieved with typical augmentation techniques. Therefore, even severely damaged teeth should always be considered for preservation during treatment planning, even when this might not lead to the most esthetic results.

If the patient presents with a major loss of tissue, all those involved in the team need to cooperate to define and implement the best possible treatment option for the particular case. In this situation, it is not just a matter of the choice of surgical techniques and prosthetic restoration, but primarily the timing of treatment and the sequence of treatment steps.

Case 3

The clinical problem in this case was advanced generalized periodontal disease with severe bone loss. The following were key factors for therapeutic success:

- Implants function as orthodontic implants (ie, as anchorage devices for the orthodontic treatment)
- Orthodontic extrusion for vertical tissue augmentation in the esthetic zone

- Root submergence technique for preserving and stabilizing the augmented tissue

A 56-year-old patient requested rehabilitation of her dentition (Figs 14-4a to 14-4d). Most of the teeth were loose and pathologically displaced because there was advanced alveolar bone loss that already affected more than two-thirds of the root length (Figs 14-4e and 14-4f). The soft tissue had attained its original level; however, most of the remaining teeth showed advanced attachment loss with deep pockets because of the extensive bone loss. Considering all the variables in this case, the decision was made to restore the entire maxilla with implants.

When the upper lip is in a resting position, the vertical dimensions are acceptable from an esthetic standpoint even though the incisors are too far facially and the alveolar bone level is greatly receded (Figs 14-4g and 14-4h). If the anterior teeth were extracted, the soft tissue would recede, and the crown length of the definitive restoration would be too great for an esthetic outcome. The ideal approach would be vertical regeneration of the alveolar bone by 3 to 5 mm without soft tissue collapse. Therefore, an orthodontic treatment was planned to correct the tooth position and augment the alveolar bone for implant placement.

After the hopeless molars were extracted, implant placement was planned. These implants would act as anchors for the orthodontic treatment, and the implant positions were estimated from the orthodontic setup model[25–27] (Fig 14-4i). Implants were placed in the posterior region in the positions planned on the orthodontic setup with simultaneous augmentation (Figs 14-4j and 14-4k). The procedure equates to the implant IO sequence. In the IO sequence, a precise assessment of the implant positions is crucial for an esthetic outcome. After the prosthetic restoration of the molar implants and anchorage devices were available, occlusion was supported, and the orthodontic treatment was begun to close the spaces horizontally and extrude the anterior teeth. To maintain adequate space conditions, the tooth forms were adapted to the altered requirements with composite during extrusion. Alveolar bone and soft tissue were augmented via extrusion over 10 months (extrusion phase). The situation was then stabilized for 6 months (retention phase). The anterior teeth had to be extruded to the ideal esthetic position. The different apicocoronal root positions after extrusion show that each anterior tooth was extruded depending on its attachment level until the necessary interdental bone height was established (Figs 14-4l to 14-4p). After a retention phase of 6 months, the implants

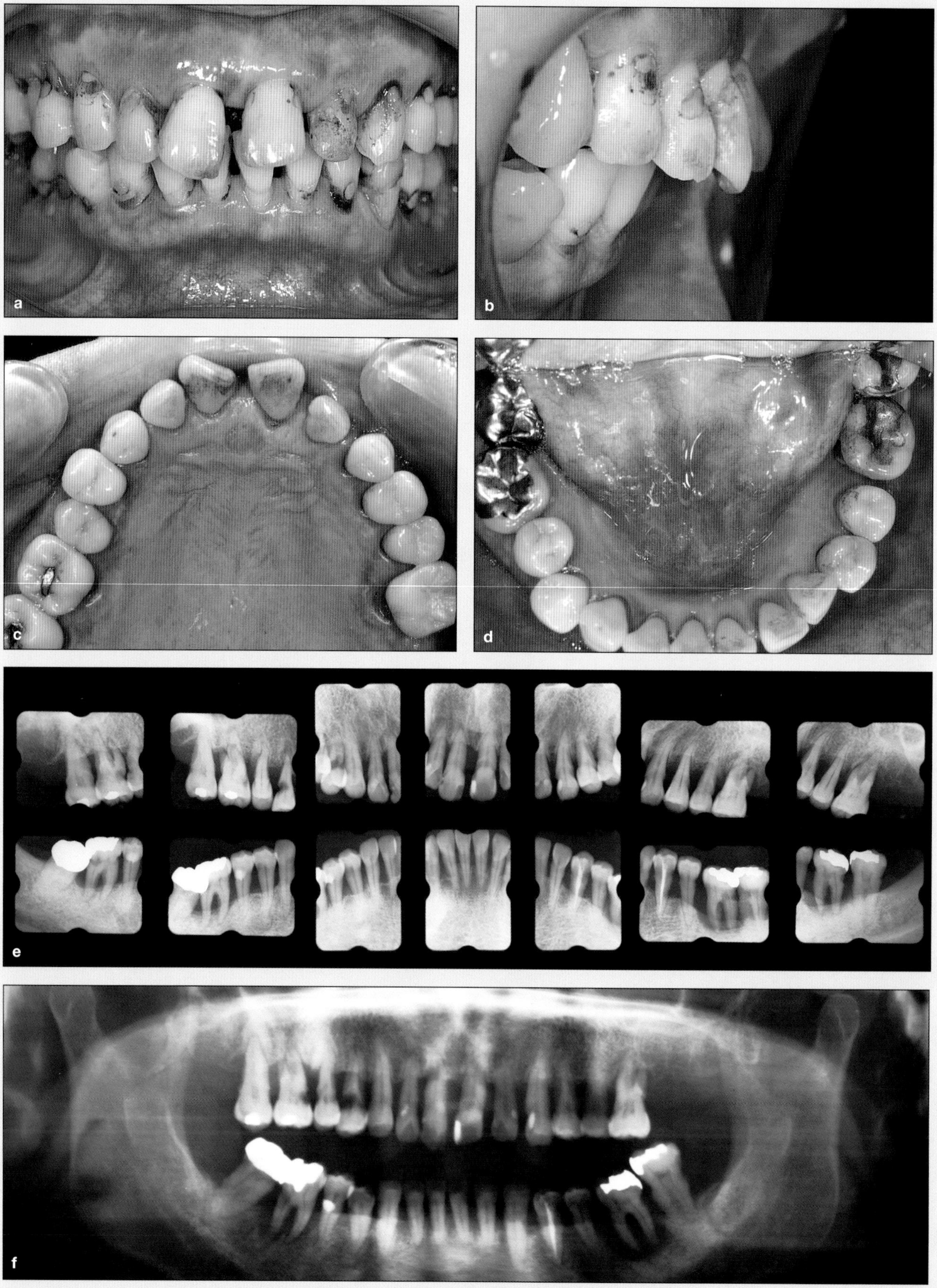

Fig 14-4 / *(a to d)* Intraoral preoperative situation. *(e and f)* Radiographs before the start of treatment.

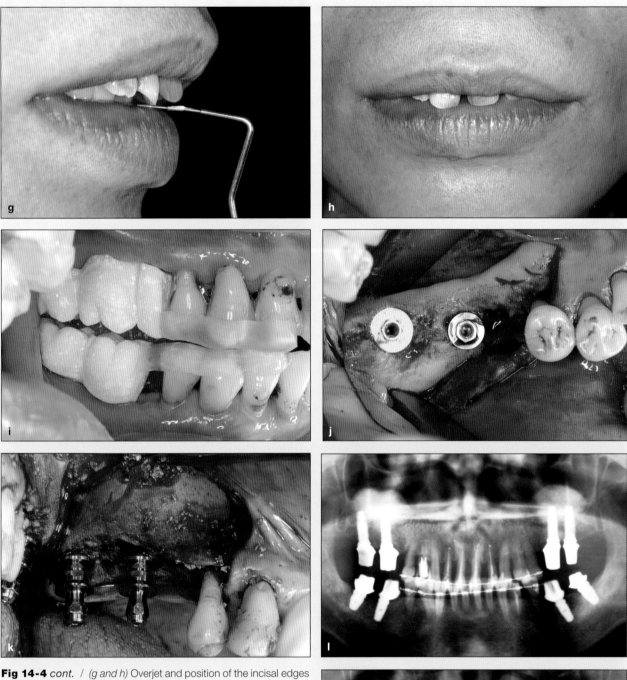

293

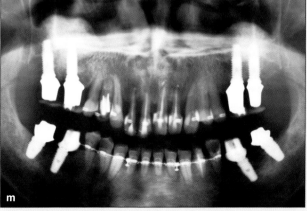

Fig 14-4 *cont.* / *(g and h)* Overjet and position of the incisal edges before treatment. *(i)* The diagnostic template indicates the implant positions that were planned after extraction of the molars not worth preserving. *(j and k)* Implants were placed in the posterior region in the positions planned on the orthodontic setup. *(l and m)* Comparison of the panoramic radiographs before and after orthodontic extrusion.

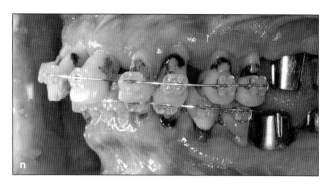 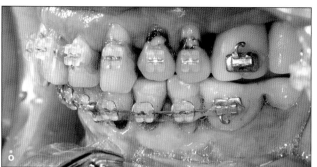

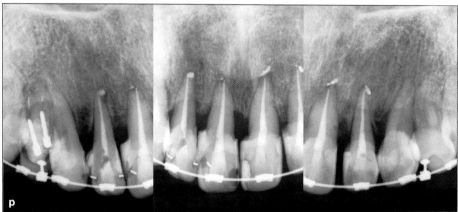

294

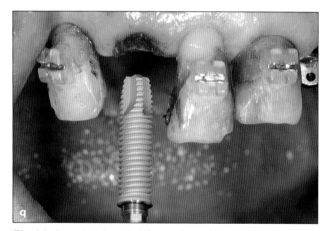 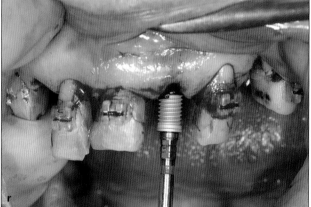

Fig 14-4 *cont.* / *(n and o)* Comparison of lateral views before and after extrusion. *(p)* Each of the incisor roots are in a different position, showing that each tooth was extruded depending on the attachment level. *(q and r)* Immediate implants were placed.

were placed in the fresh extraction sockets of the maxillary lateral incisors and first premolars in a minimally invasive procedure (Figs 14-4q to 14-4t).

The implants were placed in the ideal positions corresponding to the most palatal position within the sockets. After extrusion, the remaining teeth were capable of maintaining the soft tissue frame, but their loss of attachment was too great to support crowns or partial dentures (Fig 14-4u). Extraction of these teeth, even with ridge preservation techniques, would have led to a deterioration in the already optimized hard and soft tissue architecture.

This situation is therefore a good indication for the root submergence technique.[24] To avoid relapse of the vertical problems, it is advisable to retain the extruded teeth for as long as possible, preferably at least 6 months, before beginning the root submergence procedure. For the root submergence technique, the crowns of the teeth were cut off, and the pulp was directly capped with mineral trioxide aggregate (MTA) (Fig 14-4v). To avoid the need to harvest soft tissue from the palate, the crowns were cut off at the bony ridge level (ie, more apical than ideal) and the roots were covered with collagen sponge soaked in plasma

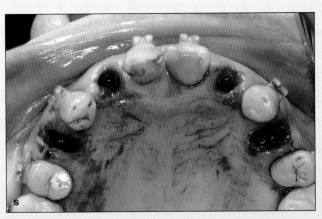

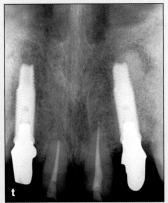

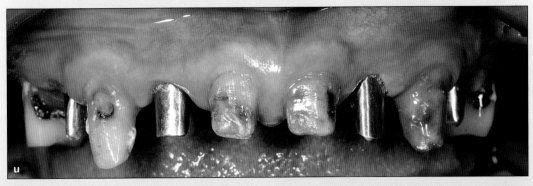

295

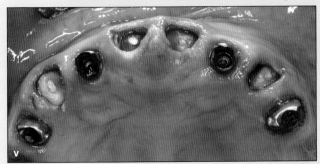

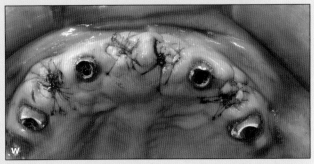

Fig 14-4 *cont.* / *(s and t)* Implants were placed in a minimally invasive procedure. *(u)* Soft tissue situation after incorporation of the implants. *(v)* The vital teeth were cut off at the bone level, and the pulps were directly capped with MTA. *(w)* The roots were sealed with collagen. *(x)* The root submergence technique conserves the bone level. *(y)* The soft tissue is supported by the submerged roots.

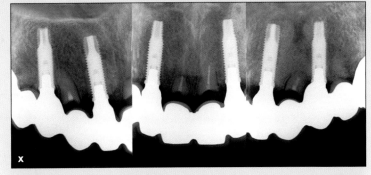

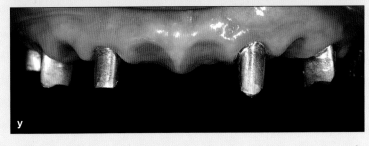

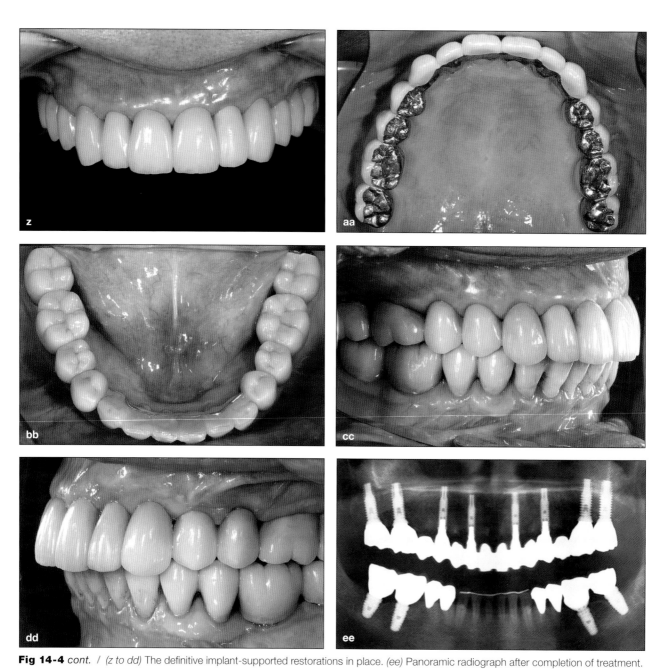

Fig 14-4 *cont.* / *(z to dd)* The definitive implant-supported restorations in place. *(ee)* Panoramic radiograph after completion of treatment.

rich in growth factors (PRGF; Fig 14-4w).[28,29] If complete sealing of the socket is not successful, a small connective tissue graft (CTG) is required. If the patient had agreed to a CTG, the crowns would have been cut about 1 mm coronal to the bony ridge so that supra-alveolar fibers of the root surface would have been preserved.

Owing to a good strategic choice of pontic positions and use of the root submergence technique, remodeling processes after extraction could be avoided and tissue

preserved (Figs 14-4x and 14-4y). This is reflected in the definitive restoration with the improved interdental bone level and an ideal vertical level caused by the submucosally preserved roots (Figs 14-4z to 14-4ee).

After completion of the treatment, professional maintenance therapy must always be matched to the patient's individual risk of periodontitis. For this patient, monthly SPT was scheduled with the dental hygienist (Figs 14-4ff and 14-4gg).

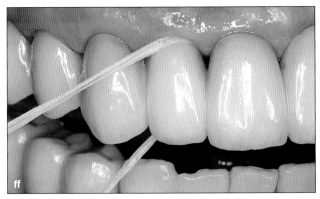 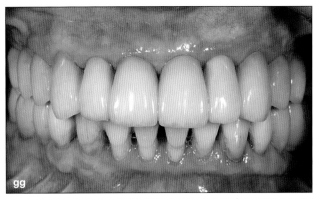

Fig 14-4 *cont.* / *(ff)* The patient is educated to clean with dental floss as part of periodontal maintenance therapy. *(gg)* Condition 2 years after completion of the treatment. (Surgery and prosthodontics performed by T. Ishikawa; orthodontics performed by K. Kida; laboratory work performed by K. Nakajima.)

Case 4

The clinical problem in this case was severe vertical tissue loss caused by trauma. The following were key factors for therapeutic success:

- Space management due to decrease in the number of teeth to be replaced
- Two-stage GBR
- Soft tissue augmentation

The 25-year-old patient had sustained a trauma in the esthetic zone in an automobile accident 10 years earlier. The tooth loss had been treated with a fixed partial denture. As the patient got older and continued to grow, the damaged abutment teeth were unable to erupt correctly, which led to an extensive vertical bone deficit and open bite (Figs 14-5a and 14-5b). Because of the high smile line, this vertical defect was much more difficult to reconstruct esthetically (Figs 14-5c and 14-5d). The full extent of the tissue defect was evident after extraction of the maxillary central incisors, which were not worth preserving (Figs 14-5e to 14-5g).

A wax-up was created, and a 3D radiologic diagnostic assessment was performed using CBCT scans. The diagnostic wax-up revealed the solution to the limited mesiodistal space and adverse gingival contour of the remaining anterior teeth: the four lost teeth could be replaced with three units, and the left first premolar could take the place of the canine (Fig 14-5h). The diagnostic

template and CBCT scans revealed the exact size of the defect (Figs 14-5i to 14-5k). It was planned to place three implants and simultaneously perform 3D bone augmentation in a single operation.

The implants were placed in the prosthetically ideal position. The shoulders of the implants projected beyond the local bone by as much as 6 mm vertically. The occlusal view after implant placement showed a favorable bone foundation for vertical augmentation (Fig 14-5l). For horizontal augmentation, a bone thickness of at least 2 mm at the platform on the buccal aspect is sufficient and counteracts any negative effects of recession and papillae loss caused by normal bone remodeling.[30]

There are three possible intraoral vertical references for bone augmentation (Figs 14-5m and 14-5n): *(1)* the bone level should lie 4 mm apical to the interproximal contact or the papilla apices; *(2)* the bone level should lie on the imaginary line through the adjacent bone apices; *(3)* the interproximal bone level should be located 2 to 3 mm coronal to the implant platform. The interproximal bone height (ie, 4 mm) and the line between the bone apices bordering the gap (*white line* in Figs 14-5m and 14-5n) show that there is a vertical augmentation requirement of 9 mm. After implant placement, the third reference (ie, 2 to 3 mm coronal to the implant platform) defined the same augmentation target (ie, 9 mm) as the other two references. This confirmed the correct relationship between the planned superstructure, the existing attachment level at the adjacent teeth, and the implant positions.[8]

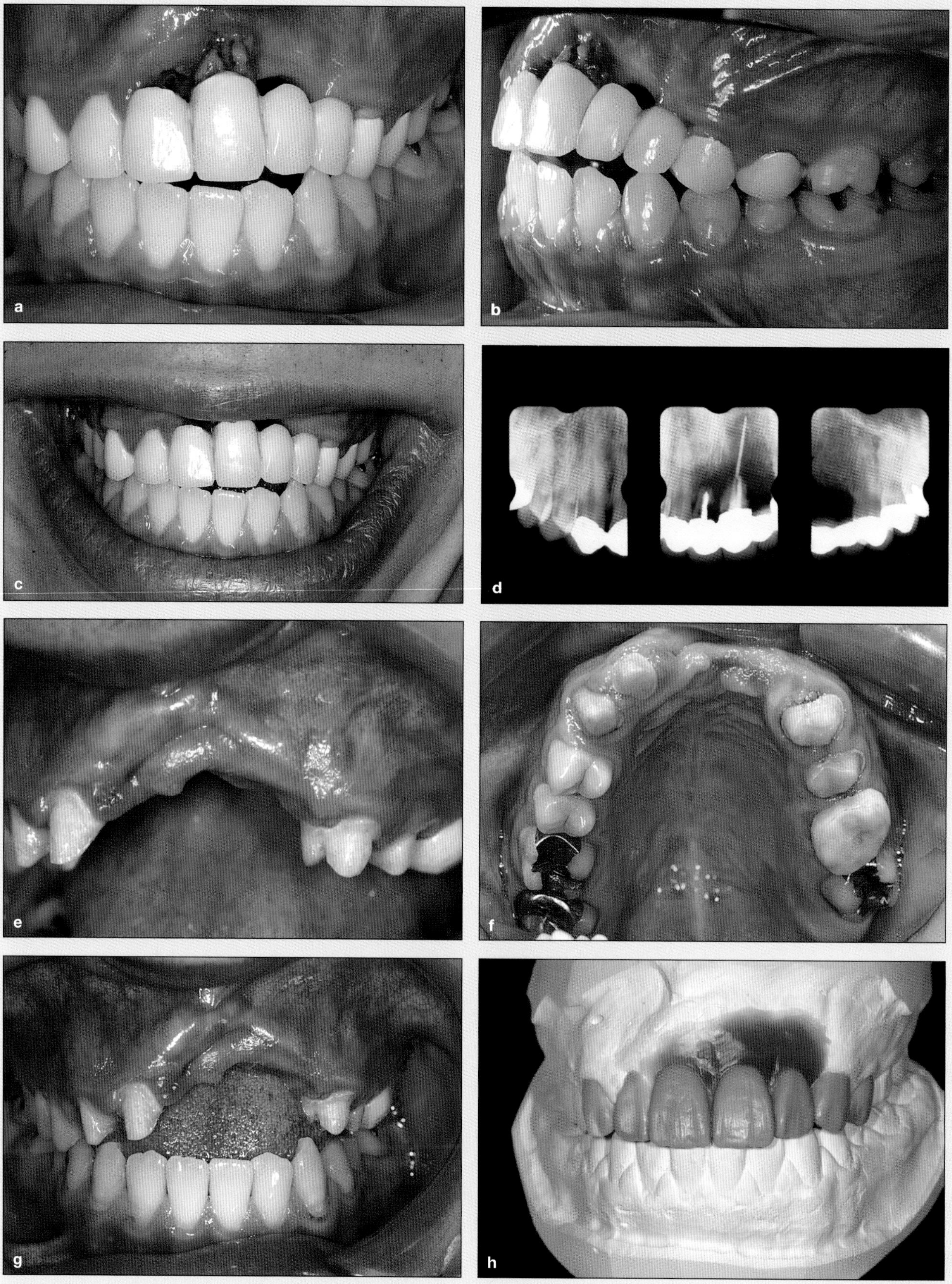

Fig 14-5 / *(a)* Initial situation with pronounced vertical tissue loss and open bite. *(b)* The extent of vertical tissue loss becomes clear in the lateral view. *(c)* The very high smile line exposes the defect, presenting another challenge. *(d)* The radiographs show the excessive vertical bone loss. *(e and f)* Frontal and occlusal views of the ridge 3 months after extraction of the central incisors. There is an extensive 3D defect. *(g)* Frontal view before bone augmentation. *(h)* Diagnostic wax-up with the left first premolar switched to the canine site. →

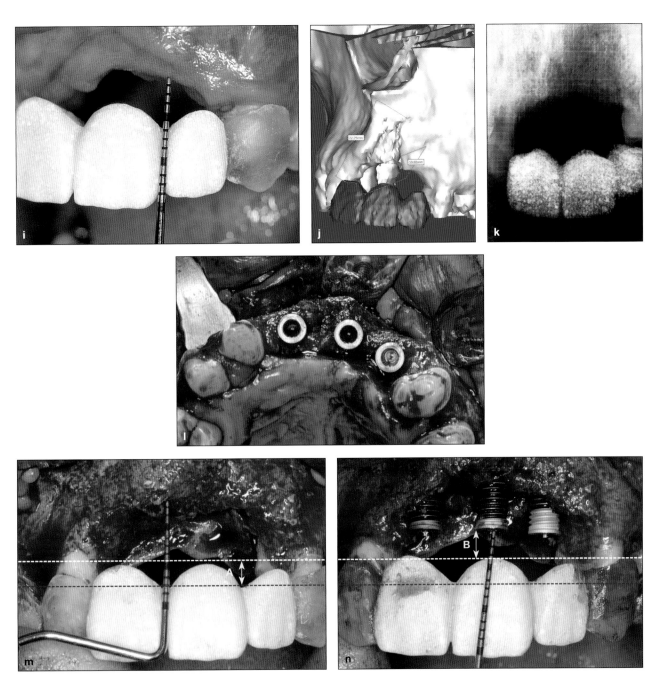

Fig 14-5 *cont.* / *(i to k)* After extraction of the teeth not being preserved, the tissue healed, and the full extent of the defect became apparent. The diagnostic template and CBCT images revealed the exact size of the defect. *(l)* The implants were placed in the prosthetically ideal positions. *(m and n)* The surgical template indicates the ideal vertical position of the implant shoulder and the target for bone augmentation. Vertical references can be used for bone augmentation in this case. The *white line* passes through the crestal bone apices of the adjacent teeth, and the *red line* passes through the papilla apices. The crestal bone should lie 4 mm apical to the papilla apex (A). The implant shoulder should lie 2 to 3 mm apical to the future soft tissue or crown margin (B).

After augmentation with autogenous bone chips and anorganic bovine bone mineral (ABBM), the augmentation material was covered with three titanium meshes followed by a collagen membrane (Fig 14-5o). After successful incorporation of the augmentation material, a distinct gain in tissue was observed so that 4 mm of bone had been regenerated buccal to the implants (Fig 14-5p).

Looking at the vertical conditions, however, it was evident when considering all three references that there was still a space of 2 to 3 mm requiring bony filling so that

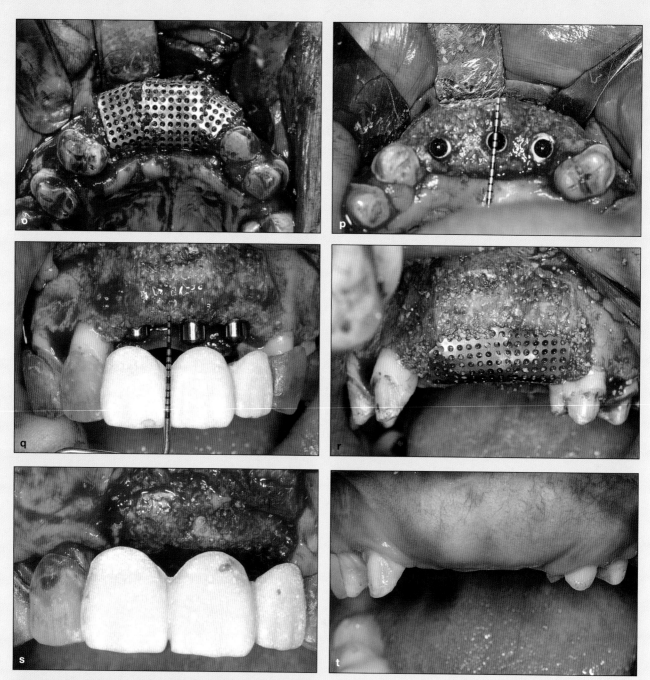

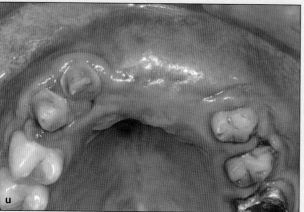

Fig 14-5 *cont.* / *(o)* The space for bone regeneration is secured with simple titanium meshes. *(p)* View after the first GBR. The implants were completely covered with regenerated tissue. After 7 months, the vestibular bone thickness was more than 4 mm. *(q)* The 3-mm-long healing abutments defined the target for the second GBR. There was still a shortage of 2 to 3 mm of bone for establishing papillae. *(r)* During the second GBR, the healing abutments served as vertical stops for the titanium mesh. *(s)* After 7 months, the surgical template showed that the regenerated tissue height fully satisfied the vertical requirements. *(t)* After bone augmentation, it becomes clear that there is insufficient keratinized tissue available. *(u)* The occlusal view reveals an insufficient vestibular ridge contour.

→

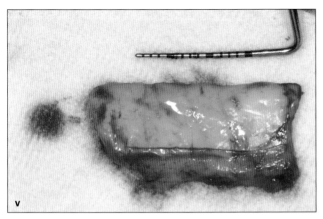

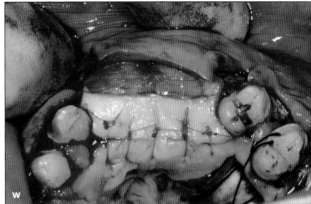

Fig 14-5 *cont.* / *(v to x)* Soft tissue augmentation was completed with a full-thickness graft with connective tissue and a keratinized strip.

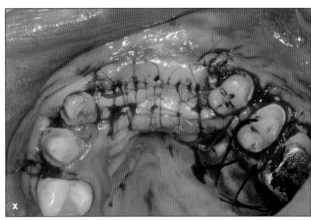

301

the esthetically important papillae could be established (Fig 14-5q). A second augmentation was performed with titanium mesh, with healing abutments providing vertical support (Fig 14-5r). After another 7 months' healing, a total of 9 mm of bone was vertically augmented in this manner (Fig 14-5s).

A deficient ridge can lose keratinized tissue as well as bone. The releasing incision of the periosteum of the mucosal area does not increase keratinized tissue—it stretches the flap and moves the mucogingival junction coronally. When vertical ridge defects are treated, bone augmentation alone is often not enough for an esthetic result.[31–33] In this case, the soft tissue contour after bone augmentation was still not ideal; there was a soft tissue deficiency despite the adequate bone ridge (Figs 14-5t and 14-5u). Therefore, soft tissue augmentation was also required. The size of the soft tissue graft was calculated on the basis of the vestibular displacement. To correct the shift of the mucogingival junction and maintain adequate soft tissue thickness, a combination graft with an 8-mm-wide band of keratinized tissue was harvested from the palate and sutured palatally in the deficient area (Figs

14-5v to 14-5x). The native keratinized tissue was shifted labially to gain thickness, maintain an esthetic appearance, and hide the grafted area from view. After the graft was incorporated and the tissue had matured, soft tissue conditioning was begun with the definitive abutments and a provisional restoration (Figs 14-5y to 14-5aa). The procedure reduces tissue loss compared with multiple abutment disconnections and reconnections and additionally helps to preserve the regenerated bony ridge.[34–36]

The esthetic prognosis increases with a strategically placed pontic instead of three adjacent implant restorations. To improve the soft tissue contour in the region of the right lateral incisor, extrusion of that tooth was planned. Extrusion started 2 months after incorporation of an implant-supported provisional restoration (Figs 14-5bb to 14-5dd). The tooth was extruded by 2 mm within 1 month, then retained for 5 months. The soft tissue was left to mature for 10 months before the definitive restoration was placed. The abutments and provisional denture were used to condition the soft tissues, creating an esthetic contour (Figs 14-5ee).

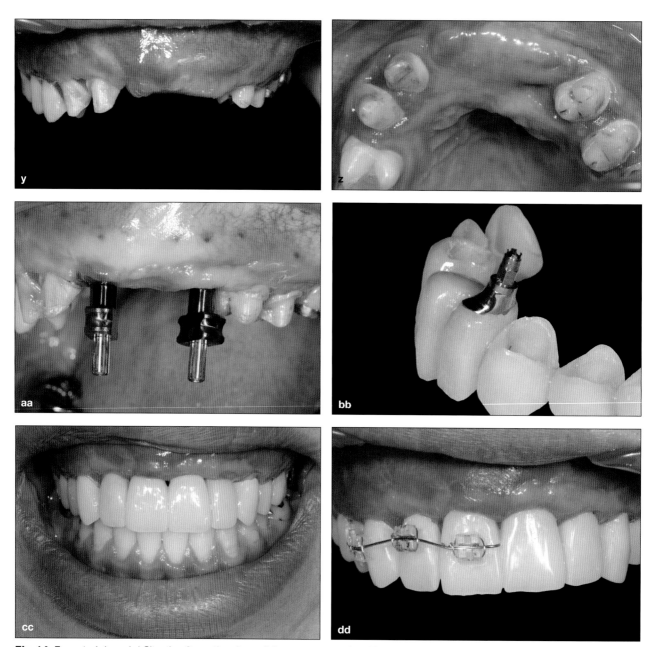

Fig 14-5 *cont.* / *(y and z)* Situation 2 months after soft tissue augmentation. The 3D ridge contour was improved; this change cannot be brought about by bone augmentation alone. *(aa)* Impressions were taken for the definitive abutments after soft tissue healing, when the healing abutments were connected. *(bb and cc)* Soft tissue conditioning was subsequently started with the definitive abutments and a provisional restoration. *(dd)* The right lateral incisor was extruded to improve the soft tissue level.

Radiographs after completion of the treatment show that the bone was regenerated up to the level of the crestal bone of the adjacent teeth (see Fig 14-5kk). The height of the tissue was preserved by using a strategically placed pontic instead of three adjacent implants. Platform switching also seems to have had a positive effect on bone preservation around functioning implants.

This case illustrates how long it can take to treat complex cases. It is essential to allow enough time to ensure good results in cases with severe defects. None of the treatment phases should be rushed. In this manner, even given an extreme preoperative situation, it was possible to achieve a very good esthetic outcome, which is still stable 6 years after treatment (Figs 14-5ff to 14-5mm).

Fig 14-5 *cont.* / *(ee)* The contoured soft tissue before the definitive restoration was placed. *(ff to jj)* End result. The anterior guidance was correctly established with the original left first premolar functioning as the left canine.

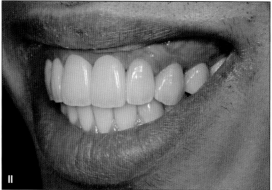

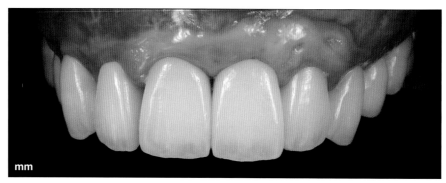

Fig 14-5 *cont.* / *(kk)* Radiographs after completion of the treatment. The bone had been regenerated up to the height of the bone apices at the teeth bordering the space. The implant at the left central incisor site was ultimately left as a "sleeping implant" to enhance the esthetic outcome. *(ll)* Lateral view of the patient smiling 3 years after completion of the treatment. *(mm)* Six years after treatment, the regenerated tissue offers satisfactory support and framing of the natural-looking restoration. (Surgery, orthodontics, and prosthodontics performed by T. Ishikawa; laboratory work performed by K. Nakajima.)

Case 5

The problem in this case was severe vertical tissue loss caused by trauma. The following were key factors for therapeutic success:

- Vertical augmentation with distraction osteogenesis
- Horizontal ridge augmentation with bone spreading and GBR
- Soft tissue augmentation

This middle-aged patient wanted esthetic rehabilitation of her anterior dentition. A vertical tissue defect had developed as a result of advanced periodontitis. The four missing maxillary incisors had been replaced by a partial denture, and the missing tissue had been replaced with a silicone gingival mask (Figs 14-6a to 14-6e). Prostheses such as these are subject to rapid color changes and will impair phonetics and the taste of food. The patient desperately wanted this situation to be improved.

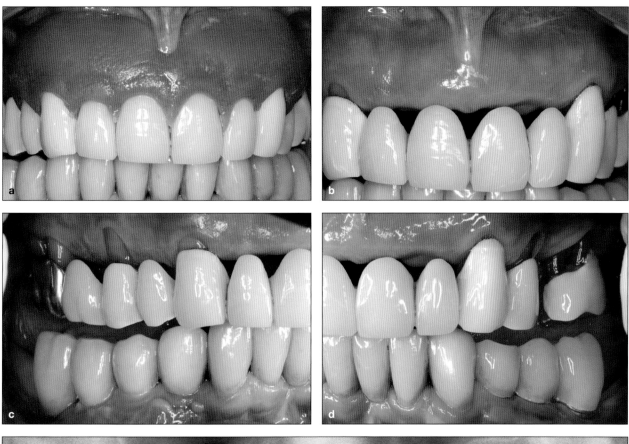

Fig 14-6 / *(a)* Silicone gingival prosthesis in the anterior maxilla. *(b)* Without the prosthesis, the vertical tissue loss in the region and gingival recessions at the canines become apparent. *(c and d)* Preoperative lateral views of the maxilla. *(e)* Panoramic radiograph of the preoperative situation. ⟶

After systematic periodontal treatment, distraction osteogenesis was performed for vertical ridge augmentation (Figs 14-6f to 14-6i; see chapter 9). After this, horizontal augmentation was additionally required and was performed by means of bone spreading and GBR (Figs 14-6j and 14-6k). Two implants were placed in the maxillary lateral incisor sites as abutments for a partial denture (Fig 14-6l). In the pontic area of the central incisors, the soft tissue was carefully conditioned with a provisional partial denture before the definitive superstructure was placed (Figs 14-6m to 14-6o).

306

Fig 14-6 *cont.* / *(f)* The distractor in place after the healing phase. *(g)* Ridge level after the distraction phase. The segment was markedly overdistracted to compensate for recession during the retention phase. *(h)* After the 2-week retention phase, a marked gain in ridge height can be seen. The distractor screw was trimmed to make the situation more comfortable for the patient. *(i)* The distractor was removed. At this stage, the ridge had been augmented vertically but not yet horizontally. *(j)* For horizontal correction of the defect, the ridge was split with a piezoelectric surgical instrument and spread and augmented with the GBR technique. *(k)* Situation 3 months later. The ridge was adequately augmented with anorganic bovine bone mineral.

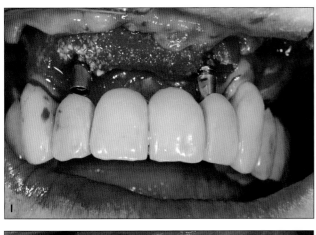
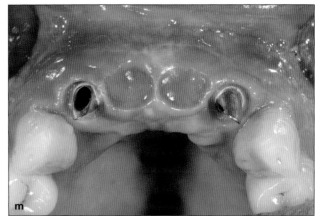
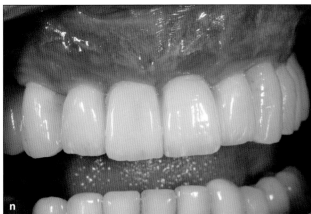

Fig 14-6 *cont.* / *(l)* Two implants were placed at the sites of the lateral incisors. *(m)* Situation 6 months later, after the tissue had matured. The soft tissue at the pontic sites had been conditioned with a provisional partial denture. *(n)* Definitive restoration with a porcelain-fused-to-metal partial denture on the lateral incisor implants. *(o)* Portrait of the patient after completion of the treatment. (Surgery and prosthodontics performed by G. Körner; laboratory work performed by K. Müterthies.)

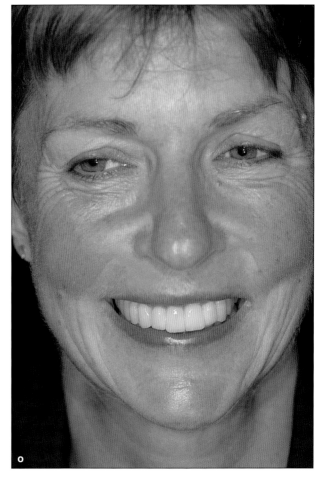

Conclusion

Complex cases often present very unfavorable preoperative situations. These may be the result of tooth agenesis, malocclusion, pathologic tooth movements, pronounced attachment loss, and extensive vertical tissue loss caused by infection or trauma. Therefore, complex cases require an unbiased interdisciplinary approach in which the attending dentists and dental technicians have to select the most appropriate therapeutic measures from the various disciplines. Good functional and esthetic results can be achieved with careful planning, open communication in an interdisciplinary team of practitioners, and the capacity to adapt to changing situations.

References

1. Keim RG. The art of interdisciplinary teamwork. J Clin Orthod 2013;47:513–514.
2. Spear FM, Kokich VG. A multidisciplinary approach to esthetic dentistry. Dent Clin North Am 2007;51:487–505.
3. Daftary F, Mahallati R, Bahat O, Sullivan RM. Lifelong craniofacial growth and the implications for osseointegrated implants. Int J Oral Maxillofac Implants 2013;28:163–169.
4. Brunsvold MA. Pathologic tooth migration. J Periodontol 2005;76:859–866.
5. Artun J, Urbye KS. The effect of orthodontic treatment on periodontal bone support in patients with advanced loss of marginal periodontium. Am J Orthod Dentofacial Orthop 1988;93:143–148.
6. Wennström JL, Stokland BL, Nyman S, Thilander B. Periodontal tissue response to orthodontic movement of teeth with infrabony pockets. Am J Orthod Dentofacial Orthop 1993;103:313–319.
7. Funato A, Ishikawa T, Kitajima H, Yamada M, Moroi H. A novel combined surgical approach to vertical alveolar ridge augmentation with titanium mesh, resorbable membrane, and rhPDGF-BB: A retrospective consecutive case series. Int J Periodontics Restorative Dent 2013;33:437–445.
8. Ishikawa T, Salama M, Funato A, et al. Three-dimensional bone and soft tissue requirements for optimizing esthetic results in compromised cases with multiple implants. Int J Periodontics Restorative Dent 2010;30:503–511.
9. Vela X, Méndez V, Rodríguez X, Segalà M, Gil JA. Soft tissue remodeling technique as a non-invasive alternative to second implant surgery. Eur J Esthet Dent 2012;7:36–47.
10. Cho-Yan Lee J, Mattheos N, Nixon KC, Ivanovski S. Residual periodontal pockets are a risk indicator for peri-implantitis in patients treated for periodontitis. Clin Oral Implants Res 2012;23:325–333.
11. Linkevičius T, Puišys A, Vindašiūtė E, Linkevičienė L, Apse P. Does residual cement around implant-supported restorations cause peri-implant disease? A retrospective case analysis. Clin Oral Implants Res 2013;24:1179–1184.
12. Pjetursson BE, Helbling C, Weber HP, et al. Peri-implantitis susceptibility as it relates to periodontal therapy and supportive care. Clin Oral Implants Res 2012;23:888–894.
13. Wilson TG Jr. The positive relationship between excess cement and peri-implant disease: A prospective clinical endoscopic study. J Periodontol 2009;80:1388–1392.
14. Blanco Carrión J, Ramos Barbosa I, Pérez López J. Osseointegrated implants as orthodontic anchorage and restorative abutments in the treatment of partially edentulous adult patients. Int J Periodontics Restorative Dent 2009;29:333–340.
15. Huang LH, Shotwell JL, Wang HL. Dental implants for orthodontic anchorage. Am J Orthod Dentofacial Orthop 2005;127:713–722.
16. Kokich VG. Managing complex orthodontic problems: The use of implants for anchorage. Semin Orthod 1996;2:153–160.
17. Smalley WM. Implants for tooth movement: Determining implant location and orientation. J Esthet Dent 1995;7:62–72.
18. Janakievski J, Kokich VO, Kinzer G. Interdisciplinary collaboration: An approach to optimize outcomes for patients with compromised dental esthetics. Int J Esthet Dent 2015;10:302–331.
19. Esposito M, Grusovin MG, Felice P, Karatzopoulos G, Worthington HV, Coulthard P. The efficacy of horizontal and vertical bone augmentation procedures for dental implants: A Cochrane systematic review. Eur J Oral Implantol 2009;2:167–184.
20. Rocchietta I, Fontana F, Simion M. Clinical outcomes of vertical bone augmentation to enable dental implant placement: A systematic review. J Clin Periodontol 2008;35(8 suppl):203–215.
21. Korayem M, Flores-Mir C, Nassar U, Olfert K. Implant site development by orthodontic extrusion. A systematic review. Angle Orthod 2008;78:752–760.
22. Salama H, Salama M. The role of orthodontic extrusive remodeling in the enhancement of soft and hard tissue profiles prior to implant placement: A systematic approach to the management of extraction site defects. Int J Periodontics Restorative Dent 1993;13:312–333.
23. Mankoo T, Frost L. Rehabilitation of esthetics in advanced periodontal cases using orthodontics for vertical hard and soft tissue regeneration prior to implants: A report of 2 challenging cases treated with an interdisciplinary approach. Eur J Esthet Dent 2011;6:376–404.
24. Salama M, Ishikawa T, Salama H, Funato A, Garber D. Advantages of the root submergence technique for pontic site development in esthetic implant therapy. Int J Periodontics Restorative Dent 2007;27:521–527.
25. Mason WE, Rugani FC. Prosthetically determined implant placement for the partially edentulous ridge: A reality today. J Mich Dent Assoc 1999;81:28–37.
26. Schneider G, Simmons K, Nason R, Felton D. Occlusal rehabilitation using implants for orthodontic anchorage. J Prosthodont 1998;7:232–236.
27. Smalley WM, Blanco A. Implants for tooth movement: A fabrication and placement technique for provisional restorations. J Esthet Dent 1995;7:150–154.
28. Anitua E. The use of plasma-rich growth factors (PRGF) in oral surgery. Pract Proced Aesthet Dent 2001;13:487–493.
29. López-Jornet P, Camacho-Alonso F, Molina-Miñano F, Vicente-Ortega V. Effects of plasma rich in growth factors on wound healing of the tongue. Experimental study on rabbits. Med Oral Patol Oral Cir Bucal 2009;14:e425–e428.
30. Grunder U, Gracis S, Capelli M. Influence of the 3-D bone-to-implant relationship on esthetics. Int J Periodontics Restorative Dent 2005;25:113–119.
31. Kan JY, Rungcharassaeng K, Umezu K, Kois JC. Dimensions of peri-implant mucosa: An evaluation of maxillary anterior single implants in humans. J Periodontol 2003;74:557–562.
32. Lee DW, Park KH, Moon IS. Dimension of keratinized mucosa and the interproximal papilla between adjacent implants. J Periodontol 2005;76:1856–1860.
33. Linkevičius T, Apse P, Grybauskas S, Puišys A. The influence of soft tissue thickness on crestal bone changes around implants: A 1-year prospective controlled clinical trial. Int J Oral Maxillofac Implants 2009;24:712–719.
34. Abrahamsson I, Berglundh T, Lindhe J. The mucosal barrier following abutment dis/reconnection. An experimental study in dogs. J Clin Periodontol 1997;24:568–572.
35. Rodríguez X, Vela X, Méndez V, Segalà M, Calvo-Guirado JL, Tarnow DP. The effect of abutment dis/reconnections on peri-implant bone resorption: A radiologic study of platform-switched and non-platform-switched implants placed in animals. Clin Oral Implants Res 2013;24:305–311.
36. Rompen E. The impact of the type and configuration of abutments and their (repeated) removal on the attachment level and marginal bone. Eur J Oral Implantol 2012;5(suppl):S83–S90.

A–Z

Index

Index

Page references followed by "f" denote figures; "b" denote boxes; and "t" denote tables.

A

313

M

N

O

P

U

V

W

Z